Biosynthetic Polymers for Medical Applications

Related titles

Durability and reliability of medical polymers
(ISBN 978-1-84569-929-1)

Shape memory polymers for biomedical applications
(ISBN 978-0-85709-698-2)

Modelling degradation of bioresorbable polymeric medical devices
(ISBN 978-1-78242-016-3)

Woodhead Publishing Series in Biomaterials:
Number 107

Biosynthetic Polymers for Medical Applications

Edited by

L. Poole-Warren, P. Martens and R. Green

ELSEVIER

AMSTERDAM • BOSTON • CAMBRIDGE • HEIDELBERG
LONDON • NEW YORK • OXFORD • PARIS • SAN DIEGO
SAN FRANCISCO • SINGAPORE • SYDNEY • TOKYO
Woodhead Publishing is an imprint of Elsevier

WP
WOODHEAD PUBLISHING

Woodhead Publishing is an imprint of Elsevier
80 High Street, Sawston, Cambridge, CB22 3HJ, UK
225 Wyman Street, Waltham, MA 02451, USA
Langford Lane, Kidlington, OX5 1GB, UK

ISBN: 978-1-78242-105-4 (print)
ISBN: 978-1-78242-113-9 (online)

British Library Cataloguing-in-Publication Data
A catalogue record for this book is available from the British Library

Library of Congress Control Number: 2015951100

For information on all Woodhead Publishing publications
visit our website at http://store.elsevier.com/

Contents

List of contributors

D. Abdelhamid Minia University, Minia, Egypt

M.R. Abidian Biomedical Engineering Department, University of Houston, Houston, TX, USA

R. Adhikari Commonwealth Scientific and Industrial Research Organisation (CSIRO) Manufacturing Flagship, Clayton, VIC, Australia

M. Asplund Freiburg Institute for Advanced Studies, Albert-Ludwigs Universität, Freiburg, Germany; IMTEK, Albert-Ludwigs Universität, Freiburg, Germany

J.A. Goding Graduate School of Biomedical Engineering, University of New South Wales, Sydney, NSW, Australia

R.A. Green Graduate School of Biomedical Engineering, University of New South Wales, Sydney, NSW, Australia

S.S. Griesser Ian Wark Research Institute, University of South Australia, Mawson Lakes, SA, Australia

H.J. Griesser Mawson Institute, University of South Australia, Mawson Lakes, SA, Australia

P.A. Gunatillake Commonwealth Scientific and Industrial Research Organisation (CSIRO) Manufacturing Flagship, Clayton, VIC, Australia

M. Haeussler CSIRO Materials Science and Engineering, Clayton, VIC, Australia

K.E.S. Locock CSIRO Materials Science and Engineering, Clayton, VIC, Australia

P.J. Martens Graduate School of Biomedical Engineering, University of New South Wales, Sydney, NSW, Australia

L. Meagher CSIRO Materials Science and Engineering, Clayton, VIC, Australia

T.D. Michl Ian Wark Research Institute, University of South Australia, Mawson Lakes, SA, Australia

E.M. Moore Duke University, Durham, NC, USA

B.A. Nsiah Duke University, Durham, NC, USA

B. Ozcelik Commonwealth Scientific and Industrial Research Organisation (CSIRO), Clayton, VIC, Australia

A.J. Patton Graduate School of Biomedical Engineering, University of New South Wales, Sydney, NSW, Australia

L.A. Poole-Warren Graduate School of Biomedical Engineering, University of New South Wales, Sydney, NSW, Australia

J.J. Roberts Graduate School of Biomedical Engineering, University of New South Wales, Sydney, NSW, Australia

L.C. Roudsari Duke University, Durham, NC, USA

H. Thissen CSIRO Manufacturing Flagship, VIC, Australia

K. Udipi Biopolymer Designs Inc., Santa Rosa, CA, USA

K.E. Uhrich Rutgers University, Piscataway, NJ, USA

N.K. Virdone Duke University, Durham, NC, USA

J.L. West Duke University, Durham, NC, USA

N. Yi Pennsylvania State University, PA, USA

Woodhead Publishing Series in Biomaterials

1 **Sterilisation of tissues using ionising radiations**
Edited by J. F. Kennedy, G. O. Phillips and P. A. Williams
2 **Surfaces and interfaces for biomaterials**
Edited by P. Vadgama
3 **Molecular interfacial phenomena of polymers and biopolymers**
Edited by C. Chen
4 **Biomaterials, artificial organs and tissue engineering**
Edited by L. Hench and J. Jones
5 **Medical modelling**
R. Bibb
6 **Artificial cells, cell engineering and therapy**
Edited by S. Prakash
7 **Biomedical polymers**
Edited by M. Jenkins
8 **Tissue engineering using ceramics and polymers**
Edited by A. R. Boccaccini and J. Gough
9 **Bioceramics and their clinical applications**
Edited by T. Kokubo
10 **Dental biomaterials**
Edited by R. V. Curtis and T. F. Watson
11 **Joint replacement technology**
Edited by P. A. Revell
12 **Natural-based polymers for biomedical applications**
Edited by R. L. Reiss et al.
13 **Degradation rate of bioresorbable materials**
Edited by F. J. Buchanan
14 **Orthopaedic bone cements**
Edited by S. Deb
15 **Shape memory alloys for biomedical applications**
Edited by T. Yoneyama and S. Miyazaki
16 **Cellular response to biomaterials**
Edited by L. Di Silvio
17 **Biomaterials for treating skin loss**
Edited by D. P. Orgill and C. Blanco
18 **Biomaterials and tissue engineering in urology**
Edited by J. Denstedt and A. Atala
19 **Materials science for dentistry**
B. W. Darvell

44 **Durability and reliability of medical polymers**
Edited by M. Jenkins and A. Stamboulis
45 **Biosensors for medical applications**
Edited by S. Higson
46 **Sterilisation of biomaterials and medical devices**
Edited by S. Lerouge and A. Simmons
47 **The hip resurfacing handbook: A practical guide to the use and management of modern hip resurfacings**
Edited by K. De Smet, P. Campbell and C. Van Der Straeten
48 **Developments in tissue engineered and regenerative medicine products**
J. Basu and J. W. Ludlow
49 **Nanomedicine: Technologies and applications**
Edited by T. J. Webster
50 **Biocompatibility and performance of medical devices**
Edited by J-P. Boutrand
51 **Medical robotics: Minimally invasive surgery**
Edited by P. Gomes
52 **Implantable sensor systems for medical applications**
Edited by A. Inmann and D. Hodgins
53 **Non-metallic biomaterials for tooth repair and replacement**
Edited by P. Vallittu
54 **Joining and assembly of medical materials and devices**
Edited by Y. (Norman) Zhou and M. D. Breyen
55 **Diamond-based materials for biomedical applications**
Edited by R. Narayan
56 **Nanomaterials in tissue engineering: Fabrication and applications**
Edited by A. K. Gaharwar, S. Sant, M. J. Hancock and S. A. Hacking
57 **Biomimetic biomaterials: Structure and applications**
Edited by A. J. Ruys
58 **Standardisation in cell and tissue engineering: Methods and protocols**
Edited by V. Salih
59 **Inhaler devices: Fundamentals, design and drug delivery**
Edited by P. Prokopovich
60 **Bio-tribocorrosion in biomaterials and medical implants**
Edited by Y. Yan
61 **Microfluidic devices for biomedical applications**
Edited by X-J. James Li and Y. Zhou
62 **Decontamination in hospitals and healthcare**
Edited by J. T. Walker
63 **Biomedical imaging: Applications and advances**
Edited by P. Morris
64 **Characterization of biomaterials**
Edited by M. Jaffe, W. Hammond, P. Tolias and T. Arinzeh
65 **Biomaterials and medical tribology**
Edited by J. Paolo Davim
66 **Biomaterials for cancer therapeutics: Diagnosis, prevention and therapy**
Edited by K. Park
67 **New functional biomaterials for medicine and healthcare**
E. P. Ivanova, K. Bazaka and R. J. Crawford

68 **Porous silicon for biomedical applications**
Edited by H. A. Santos
69 **A practical approach to spinal trauma**
Edited by H. N. Bajaj and S. Katoch
70 **Rapid prototyping of biomaterials: Principles and applications**
Edited by R. Narayan
71 **Cardiac regeneration and repair Volume 1: Pathology and therapies**
Edited by R-K. Li and R. D. Weisel
72 **Cardiac regeneration and repair Volume 2: Biomaterials and tissue engineering**
Edited by R-K. Li and R. D. Weisel
73 **Semiconducting silicon nanowires for biomedical applications**
Edited by J. L. Coffer
74 **Silk biomaterials for tissue engineering and regenerative medicine**
Edited by S. Kundu
75 **Biomaterials for bone regeneration: Novel techniques and applications**
Edited by P. Dubruel and S. Van Vlierberghe
76 **Biomedical foams for tissue engineering applications**
Edited by P. Netti
77 **Precious metals for biomedical applications**
Edited by N. Baltzer and T. Copponnex
78 **Bone substitute biomaterials**
Edited by K. Mallick
79 **Regulatory affairs for biomaterials and medical devices**
Edited by S. F. Amato and R. Ezzell
80 **Joint replacement technology Second edition**
Edited by P. A. Revell
81 **Computational modelling of biomechanics and biotribology in the musculoskeletal system: Biomaterials and tissues**
Edited by Z. Jin
82 **Biophotonics for medical applications**
Edited by I. Meglinski
83 **Modelling degradation of bioresorbable polymeric medical devices**
Edited by J. Pan
84 **Perspectives in total hip arthroplasty: Advances in biomaterials and their tribological interactions**
S. Affatato
85 **Tissue engineering using ceramics and polymers Second edition**
Edited by A. R. Boccaccini and P. X. Ma
86 **Biomaterials and medical-device associated infections**
Edited by L. Barnes and I. R. Cooper
87 **Surgical techniques in total knee arthroplasty (TKA) and alternative procedures**
Edited by S. Affatato
88 **Lanthanide oxide nanoparticles for molecular imaging and therapeutics**
G. H. Lee
89 **Surface modification of magnesium and its alloys for biomedical applications Volume 1: Biological interactions, mechanical properties and testing**
Edited by T. S. N. Sankara Narayanan, I. S. Park and M. H. Lee

90 **Surface modification of magnesium and its alloys for biomedical applications Volume 2: Modification and coating techniques**
Edited by T. S. N. Sankara Narayanan, I. S. Park and M. H. Lee
91 **Medical modelling: the application of advanced design and rapid prototyping techniques in medicine Second edition**
Edited by R. Bibb, D. Eggbeer and A. Paterson
92 **Switchable and responsive surfaces and materials for biomedical applications**
Edited by Z. Zhang
93 **Biomedical textiles for orthopaedic and surgical applications: fundamentals, applications and tissue engineering**
Edited by T. Blair
94 **Surface coating and modification of metallic biomaterials**
Edited by C. Wen
95 **Hydroxyapatite (HAP) for biomedical applications**
Edited by M. Mucalo
96 **Implantable neuroprostheses for restoring function**
Edited by K. Kilgore
97 **Shape memory polymers for biomedical applications**
Edited by L. Yahia
98 **Regenerative engineering of musculoskeletal tissues and interfaces**
Edited by S. P. Nukavarapu, J. W. Freeman and C. T. Laurencin
99 **Advanced cardiac imaging**
Edited by K. Nieman, O. Gaemperli, P. Lancellotti and S. Plein
100 **Functional marine biomaterials: properties and applications**
Edited by Se-Kwon Kim
101 **Shoulder and elbow trauma and its complications: Volume 1: The Shoulder**
Edited by R. M. Greiwe
102 **Nanotechnology-enhanced orthopedic materials: Fabrications, applications and future trends**
Edited by L. Yang
103 **Medical devices: Regulations, standards and practices**
Edited by S. Ramakrishna, L. Tian, C. Wang, S. L. and T. Wee Eong
104 **Biomineralisation and biomaterials: fundamentals and applications**
Edited by C. Aparicio and M. Ginebra
105 **Shoulder and elbow trauma and its complications: Volume 2: The Elbow**
Edited by R. M. Greiwe
106 **Characterisation and design of tissue scaffolds**
Edited by P. Tomlins
107 **Biosynthetic polymers for medical applications**
Edited by L. Poole-Warren, P. Martens and R. Green

Part One

Introduction and fundamentals

Introduction to biomedical polymers and biocompatibility

1

L.A. Poole-Warren, A.J. Patton
Graduate School of Biomedical Engineering, University of New South Wales, Sydney, NSW, Australia

1.1 Introduction

The key feature of polymers that allows them to be so effectively applied to medical devices is their versatility in terms of the plethora of structures, properties and functions exhibited. Unlike metals and ceramics, polymers can be fabricated in forms that range from soft gels to flexible fibres and porous forms to hard, non-porous bulk materials. Polymers can be classified broadly into those that are biologically derived, or natural polymers, and those that are manufactured or synthetic. Both of these two broad classes of polymers are widely used in biomedical device applications.

Where natural polymers are as old as life itself, synthetic polymers or plastics are man-made materials that have a history of less than 100 years. Over that relatively short period, synthetic polymers have become ubiquitous in commodity products today. Synthesised via covalent linking of multiple small chemical structures called 'mers' to form long-chain molecules or polymers, these materials have an extraordinary range of physical properties that allow them to be utilised in almost any application.

> Chapter 2 outlines the non-degradable, synthetic materials that are typically used for biomedical applications. Advancements over the past decade are covered with a specific focus on poly(olefins), poly(urethanes), poly(carbonates), poly(siloxanes), poly(amides), poly(ethers) and poly(sulphones). A brief introduction to the chemistry, physical properties, biocompatibility and biostability of seven major classes of synthetic polymers is given. The term 'non-degradable' is used to imply that the polymers are resistant to degradation by hydrolytic and other mechanisms operating in biological environments.
>
> Chapter 3 covers degradable polymers commonly used in biomedical applications with a focus on synthetic materials. Degradable polymers are classified into two key groups. The first is biodegradable polymers, which break down under physiological conditions. Biodegradation is a biologically based process that leads to degradation. Biological processes encompass human enzymes, microbial enzymes and even hydrolysis. Degradation refers to bond cleavage and includes

Continued

Biosynthetic Polymers for Medical Applications. http://dx.doi.org/10.1016/B978-1-78242-105-4.00001-8

hydrolysis of ester bonds or ultraviolet-promoted cleavage of C−C bonds. Typically, biodegradable polymers would include hydrolytically and/or enzymatically susceptible bonds such as polyesters, polyanhydrides, polycarbonates, polyamides and polyurethanes. The second group, bioerodible polymers, in which the chemistry of the polymer is not fundamentally changed during degradation, rather, the physical state changes from a solid structure to a solubilized polymer. 'Bioresorbable' is a synonym of bioerodible and the implication is that the polymer is resorbed, or adsorbed, into the surrounding tissue.

Based on excerpts from Chapters 2 and 3.

In this chapter, the natural polymers will be described followed by consideration of the benefits and limitations of both synthetic and natural polymers relating to their application in medical devices. Finally, the critical factors that impact on biocompatibility of both polymer classes will be evaluated. Combining polymers from the two classes to form biosynthetic materials has been proposed to overcome some of the limitations that each type presents for medical device development and this concept forms the basis of this book.

1.2 Natural or biological polymers

All living organisms are made up of proteins, carbohydrates, lipids and nucleic acids, the four key macromolecular building blocks of life. These molecules comprise the natural polymers that have evolved over the ages into the most elegant molecules known to man. To be exploited as materials for biomedical devices, natural polymers are either sourced from tissues derived from living organisms or are synthesised and processed using in vitro techniques via cell culture, recombinant approaches or using cell-free synthetic systems (reviewed in Refs [1,2]).

Biological polymers are capable of supporting complex higher order biological functions and are able to be synthesised by organisms in situ. It is this group of complex, functional polymers that inspire the quest of biomaterials researchers to produce materials capable of repairing, replacing or the ultimate, regenerating tissues and organs in humans. Table 1.1 outlines the four main types of natural polymers and their characteristics and functions.

Looking to the past it is clear that humans have always modified available biological materials as ready resources for producing tools, clothing, medicines, food and shelter. The use of animal hides for clothing, building shelters and constructing watercraft are examples of how these versatile biological polymers have been manipulated for thousands of years to produce useful items. Although lipids, such as autologous fat, and deoxyribose nucleic acids (DNA) have been explored for surgical and pharmaceutical applications, there are limited examples of commercialisation of medical devices based on these polymers. The focus herein will be on protein and carbohydrate polymers, the primary constituents of extracellular matrix (ECM), which are the most commonly applied in biomedical devices.

Table 1.1 Four main types of natural polymers and their characteristics and functions

Polymer	Sources	Characteristics/ functions	Device/medical applications
Proteins	Animal tissue such as from bovine, porcine and ovine sources Tissue used includes skin, tendon, pericardium, vasculature and intestine Recombinant expression systems for proteins such as collagen and elastin also used	Long chain 1° poly-amino acid structure. 2° structure formed by folding and coiling producing characteristic α-helices and β-sheets Heterogeneous molecules with highly variable polar and non-polar regions Multiple roles in structure and function of tissues and cells. Major structural component of connective tissue. Key role in cell communications and immune functions.	Dermal fillers Major structural component of surgical meshes Sutures Tissue engineered skin Drug applications (antibodies and cytokines)
Carbohydrates	Animal tissue such as rooster combs (avian) and marine exoskeleton (crustacean) Plant tissue such as algae and potatoes Bacterial fermentation (e.g. *Streptococcus* and *Bacillus* species) Cell culture supernatant	Long-chain molecules made up of saccharide monomers Highly polar Key energy storage macromolecule (in plants, primarily starch, and in animals glycogen) Role in structure and mechanics of tissues and in biological functions including cell and growth factor signalling	Dermal fillers Haemostatic agents Wound dressings Component of acellular dermal matrix (ADM) Tissue engineered cartilage Vitreous humor Drug applications (heparin)
Lipids	Usually autologous sources for transplant	Insoluble in water Key function long term energy storage and insulation Primary constituent of cell membranes in animals	Autologous fat used as a tissue filler

Continued

Table 1.1 Continued

Polymer	Sources	Characteristics/ functions	Device/medical applications
Nucleic acids	Located in the nucleus of cells Typically synthesised	Two main types, deoxyribonucleic acid (DNA) and ribonucleic acid (RNA) Composed of nucleotides made up of sugar, base and phosphate groups	Drug applications (siRNA)

1.2.1 Extracellular matrix

Composed primarily of water, proteins and polysaccharides, soft-tissue ECM is a hydrogel with a variable water content dependent on the specific tissue. Although ECM is often termed the non-cellular or acellular component of tissue, it is exquisitely designed and synthesised by different cell types for structural support and cellular communications [3]. ECM is an extraordinarily dynamic component of tissue due first to its critical support of cell functions and second to the constant remodelling that it undergoes in order to maintain its function (see Ref. [3] for a poster summarising ECM structure and function).

The three primary functions of ECM are structural and mechanical support, maintenance of homeostasis and support of critical cellular functions such as adhesion, signalling, motility, proliferation and differentiation. ECM is tailored for each tissue during development and thus has considerable heterogeneity. Although ECM is tissue-specific, in mammalian connective tissue, the fibrous proteins comprise the bulk of the polymer content with polysaccharides making up a smaller proportion [4].

Collagen and elastin are the major structural proteins with laminin and fibronectin being found in smaller amounts. The polysaccharides in ECM are the glycosaminoglycans (GAG), most of which decorate proteins to form the proteoglycans (PGs) [5]. Chondrotin sulphate is the most abundant PG in ECM. Hyaluronic acid (HA) is a non-sulphated GAG that does not associate with proteins to form PGs [5].

1.2.2 Isolation and processing of natural polymers

Animal and plant tissue from which proteins and polysaccharides are isolated must be processed through a series of conditions for purification of the extracts and may also require further modification to yield a manufacturable product. Figure 1.1 illustrates generic processing steps that are required to manufacture medical materials derived from natural tissues. Where selection of natural polymers is a preferred option for medical device application, potential bioburden sources and processes required for their removal are vital factors that should be considered. The following sections outline

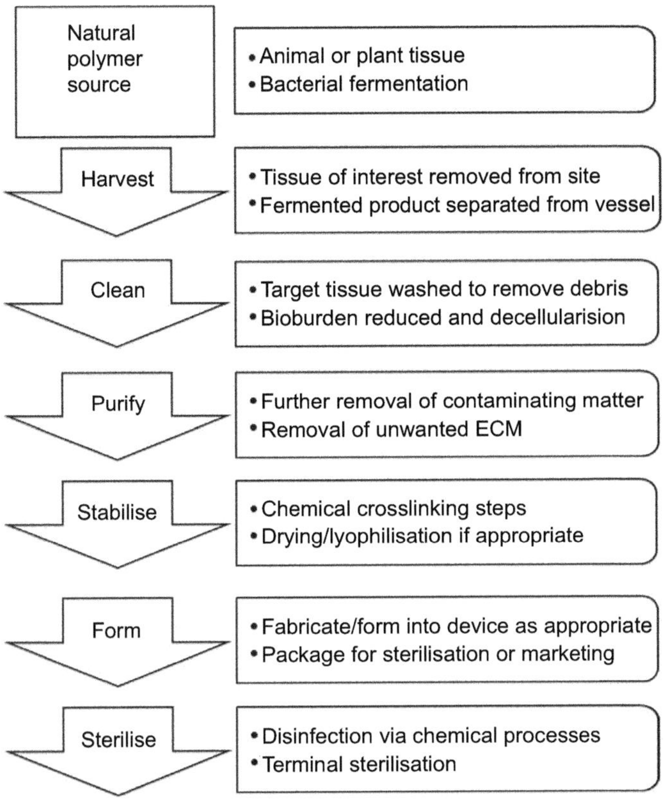

Figure 1.1 Generic processing steps for production of biologically derived polymeric materials.

in more detail the proteins and polysaccharides, two key classes of polymers that comprise ECM and are a major source of these two types of polymers.

1.2.3 Protein polymers

Proteins are polymers of amino acids with primary structures linked together by amide bonds. More complex secondary and tertiary structures occur as a result of folding in combination with peptide bonding and other forms of molecular association such as ionic and hydrophobic interactions and van der Waals forces. As expected for the most abundant natural polymer in animals, proteins are produced in numerous forms and have a multitude of functions. They are classified as the insoluble or fibrous proteins or as soluble proteins with specialised biochemical functions such as enzymatic activity. The fibrous proteins are not only in the highest proportion comprising up to 30% of the solid content of ECM, they are the most studied of the natural polymers for biomaterials applications [6].

While many proteins have been selected for fabrication of biomedical devices, the most prevalent in commercial use are collagen and its derivatives, and fibrin. Although not yet commercially available, recombinant forms of tropelastin have been produced and clinical trials of its use as a dermal filler have been reported by the Australian company Elastagen [7]. As the most abundant connective tissue protein in mammals, collagen holds the position as one of the most commonly used natural polymers for biomedical applications. The primary structure of collagen is characterised by an amino acid composition rich in glycine, proline and hydroxyproline and it has a triple helical tertiary structure. The key properties that are desirable for medical applications include the ability to be remodelled and degraded in animals via collagenase digestion and the capacity for interacting with many different cell types via adhesion sequences. This complex fibrillar protein has a long and successful history as a biomaterial for applications such as bioprosthetic heart valves, as biological meshes for tissue and organ supports and as injectable materials for dermal fillers [8].

Collagen used for biomedical devices is typically sourced from bovine skin or other animal tissues, including human tissues sourced from cadavers, which are abundant in the protein. Of key importance for biomedical uses of proteins is minimising the risk of prion contamination via using sources free of bovine encephalitis and the removal of components that may be antigenic or infectious. Thus processes typically include steps for removal of cells and highly antigenic epitopes on biological polymers and removal of other organic contaminants such as bacteria and viruses. The extent of processing that occurs following the cleaning and purification steps in the process is dependent on the type of product being developed. Examples of the range of processing approaches that are conducted can be found by comparison of biological meshes, which are typically based on insoluble structural connective tissues, and collagen-based dermal fillers which are mainly soluble, injectable materials. Following tissue processing, the final product may be provided dry or hydrated and additional preservation steps are typically conducted for those supplied in hydrated form. An example of the latter is bioprosthetic heart valves which tend to be fixed in glutaraldehyde to reduce immunogenicity and stabilise the tissue to expand both its shelf life and in vivo persistence [9].

A biological mesh that is minimally processed is AlloDerm®, which is sourced from human cadaver skin. Although manufacture of this product is far from simple, the objective of the processing steps is to remove antigenic and cellular components while causing minimal disruption to the native ECM [10]. Table 1.2 (modified from Refs [6,11,12]) lists the major types of biological meshes commercially available today. AlloDerm®, Permacol™ and Surgisis® are among the most common biological meshes used for applications such as hernia repair. Comparison of the performance of these three meshes suggested that although all experience significant recurrence rate, higher rates occur in more complex surgical sites and usually are associated with infected or highly compromised sites [12]. The finding that Permacol™, derived from crosslinked porcine dermis, was associated with the lowest complication rates was not supported by a study comparing this mesh with a similar non-crosslinked mesh Strattice™ [13]. The retrospective study suggested that although both meshes had similar recurrence rates, Strattice™ was associated with significantly lower infection rates [13]. The conflicting reports on biological functional performance highlight the current unmet need for meshes that address criteria for repair and replacement of specific tissues.

Table 1.2 Biological meshes

Source	Tradename/ Manufacturer	Form and processing	Sterilisation
Bovine pericardium	Tutopatch™/ Tutogen™	Processed, solvent dehydrated and preserved. Three-dimensional collagen framework maintained during processing. No crosslinking agents added.	Gamma irradiation
Bovine pericardium	Veritas®/Synovis Inc.	Processed with propylene oxide to decellularize and stabilize end product by capping free amine groups. Multidirectional collagen fibres and minimal elastin content. No crosslinking agents added.	Electron beam radiation (E-beam)
Bovine pericardum	Peri-guard®/Synovis Inc.	Pericardium procured from cattle originating in the United States. Treated with 1 M sodium hydroxide for 60–75 min at 20–25 °C and crosslinked using glutaraldehyde.	Ethanol and propylene oxide
Fetal bovine dermis	SurgiMend®/TEI Biosciences Inc.	Dermal collagen is decellularised. Product contains five times more type III collagen than any other biological matrix. No crosslinking agents added. Shipped dehydrated.	Ethylene oxide (EtO)
Human dermis	AlloDerm®/LifeCell™ Corp.	Aseptic proprietary process, removal of epidermis by incubating the skin overnight in 1 M NaCl at 37 °C. Processed to remove cells and freeze-dried to dehydrate and 'preserve'. Refrigeration required until ready for use. No crosslinking agents added. Not terminally sterilized.	
Human dermis	AlloMax™/Davol Inc./ RTI Surgical Inc.	Dried product rehydrated to desired consistency. Not freeze-dried, does not require refrigeration for storage. No crosslinking agents added.	Gamma irradiation
Human dermis	Derma-Matrix™/ DePuy Synthes	Decellularised matrix. Integrity of the matrix maintained. No crosslinking agents added.	Bacterially inactivated
Human dermis	Repriza®/Promethean LifeSciences Inc.	Provided sterile and prehydrated in a double-peel pouch. No crosslinking agents added. Not terminally sterilized.	
Human dermis	DermaSpan™/Bliss GVS Pharma	Processing via a unique protocol that includes a terminal irradiation step. Precision dose sterilization, provides sterility without disrupting the delicate collagen integrity. No crosslinking agents added.	Precision dose sterilization

Continued

Table 1.2 Continued

Source	Tradename/ Manufacturer	Form and processing	Sterilisation
Human dermis musculoskeletal transplant	FlexHD®/ Musculoskeletal transplant Foundation/ Ethicon Inc.	Minimally processed to remove epidermal and dermal cells and packaged in an ethanol solution. No terminal sterilization process is used, but the product does pass sterility testing in accordance with United States Pharmacopeia. No refrigeration and no rehydration necessary. No crosslinking agents added.	Aseptic processing
Porcine dermis	Collamend™/C. R. Bard Inc.	Processing technique decellularises and preserves tissue strength and structure. Crosslinked collagen and elastin using 1-ethyl-3-(3-dimethylaminopropyl) carbodiimide (EDAC)	Ethylene oxide (EtO)
Porcine dermis	Strattice™/LifeCell™	Processing removes cells and the α-gal antigen to decrease host immune response and improve tissue integration. Packaged in a phosphate-buffered saline solution with matrix stabilizers. No crosslinking agents added.	E-beam
Porcine dermis	XenMatrix™/C. R. Bard Inc.	Proprietary process which removes cells while maintaining tissue structure and strength. No crosslinking agents added.	E-beam
Porcine dermis	Permacol™/Covidien©	Processing leaves the matrix and elastic fibres intact. Crosslinked with noncalcifying hexamethylene diisocyanate (HMDI) to increase strength and durability. This method of crosslinking further makes the material highly resistant to breakdown by naturally occurring collagenases.	Gamma irradiation
Porcine intestine	FortaGen®/ Organogenesis Inc.	Little information on processing and sterilisation available. Low level of crosslinking. Not terminally sterilized.	
Porcine intestine	Surgisis®/Cook Biotech	Harvested from the submucosa of porcine intestine. The product is terminally sterilized and shipped dehydrated. No crosslinking agents added.	Ethylene oxide (EtO)

Highly purified, soluble collagen materials such as the injectable dermal filler Zyderm® are at the other end of the scale since they undergo more significant processing than most of the above-mentioned biological meshes. Table 1.3 outlines the range of biological polymer-based fillers used in medical applications. Collagen has the longest history of use and remains the most successful in terms of the longevity of the device. These fillers are largely supplied as a solution of Type I collagen that is isolated and purified using a series of techniques depending on the source. As noted above, animal tissue sources require significant processing that may include protease treatment to produce the final product. Other sources of collagen include human collagen isolated from fibroblast cell culture [14]. Although specific processing steps and information on composition for these fillers are often proprietary, similar soluble Type I collagen products available for research are soluble in weak acids at relatively low concentrations. For example, PureCol® is supplied by Advanced BioMatrix as a 0.3% aqueous solution in 0.01 M HCl at pH $\sim$2.0 [15]. To form a gel, the product is typically diluted and the pH neutralised prior to warming to 37 °C at which temperature the collagen spontaneously forms a gel. The processing steps for production of soluble collagen removes potentially immunogenic telopeptides and produces formulations that have appropriate stability and are able to be delivered surgically or easily injected [16].

Gelatin is a derivative of collagen that is sourced mainly from animal skin or bones. Typically processing involves isolation and partial hydrolysis of collagen via acid and/or alkaline (lime) treatment. These treatments may be augmented by heating and together the processes act as both disinfecting and hydrolysis steps, reducing the bioburden and the molecular weight. Molecular weight of gelatin is one or two orders of magnitude lower than native collagen or soluble collagen forms depending on the extent of hydrolysis [17,18]. In 1997, the Food and Drug Administration (FDA) determined that simple acid or alkali treatment was not sufficient to assure deactivation of prions and produced additional guidance to manufacturers requiring assurance that animal collagen sources were free from prion contamination [19].

Medical device applications of gelatin are predominantly for haemostasis although they have been used in the past as dermal implants for aesthetic use. The forms used are all absorbable and range from porous sponges and powders through to gels. In the biomaterials research literature, gelatin has been extensively used as a tissue engineering scaffold due to its cell compatibility, water solubility and the capacity to be degraded via enzymatic hydrolysis [20].

Fibrin is polymerised in response to activation of the coagulation cascade. The polymer is formed following thrombin catalysed enzymatic cleavage of peptides of the plasma glycoprotein fibrinogen. Fibrinogen has a high molecular weight of the order of 340 kDa and is composed of disulphide bridged Aa-, Bb-, and c-chains [21]. In its native form in mammals, this biological polymer is the pre-polymer of fibrin, which is the critical structural component of the provisional matrix for haemostais and wound healing. Fibrin binds heparin and has a role in cell-matrix signalling due to amino acid sequences that present several growth factors such as fibroblast growth factor-2 and vascular endothelial growth factor (VEGF) that play a critical role in cell signalling in would healing [21,22].

Table 1.3 Dermal fillers based on natural polymers approved by the Food and Drug Administration, USA

Material type/ source	Tradename/ approval date	Approved uses	Potential reasons/ sites to avoid use
Collagen/human tissue	Cosmoderm® 1 Human-Based C 3/11/2003	Superficial papillary dermis for correction of soft tissue contour deficiencies, such as wrinkles and acne scars. Mid-to-deep dermis for correction of soft tissue contour deficiencies, such as wrinkles and acne scars.	History of anaphylaxis. Known lidocaine hypersensitivity. Breast augmentation, and for implantation into bone, tendon, ligament, or muscle.
Collagen/porcine collagen	Evolence™ Collagen Filler 6/27/2008	Correction of moderate to deep facial wrinkles and folds such as nasolabial folds.	Known hypersensitivity to any collagen products. History of anaphylaxis. Implantation in spaces other than the dermis of the face. Implantation in patients with bleeding disorders.
Collagen/bovine dermal collagen	Zyderm® Collagen Implant/ Zyplast® 9/18/1981	Indicated for the correction of contour deformities of the dermis in non-weight bearing areas. Should be injected into the superficial papillary dermis.	Severe allergies manifested by a history of anaphylaxis. Known lidocaine hypersensitivity. History of allergies to any bovine collagen product. Breast augmentation, and for implantation into bone, tendon, ligament, or muscle.

Table 1.3 **Continued**

Material type/ source	Tradename/ approval date	Approved uses	Potential reasons/ sites to avoid use
Hyaluronic acid	Belotero Balance®, Juvederm® 24HV, Juvederm® 30 and Juvederm® 30HV 6/02/2006	Indicated for injection into the mid-to-deep dermis for correction of moderateto-severe facial wrinkles and folds such as nasolabial folds.	Severe allergies manifested by a history of anaphylaxis, or history or presence of multiple severe allergies. History of allergies to gram-positive bacterial proteins Implantation into blood vessels, implantation into dermal vessels may cause vascular occlusion, infarction, or embolic phenomena.
Hyaluronic acid/ avian sourced	Captique™ Injectable Gel 11/12/2004		
Hyaluronic acid/ *Streptococcus* species of bacteria	Restylane® Injectable Gel 10/11/2011	Indicated for mid-to-deep dermal implantation for the correction of moderate-to-severe facial wrinkles and folds, such as nasolabial folds. Restylane is indicated for submucosal implantation in patients over the age of 21 for lip augmentation.	Severe allergies manifested by a history of anaphylaxis. History of allergies to gram-positive bacterial proteins Breast augmentation, and for implantation into bone, tendon, ligament, or muscle. Implantation into blood vessels. Implantation into dermal vessels may cause vascular occlusion, infarction, or embolic phenomena.

Continued

Table 1.3 Continued

Material type/ source	Tradename/ approval date	Approved uses	Potential reasons/ sites to avoid use
Hyaluronic acid with lidocaine	Juvederm® Volumna XC, Prevelle Silk, Restylane® Silk, Restylane-L® Injectable Gel, Elevess™ 2/26/2008	Indicated for deep (subcutaneous and/or supraperiosteal) injection for cheek augmentation to correct age-related volume deficit in the mid-face in adults over the age of 21.	Severe allergies manifested by a history of anaphylaxis. History of allergies to gram-positive bacterial proteins. Known lidocaine hypersensitivity. Bleeding disorders.
Modified hyaluronic acid derived from a bird (avian) source/Avian sourced	Hylaform® (Hylan B Gel) 4/22/ 2004	Indicated for injection into the mid-to-deep dermis for correction of moderate-to-severe facial wrinkles and folds (such as nasolabial folds).	Use in breast augmentation, or for implantation into bone, tendon, ligament, or muscle. History of known hypersensitivity to avian proteins. Must not be injected into blood vessels. Introduction of gel into the vasculature may occlude the vessels and could cause infarction or embolization.

Fibrin-based polymers have been used largely as surgical sealants or haemostatic agents, either alone or in combination with dressings. Commercially available fibrin-based surgical sealants are usually based on human fibrinogen and thrombin. The two component fibrin sealants can be mixed and applied as a liquid solution that directly polymerises in situ. The components have also been embedded in patches for preventing peri-surgical bleeding such as Evarrest®. This mesh is fabricated from 90% glycolide and 10% L-lactide (Vicryl) underlying a flexible oxidised cellulose layer (EVARREST® Fibrin Sealant Patch, Ethicon, NJ).

Elastin is a critical structural protein in mammalian connective tissues conferring compliance and elasticity to tissues such as that making up arterial wall, skin and lung tissues. It is a component of the basal lamina and provides sequences that support cell adhesion, proliferation and signalling that drives other cell functions such as matrix synthesis and remodelling [23]. In its native state, elastin is a high-molecular weight, highly crosslinked, hydrophobic protein. As a result of its high level of crosslinking, it is difficult to isolate as a soluble product without using harsh chemical treatment or enzymatic hydrolysis to break down the peptide bonds [24]. The resulting product is typically fragmented and does not represent the native 60 kDa tropoelastin polymer that is the primary structural unit of elastin. Although not as abundant as collagen, the attractive properties of elastin have led to significant research focused on potential biomedical applications. The focus of much research over the past few decades has been on recombinant approaches for producing tropoelastin although to date, biomedical devices based on elastin have not been commercialised [25,26].

1.2.4 Carbohydrate-based polymers

Complex carbohydrates, also called polysaccharides, are polymers built from sugar monomers. Simple sugars are typically water-soluble polar molecules that exist in different chiral forms denoted as D and L. When polymerised into long chains, an almost unlimited range of properties can be achieved, from hydrophilic water-soluble molecules such as heparin through to water insoluble structural materials such as cellulose and chitin. Structurally, polysaccharides are characterised by sugars covalently linked with glycoside bonds either as homopolymers composed of a single repeating saccharide molecule or heteropolymers comprising two or more sugar monomers or oligomer blocks. The functions of polysaccharides in living organisms are wide ranging from the core functions of energy storage and as structural supports, through to complex roles in cell signalling such as those exhibited by the GAG [5,27].

In the biomedical field polysaccharides are isolated from several sources including porcine, bovine and avian tissues and from plant and algal tissues such as those sourced from potatoes and seaweed, respectively. Polysaccharides from animal sources are typically isolated from the ECM of connective tissue with key examples being heparin (porcine mucosa), HA (rooster combs) and chitosan (crustaceans). Carbohydrates from plant sources are mainly used in the plant as an energy source, for example, starch in potato and corn and as structural materials such as cellulose in plant cell walls. Bacterial fermentation and isolation from cell culture media have also been used to synthesise polysaccharides for biomaterial applications [28], and removal of bioburden and contaminating bacterial products is a critically important part of such manufacturing processes (see Figure 1.1).

> The antibacterial properties of chitosan are highlighted in Chapter 4. Commercial products based on chitosan include HemCon® bandages and ChitoFlex wound dressings (HemCon Medical Technologies, UK) and CELOX™ (Medtrade Products, UK). Selection for these uses, however, is due to its excellent biocompatibility, biodegradability, non-toxicity and low immunogenicity rather than its antimicrobial properties.
>
> Chapter 5 introduces the use of plasma-based surface modification for the control of biointerfacial interactions. Plasma-based surface modification methods

Continued

have been extraordinarily successful in providing improved biocompatibility and cellular responses. The effectiveness, reproducibility, convenience and environmental benefits of using a plasma process compared with alternatives, such as solution-based processes, will ensure that this class of surface modification procedures will remain attractive to manufacturers in the future. However, the requirement of a vacuum process and the associated fact that a batch process is required has prevented even wider applications. It is therefore likely that the focus will shift further to plasma treatment options that do not require a vacuum and/or batch processing.

Based on excerpts from Chapters 4 and 5.

The most prevalent polysaccharides that have been used for commercially available biomedical devices are alginate, cellulose and starch-based materials, chitosan and the GAG HA. Key features of alginate, starch and selected GAGs and their use in biomedical devices will be detailed below. The specific GAGs that will be discussed are HA and heparin, two polymers that are common in biomedical device applications. Key features that are evident in these structures are the charged nature of the molecules and their low heterogeneity in comparison with protein structures.

Alginate, a copolymer based on blocks of mannuronic (M) and guluronic acid (G), is among the most commonly cited polysaccharide biomaterials and it has a long history of use in food processing. The glycoside-bonded M and G blocks in alginate are composed of β-1,4 linked D-mannuronic acid and α-1,4-linked L-guluronic acid [29,30]. Alginates from different algal species have variability in their proportions of M blocks and G block and different block configurations, and these variations in the assembly of the polymer produce the characteristic variability in alginate properties [31]. When produced as a biomaterial, alginate polymer forms a gel via complex formation with divalent cations in aqueous, cell compatible conditions. However mammals do not have appropriate enzymes to break down the polymer and although much research has been conducted on modifying and blending alginates with other materials, it is largely used in surface contacting devices [29].

Alginate gels have characteristically low polymer contents of up to 2%. The mechanical strength is typically weak, in the low kilopascal range and is dependent on the M/G ratio with gels having higher G contents being stronger and having higher elastic moduli [30,32]. Additionally, the alginate complex can dissociate in electrolyte solutions such as those in vivo resulting in dissolution of the gel. One of the key properties of alginate is its capacity to absorb many times its weight in water. As a consequence, alginate has been used as an absorbant dressing for wounds associated with high levels of exudate. Since wounds that are heavily exudating may be susceptible to infection, many alginate dressings have also been produced with silver particles or ionic silver compounds added. An example is Luofucon Silver Alginate Dressings, which is indicated for 'the management of moderate to heavily exuding partial to full thickness wounds, including, postoperative wounds, trauma wounds, leg ulcers, pressure ulcers, diabetic ulcers, graft and donor sites' [33]. Addition of 50 μg silver particles per cm^2 of the alginate dressing confers antimicrobial activity.

Starch is a homopolymer that is an important polysaccharide in energy storage for plants and is based on repeating units of glucose linked by α-1,4-glycosidic bonds. Although insoluble in cold water, this polysaccharide can be digested by amylases that hydrolyse the glycoside bond in the human gastrointestinal tract. Similar to alginate, starch is regarded as safe for consumption in food products, and as a result of its low toxicity has long been applied in biomedical uses such as for powder used in surgical gloves. Few starch-based products have been developed for surgical devices although there is a large volume of research being conducted on these materials as components of composite biomaterials [34]. One example of medical device applications using potato starch is a bioabsorbable haemostatic agent based on dry starch particles [35]. Since starch can be enzymatically broken down in humans, these particles are typically resorbed within 2 days post-surgery.

Cellulose is another glucose polymer that is used in medical applications. It differs from starch in that it is linked via β-1,4-glycosidic bonds, is a highly crystalline linear polymer that is insoluble in water and is not able to be digested by humans. Several animal species such as the ruminants are able to digest this polysaccharide due to the presence of specialist microbial populations in the gastrointestinal tract. Historically, cellulose found widespread use in hollow fibre membranes for haemodialysis; however it was replaced by alternate materials after reports of complement mediated leukopenia were associated with these membranes [36]. A water soluble derivative of cellulose, carboxymethylcellulose (CMC), is in widespread use today as a food additive, as a viscosity modifier in pharmaceuticals and as a lubricant in artificial tears. In medical device applications CMC has been used blended with dressings or bandages to provide moist healing environments and absorb exudate. Transformation of cellulose to starch has been demonstrated through a chemical process which is potentially significant given the abundance of cellulose as a discardable by-product of many manufacturing processes involving plant matter [27].

The GAGs are a specialised family of molecules that are key components of mammalian ECM. The two types of GAGs are those that are sulphated and decorate proteins to form the proteoglycans and HA, a GAG that does not bind with proteins. The most abundant of the sulphated GAGs in ECM is chondroitin sulphate with other members including dermatan, heparin/heparin and keratin comprising the remainder of the group.

Chapter 6 outlines approaches to producing anti-thrombogenic coatings on vascular stents. One of the most studied approaches is using heparin given its function as a potent anticoagulant. Heparin forms a complex with antithrombin III and binds with thrombin to produce the non-thrombogenic effect. Nonthrombogenic coatings can be prepared by either immobilizing heparin on the surface by strong ionic binding or by chemical grafting.

Continued

Blood compatibility of coatings can be evaluated in vitro and in vivo as outlined in Chapter 6. Typically in vitro tests tend to be of shorter duration and the results are influenced by the blood source, the manner in which they are handled and the level of anticoagulants used.

Based on excerpts from Chapter 6.

Unlike other GAGs in ECM, HA is non-sulphated with a very high-molecular weight of the order of 10^6 Da. It has a linear unbranched backbone structure based on disaccharide units of D-glucuronic acid and D-*N*-acetylglucosamine linked via alternating β-1,4 and β-1,3 glycosidic bonds [37]. In medical devices HA has been used in multiple applications including as an anti-adhesive material, for joint pain and as a dermal filler [38]. As shown in Table 1.3, about half of the dermal fillers approved for use by the USA FDA are based on HA [39]. The major sources of HA in dermal fillers are from avian tissue (rooster combs) and bacterial fermentation exemplified by Hylaform® and Restylane®, respectively.

Restylane® is produced via bacterial formation using Gram-positive streptococcal species and is supplied as a 2% solution in a physiological buffer. The gel is stabilised using the chemical crosslinker 1,4-butanediol diglycidyl ether (BDDE). Another similar HA-based product is Hylaform®, which is similarly a crosslinked formulation but differs from Restylane® in that it is sourced from avian tissue. The stated advantages of the HA-based fillers are that there is less likelihood of allergic reactions that can be associated with collagen-based fillers and that they are associated with greater ease of use [40].

Another very commonly used GAG in biomedical applications, as an anticoagulant drug, is heparin. Heparin is a highly heterogeneous sulphated molecule based primarily on the disaccharide 2-*O*-sulfo-α-L-iduronic acid and 6-*O*-sulfo-*N*-sulfo-α-D-glucosamine linked via β-1,4 glycoside bonds. It is typically sourced from porcine mucosal tissue and is made up of a polydisperse solution with an average molecular weight of 17 kDa. Heparin has been used extensively as a modifying biologic on commercially available blood contacting devices such as haemodialysis catheters [41]. In biomaterials research, heparin has also been the subject of investigation of its growth factor binding capacity with the objective of exploiting this for drug or device applications. Heparin–VEGF modification of decellularised bioprothetic heart valves using a multilayer coatings was shown to have a dual effect as an anticoagulant as well as encouraging cell proliferation in vitro [42]. Much of the research on utilising these specialised properties of GAGs has not yet been commercially applied.

1.3 Advantages and disadvantages of natural polymers

Biological polymers are the ultimate in custom-designed materials since they are synthesised by living organisms in situ to fit very specific forms and create specific niches for supporting cell, tissue and organ functions. They are thus ideally designed for their original purpose. As preceding sections have outlined, there is a wide variety of biological polymers that have been used as materials in medical devices. The rationale for selection of these polymers relate in the most part to their biological properties rather than inherent physical, mechanical or chemical attributes. Although providing ideal structure and support when in their native form, when isolated, physical and mechanical properties of natural polymers can deteriorate. Examples of this are collagen and elastin, which together confer strength and elasticity to dermal tissue; however when isolated and purified experience significant deterioration in mechanical properties. Additionally, if processed tissue itself is used as a biomaterial scaffold, removal of antigenic components such as cell components and antigenic epitopes on proteins can result in a significant reduction of mechanical properties. For example, bone synthesised by vertebrates is a composite of a collagen organic matrix and a hydroxyapatite inorganic matrix. The collagen component of the composite confers flexibility and toughness and the mineral component supports stiffness; however it is the two components working together confers to the composite ideal strength under loading and bending [43]. When bone is subject to fixation or irradiation both of which alter the native structure of collagen, or collagen is removed from the composite, significant loss of toughness and flexibility occurs [44,45]. Despite decades of research on collagen–Hap composites, a bone replacement material that can match the properties of native bone tissue remains elusive.

1.3.1 Biological polymer benefits

Proteins and polysaccharides have many features that render them attractive for use in medical devices. However, the primary use of these polymers as medical materials is not based on the premise that they will provide ideal structures that exactly match native tissue. Following isolation properties can be fundamentally altered and although not able to replicate or regenerate tissue, biomimetic features of isolated natural polymers can promote cell and tissue integration. The major benefits of biological polymers should be considered in terms of the functional performance of isolated polymers and their biological performance.

Functional performance refers to the capacity of the material to fulfil its requirements in the specific device application. For example, in one type of wound healing device the material specifications may include flexibility, breathability and the ability to absorb fluid, whereas in another the materials may be required to be transparent, adhesive and occlusive. For both of these applications, different materials and forms of these materials will need to be selected. In active implantable medical devices such as pacemakers, the different materials selected need to meet requirements as wide ranging as being conductive, to being insulators and supporting hermetic sealing of electronics and electrode connections.

> Chapter 10 introduces conducting polymers, which add to the versatility of polymers by adding electroactivity to the repertoire of properties possible. Polymers are typically used as insulators. Wires are coated with plastics, and switches are

Continued

made of plastics for insulation purpose. But in fact, not all polymers are insulators. They can be just as conductive as metals. Mechanisms of conduction, how conducting polymers (CPs) are polymerised and specific applications are covered in this chapter.

Chapter 11 addresses the biosynthetic approach to producing conducting polymers with the capacity to integrate with cells and tissues. Incorporation of bulky biological molecules tends to cause deterioration of CP mechanical and electrical properties driving the need to explore a range of alternate composite CP materials. Composites based on CPs have included blends, hybrids, double networks and layered structures which aim to preserve the electrical benefits of CPs but use additional polymer components to impart more control over mechanical and biological properties. It has been proposed that this new range of soft, organic electroactive materials can meet the needs of being more tissue compatible through proving a softer interface while maintaining the electronic interface between tissues and devices.

Chapter 12 outlines the degradable conjugated conducting polymers and their application in nerve guidance. Conjugated polymers themselves are not biodegradable; however, this can be addressed either by degrading a fraction of the resulting scaffold or by synthesising new families of degradable conducting polymers. Maintaining electrical conductivity is a major challenge for these materials; however, it is equally important to investigate incorporation of biomolecular and topographical cues for guidance, especially without compromising the conducting properties.

Based on excerpts from Chapters 10, 11 and 12.

Natural polymers have many characteristics that support their functional performance in a variety of applications including their ability to be produced in multiple forms in physiological milieu, their water solubility and their capacity for biodegradation and clearance from the host system. Proteins such as collagen can be degraded following implantation by native collagenases present in both inflammatory and connective tissue cells at the site of the implant. Collagen, which provides a matrix for cell adhesion via its ligands for integrin receptors, is also typically remodelled so that the introduced material is replaced by ECM deposited by connective tissue cells at the site. This is a characteristic that no purely synthetic polymer can fulfil since enzymes have not evolved to breakdown the bonds present in these man-made polymers.

Biological performance of a material is comprised of the host response to the material as well as the material response, which is the way in which the material is altered following contact with the living system, or the 'host' environment. The latter can in turn elicit subsequent host responses. The host response is typically evaluated by subjecting individual materials to specific preclinical tests such as those outlined in ISO10993-1 [46]. Selection of the types of preclinical tests that are required by regulatory authorities is based on the nature and duration of exposure of the host

Table 1.4 Types of host contact and nature and duration of contact that determine the types of biological performance tests required for preclinical evaluation of medical devices. The less invasive the contact and the shorter duration translates to lower risk and thus lower levels of testing required

Category of contact	Nature of contact	Duration
Surface	Intact skin	
	Mucosal membrane	↑
	Breached or compromised surface	<24 h
Externally communicating	Blood path, indirect	>24 h–30 days
	Tissue/bone/dentin	>30 days
	Circulating blood	↓
Implant	Tissue/bone	
	Blood	

to the device. Table 1.4 shows the classification of the type or degree of contact and the nature of contact used in ISO 10993. With lower levels of contact, such as those only contacting undamaged skin or mucosal membranes there is a minimal level of testing required. With higher levels of contact, for example, fully implanted devices the extent of testing required expands with increasing risk associated with the device application. Given the high risks associated with critical life supporting devices implanted in blood, the most stringent testing programs are implemented in these cases.

Host response, material response and the functional performance together are also evaluated by subjecting the whole device to a series of functional in vitro, ex vivo and in vivo tests. These are generally not governed by ISO 10993 preclinical testing regimes, rather they involve specifically designed evaluations conducted in animal models. If used as submission for supporting regulatory approval of a device, there may be a requirement for the evaluations to be conducted according to good laboratory practices [47]. Finally, the ultimate assessment of safety typically requires clinical trial as appropriate to the specific application. This is conducted under the prevailing clinical trials governance required by regulatory authorities.

A generally accepted overarching definition of biocompatibility is provided in the Williams dictionary of Biomaterials, 'The ability of a material to perform with an appropriate host response in a specific application' [48]. Further to this, it is important to note that biocompatibility is not as simple as a single

Continued

measure. There are numerous tests provided for biocompatibility by the ISO standards [46]. These include:

1. Cytotoxicity
2. Sensitization
3. Haemocompatibility
4. Pyrogenicity
5. Implantation
6. Genotoxicity
7. Carcinogenicity
8. Reproductive and developmental toxicity
9. Biodegradation testing

Therefore, it is fairly clear that biocompatibility is not a simple or straightforward matter, it is made up of numerous properties of a material: its manufacture, storage and structure. All of these issues must be considered before a device is to be implanted.

Furthermore, the United States FDA states that biocompatibility is not a matter as simple as assessing the materials the device is constructed from:

The biocompatibility of a final device depends not only on the materials but also on the processing of the materials, manufacturing methods (including the sterilization process), and the manufacturing residuals that may be present on the final device [49].

Biological polymers clearly have beneficial biological performance in terms of their biodegradability as outlined, however their key advantages can be explained in terms of their compatibility with human cells and tissue, in terms of both low toxicity and bioactive capacity. In relation to bioactivity, a key benefit is the ability of proteins and polysaccharides to directly support cell growth and differentiation. By presentation of growth factors and signalling cells they are also able to indirectly support and direct a multitude of cell functions. Finally, their mechanics although not ideal may be more appropriately matched to tissue mechanics than many synthetic materials.

1.3.2 Limitations of natural polymers

When selecting materials for implantable medical devices, several factors must be considered as outlined in Table 1.5. In broad terms these factors include the chemical, physical, electrical and biological materials properties that impact on the functional and biological performance of the material in the specific device application. However, there are some properties of natural polymers that are specific to this class of materials that need to be considered. These properties include features that may result in deterioration of functional performance such as control of chemical structure and stability, challenges with physical and mechanical properties, sterilisation and shelf-life. More critically, those material properties that may elicit a detrimental host response such as

Table 1.5 **Factors for consideration in selecting natural polymers**

Design requirement	Considerations when selecting biological polymers
Chemical	**1.** Reproducibility/quality control **2.** Chemical stability/degradability **3.** Solubility **4.** Sterilisability
Physical/mechanical	**1.** Mechanics **2.** Topography **3.** Dimensional stability **4.** Shelf-life
Electrical	**1.** Insulation **2.** Conductivity/electroactivity
Biological	**1.** Immunogenicity **2.** Transmission of infectious agents and prions

immunotoxicity and transmission of infectious agents and prions must be considered. It is these properties that need to be a particular focus when selecting natural polymers for device applications.

Considering first the functional performance, durability and dimensional stability will be the two key factors considered here. Most natural polymers are typically less durable in vivo than many of their synthetic counterparts. Heart valves are a good example of this exemplified by bioprosthetic valves being less durable than their mechanical counterparts fabricated using combinations of metals, polymers and pyrolytic carbon. Despite their advantages in requiring lower or no anticoagulation therapy, enzymatic degradation and calcification of the largely collagenous tissue used in bioprosthetic valves can lead to high failure rates [50]. Although a secondary issue, calcification which occurs due to deposition of calcium salts in the tissue component of the device has been a significant cause of valve failure in the past [51]. Use of glutaraldehyde fixatives and specific tissue processing steps to remove fats and other contaminants has yielded significant increases in the implant life of these valves, and they remain the implant of choice primarily in people who cannot tolerate the anticoagulation treatment that is required for recipients of mechanical valves [52].

Dimensional stability is another key issue that can impact on the functional performance of biological polymers. Most materials that are sourced from natural tissues have high water content and are by definition hydrogels. ECM is based on a highly swollen, crosslinked networks of natural polymer chains and in healthy individuals it maintains equilibrium hydration through natural homeostatic mechanisms. Another important factor is the mechanical stress under which the tissue exists in physiological conditions. This mechanical stress is particularly evident when tissue such as blood vessels or skeletal muscle are isolated from the host. The resected tissue undergoes shrinkage since the native tissue normally exists in tension. Further dimensional change occurs with loss of fluid from the tissue following exposure to different processing conditions and due to disruption of crosslinking within the ECM during processing. Finally, both chain scission and crosslinking can occur during sterilisation processes and this can further alter properties and result in an inability to predict the likely dimensional stability in vivo. Thus the native structure of crosslinked ECM is critical to its dimensional stability and predictability of other physical properties. When tissue is isolated and the natural crosslinks are broken and new crosslinks are formed, the physical characteristics of the 'material' produced will clearly be affected.

The complex biochemistry and structure of collagen are perfectly designed for its use in the tissue architecture. However, a key limitation of isolated soluble collagen in applications where cell delivery is required is the significant shrinkage that occurs when cells are encapsulated within the gel. Contraction of collagen gels is a well-known phenomenon that is related to both cell loading and collagen concentration [53]. In a review, the importance of cell density and polymer content in contracture has been reiterated and the utility of these gels as versatile models for studying tissue behaviour and cell–tissue interactions confirmed [54]. However, this dimensional instability and variability in physical and mechanical properties does not lend itself to future medical device applications.

Both dimensional stability and unpredictability or lack of control of the degradation rate of natural polymers can be managed to a degree by use of chemical preservatives and stabilisers. Chemicals, such as glutaraldehyde and BDDE (noted previously as being applied in commercial medical devices), act via reaction with nucleophiles in protein components of natural polymers. While this form of chemical crosslinking has the effect of modifying the degradation rate of implanted materials, residual chemicals can be toxic if released into the body. Since their mechanism is to crosslink nucleophiles, the chemicals can act directly on host tissue and thus residuals must be kept below a minimum level to reduce the probability of adverse host responses.

Hydrogels are versatile high water content tissue-like materials that are conducive to development of biosynthetic hybrid materials. Chapter 7 details degradable hydrogel systems and described these systems in the context of physico-chemical properties required for successful application to medical products. These include (1) three-dimensional (3D) structural support; (2) a permeable/interconnected porous structure; (3) suitable and controllable biodegradation rates; (4) low toxicity and immunogenicity of both the hydrogel and its degradation products; and (5) good mechanical properties for maintenance of the 3D shape during degradation and function.

Chapter 8 covers the use of hydrogels and associated angiogenesis. Designing hydrogel materials that can support and promote establishment of functional vasculature is attractive due to hydrogel mechanical properties, which can often be 'tuned' to match tissue properties, the excellent biocompatibility of many hydrogel materials, and the ability to spatially localize angiogenic activity. In order to address the need for functional vasculature, tissue engineers and biomaterials scientists are taking clues from the biology of the angiogenesis process and developing methods to mimic nature when designing proangiogenic hydrogel materials.

Chapter 9 presents an overview of the design considerations and materials for hydrogel preparation, focusing on natural and synthetic polymers and how they are combined into biosynthetic systems. By combining natural and synthetic materials researchers can present structural (e.g., topography, degradation, fibrous structural hierarchy) and biochemical cues (e.g., adhesion molecules, growth factors) in order to better understand the effects of extracellular microenvironments on phenotypic activities of cells. Thoughtful selection of hydrogel base materials is required to achieve the appropriate level of property control and achieve the desired cellular response that is inherent to each application.

Based on excerpts from Chapters 7, 8 and 9.

With reference to host response, key areas of concern intrinsic to natural polymers include immunogenicity and transmission of infectious agents and prions. The former occurs in cases where the material implanted has antigenic components, which are immunogenic and thus can activate the host immune system. The latter is an inherent risk associated with sourcing medical products from animal tissue, which may have bacterial or viral loads that are not removed via a sterilisation process or prions that are not sensitive to typical sterilisation techniques.

Both proteins and to a lesser extent polysaccharides can be immunogenic although proteins tend to be stronger antigens and typically have multiple epitopes that invoke antibody formation. The adverse host responses of biomaterial interactions with the immune system are a result of either immunostimulation or immunosuppression and can range from minor allergic reactions through to anaphylaxis and death. The consequences of adverse responses to antigen exposure occur on a range of timescales from immediate and acute through to chronic rejection [55]. Such adverse immune responses occur due to the presence of native antibodies or induction of circulating or cell surface antibodies that can bind to antigens present on implanted materials and either directly activate cells in the immune system or activate the complement cascade. The latter biological cascade forms a critical arm of the immune system and its activation results in the production of several complement fragments with biological activities and ultimately formation of a membrane attack complex that can cause cell lysis and death [56]. Although designed to protect the host against foreign agents like bacteria, unintended activation such as that which occurs after exposure to biomaterial antigens can lead to significant morbidity and mortality. Complement is classically activated by exposure to antigen–antibody complexes as part of the acquired immune system.

Preclinical studies for examining the potential for immunotoxicity are classed as tests evaluating either immunostimulation or immunosuppression and are outlined in the Biological performance standards ISO 10993-10 [57] and ISO 10993-20 [58].

In vitro tests measuring antibody formation and in vivo tests such as the guinea pig maximisation test for evaluation of hypersensitivity have been most commonly used in preclinical testing repertoires. Approximately 3% of the population is thought to be allergic to bovine collagen used in aesthetic surgery. The majority of reactions are delayed type hypersensitivity, however in some cases immediate, anaphylactic responses have occurred due to the presence of circulating antibodies against collagen epitopes [59].

Although proteins may act as stronger antigens, carbohydrate antigens are critical activators of complement via the so-called lectin pathway, which is a component of host repertoire of innate immunity. Typically activated by protein receptors or lectins that recognise carbohydrates on bacterial cell surfaces, or pathogen-associated molecular patterns (PAMPs), this arm of innate immunity can produce immediate response to challenge by introduced antigens. Examples of this are in the immediate or hyperacute responses to transplanted tissues that occur due to the presence of natural antibodies to carbohydrate antigens that decorate cell-associated proteins [60]. The specific mechanism for recognition and rejection of foreign xenogeneic tissues is via reaction between natural circulating antibodies in the host that recognise alpha-galactose (α-gal) antigens associated with constituent carbohydrate molecules [60]. This type of activation of the immune system via such PAMPS can also be biomaterial associated. Synthetic polymers with pendant carbohydrates, or glycopolymers, conjugated with protein have been synthesised using bovine serum albumin (BSA) as a model protein. These conjugates are able to activate the immune system in a manner that does not occur with BSA alone via a hapten-like mechanism [61]. While polysaccharide materials can induce immune responses, materials such as HA do not appear to be immunogenic and are often used as an alternative to protein based fillers where there is a known allergy to collagen. However, because many HA products such as Restylane® are manufactured via bacterial fermentation, immune reactions and allergy to Gram-positive bacterial cell components may occur and this is a common contraindication for use of these implants (see Table 1.3).

Transmission of infectious agents is another key risk when considering use of biologically derived materials. Microbial contamination of devices can have significant consequences in terms of infection, loss of the implanted device and mortality. Key issues with biological materials include the potential for high bioburden, the presence of contaminating bacteria or viruses that can be transmitted to humans and the difficulties presented in applying sterilisation processes to natural polymers. As shown in Figure 1.1, the processing for naturally derived materials must include steps for removal of contaminating matter and ensuring that the tissue has been disinfected and where possible terminally sterilised. With the increasing use of human cadaver materials which are not terminally sterilised (see Table 1.2), bacterial and viral contamination and transfer to recipients of these implants may occur.

Prions are also an area of concern with regard to implantable animal-derived materials. These aberrant proteins based on normal proteins which are misfolded have been confirmed as infectious agents in a variety of animal models [62]. Because prions are not cellular organisms or viruses they are differentiated from classical infectious agents in that they cannot be easily removed by standard sterilisation protocols.

The observation in the 1980 and 1990s that severe neurodegenerative disease occurred following consumption of human or animal tissue [63] led to concerns that use of animal-derived tissue in medical devices may be problematic. In 1998, the United States FDA subsequently released a guidance that has since been updated [64]. The updated guidance covers the range of issues that need to be evaluated when materials from animal sources are used in medical products. In addition to prion contamination, these issues include the aforementioned transmission of infectious agents including bacteria and viruses. The guidance also recommends that the source of the animal tissue is appropriately tracked and that inactivation of viruses is measured.

1.4 Biosynthetic polymers

Although versatile and able to provide a controlled platform for medical device fabrication, synthetic polymers do not have the inherent properties that can meet end-use requirements in applications where cell support and interactions are required. Biological polymers, as outlined in the sections above, also suffer from limitations despite their many advantages. These limitations fundamentally relate to modification following isolation and manufacture resulting in significant changes in structure and mechanics.

Much research has focused on biosynthetic polymers to meet the ever increasing demand for materials that can fulfil the range of specifications for next generation medical devices, in particular tissue engineered solutions. These hybrid polymers are formed when a natural polymer and a synthetic polymer are combined to produce a material with desirable qualities of both classes of polymer. Figure 1.2 illustrates the concept of synergistic outcomes when a biological polymer is used in conjunction with a synthetic polymer.

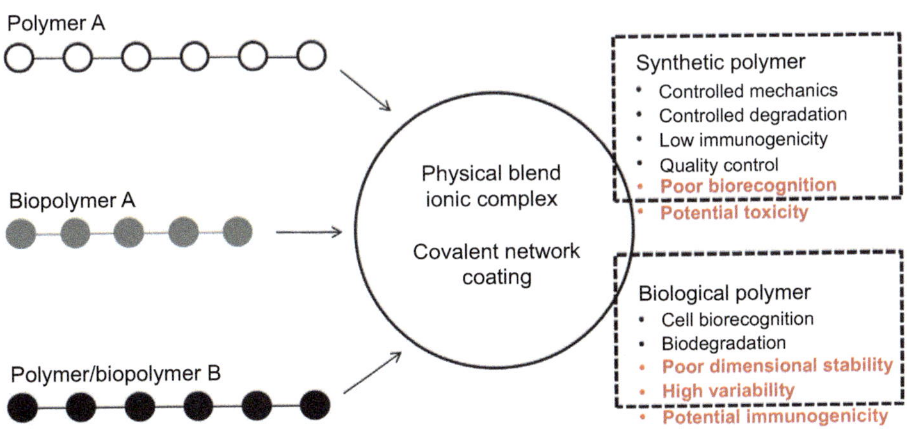

Figure 1.2 Biosynthetic polymers are formed from combinations of biological or natural polymers and synthetic polymers.

Different approaches for integration of biological and synthetic polymers can be used including physical blends, coatings, ionic complexes and covalently linked pendants or networks. While physical blends and physically adsorbed coatings present the lowest complexity in design, issues relating to diffusion and unpredictable release of components limit their use. The greatest effort in research and development of biosynthetic materials is focused on producing stable hybrids or covalently bound coatings that maintain their intended function for the required period of use. Clearly much research is still required to achieve elegant biomimetic structures that can support replacement or regeneration of native tissue.

While integrating biological and synthetic polymers has the advantage merging the benefits of both polymer types, it is not currently possible to negate all disadvantages presented by introduction of foreign materials into the body. As suggested in Figure 1.2, biosynthetic polymers can provide biorecognition, dimensional stability and control of quality not afforded by synthetic and biological polymers individually. However any potential toxicity, including immunotoxicity must still be evaluated, as both natural and synthetic polymers can be associated with these adverse effects. In theory, by minimising the concentration of biological polymers incorporated and ensuring stable integration with synthetic materials of low toxicity, the impact of any potential toxicity will be decreased substantially.

1.5 Conclusion

There remain many challenges in delivering biosynthetic materials for incorporation in therapeutic devices. These primarily relate to managing the limitations presented by each of the synthetic and natural polymer groups and to devising approaches for combining the two polymer types that minimise their disadvantages while magnifying or exploiting their advantages.

Future medical devices that allow more intimate integration of device components and tissues will rely on providing innovative materials to support development of solutions to these challenges. Development of materials that more closely mimic tissue or support in situ regeneration of damaged tissue will rely on expanding and learning from the body of knowledge on both synthetic and natural polymers and their hybrids.

References

[1] J.E. Gagner, W. Kim, E.L. Chaikof, Designing protein-based biomaterials for medical applications, Acta Biomater. 10 (4) (2014) 1542–1557.

[2] J.W. Whittaker, Cell-free protein synthesis: the state of the art, Biotechnol. Lett. 35 (2) (2013) 143–152.

[3] C. Frantz, K.M. Stewart, V.M. Weaver, The extracellular matrix at a glance, J. Cell Sci. 123 (Pt 24) (2010) 4195–4200.

[4] J. Schiller, D. Huster, New methods to study the composition and structure of the extracellular matrix in natural and bioengineered tissues, Biomatter 2 (3) (2012) 115–131.

[5] R.V. Iozzo, L. Schaefer, Proteoglycan form and function: a comprehensive nomenclature of proteoglycans, Matrix Biol. (2015).
[6] B.N. Brown, S.F. Badylak, Extracellular matrix as an inductive scaffold for functional tissue reconstruction, Transl. Res. 163 (4) (2014) 268–285.
[7] Elastagen Ltd, Elastagen | Next generation medical and cosmetic treatments [Online]. Available: http://www.elastagen.com/ (accessed 09.06.15).
[8] J.A.M. Ramshaw, Y.Y. Peng, V. Glattauer, J.A. Werkmeister, Collagens as biomaterials, J. Mater. Sci. Mater. Med. 20 (Suppl. 1) (2009).
[9] A. Jayakrishnan, S.R. Jameela, Glutaraldehyde as a fixative in bioprostheses and drug delivery matrices, Biomaterials 17 (5) (1996) 471–484.
[10] P.A. Rubin, A.M. Fay, H.D. Remulla, M. Maus, Ophthalmic plastic applications of acellular dermal allografts, Ophthalmology 106 (11) (1999) 2091–2097.
[11] H.R. Moyer, A. Losken, The science behind tissue biologics, QMP Plast. Surg. Pulse News (1997) 8–11.
[12] N.J. Smart, M. Marshall, I.R. Daniels, Biological meshes: a review of their use in abdominal wall hernia repairs, Surgeon 10 (3) (2012) 159–171.
[13] A.W. Cheng, M.A. Abbas, T. Tejirian, Outcome of abdominal wall hernia repair with permacol™ biologic mesh, Am. Surg. 79 (10) (2013) 992–996.
[14] H. Sage, R.G. Woodbury, P. Bornstein, Structural studies on human type IV collagen, J. Biol. Chem. 254 (19) (1979) 9893–9900.
[15] Advanced Biomatrix Inc., PureCol® – Directions for use [Online]. Available: https://www.advancedbiomatrix.com/images/PureCol-Directions-for-Use.pdf (accessed 10.06.15).
[16] A.K. Lynn, I.V. Yannas, W. Bonfield, Antigenicity and immunogenicity of collagen, J. Biomed. Mater. Res. – Part B Appl. Biomater. 71 (2) (2004) 343–354.
[17] S.K. Kim, Y.T. Kim, H.G. Byun, K.S. Nam, D.S. Joo, F. Shahidi, Isolation and characterization of antioxidative peptides from gelatin hydrolysate of Alaska pollack skin, J. Agric. Food Chem. 49 (4) (2001) 1984–1989.
[18] Z. Zhang, G. Li, B. Shi, Physicochemical properties of collagen, gelatin and collagen hydrolysate derived from bovine limed split wastes, J. Soc. Leather Technol. Chem. 90 (1) (2006) 23–28.
[19] FDA, The Sourcing and Processing of Gelatin to Reduce the Potential Risk Posed by Bovine Spongiform Encephalopathy (BSE) in FDA-Regulated Products for Human Use. Office of the Commissioner [Online]. Available: http://www.fda.gov/regulatoryinformation/guidances/ucm125182.htm (accessed 26.05.15).
[20] J.L. Drury, D.J. Mooney, Hydrogels for tissue engineering: scaffold design variables and applications, Biomaterials 24 (24) (2003) 4337–4351.
[21] M.W. Mosesson, Fibrinogen and fibrin structure and functions, J. Thromb. Haemost. 3 (8) (2005) 1894–1904.
[22] M.M. Martino, P.S. Briquez, A. Ranga, M.P. Lutolf, J.A. Hubbell, Heparin-binding domain of fibrin(ogen) binds growth factors and promotes tissue repair when incorporated within a synthetic matrix, Proc. Natl. Acad. Sci. U.S.A. 110 (12) (2013) 4563–4568.
[23] J.F. Almine, S.G. Wise, A.S. Weiss, Elastin signaling in wound repair, Birth Defects Res. Part C – Embryo Today Rev. 96 (3) (2012) 248–257.
[24] R.P. Mecham, Methods in elastic tissue biology: elastin isolation and purification, Changes 29 (6) (2012) 997–1003.
[25] Z. Indik, W.R. Abrams, U. Kucich, C.W. Gibson, R.P. Mecham, J. Rosenbloom, Production of recombinant human tropoelastin: characterization and demonstration of immunologic and chemotactic activity, Arch. Biochem. Biophys. 280 (1) (1990) 80–86.

[26] S.L. Martin, B. Vrhovski, A.S. Weiss, Total synthesis and expression in *Escherichia coli* of a gene encoding human tropoelastin, Gene 154 (2) (1995) 159–166.
[27] C. You, H. Chen, S. Myung, N. Sathitsuksanoh, H. Ma, X.-Z. Zhang, et al., Enzymatic transformation of nonfood biomass to starch, Proc. Natl. Acad. Sci. U.S.A. 110 (18) (2013) 7182–7187.
[28] P. Nguyen, L. Phan, B. Tran, US Patent Application Publication, US Pat. Appl. Publ., vol. 13/353,316, no. 19, 2013.
[29] A.D. Augst, H.J. Kong, D.J. Mooney, Alginate hydrogels as biomaterials, Macromol. Biosci. 6 (8) (2006) 623–633.
[30] S.N. Pawar, K.J. Edgar, Alginate derivatization: a review of chemistry, properties and applications, Biomaterials 33 (11) (2012) 3279–3305.
[31] C.K. Kuo, P.X. Ma, Ionically crosslinked alginate hydrogels as scaffolds for tissue engineering: Part 1. Structure, gelation rate and mechanical properties, Biomaterials 22 (6) (2001) 511–521.
[32] M. Matyash, F. Despang, C. Ikonomidou, M. Gelinsky, Swelling and mechanical properties of alginate hydrogels with respect to promotion of neural growth, Tissue Eng. Part C Methods 20 (5) (2013).
[33] Huizhou Foryou Medical Devices Co Ltd., 510(k) Summary: Luofucon Silver Alginate Dressing. FDA 510(k) Summary [Online]. Available: http://www.accessdata.fda.gov/cdrh_docs/pdf12/K120181.pdf.
[34] A.P. Marques, R.L. Reis, J.A. Hunt, The biocompatibility of novel starch-based polymers and composites: In vitro studies, Biomaterials 23 (6) (2002) 1471–1478.
[35] PMA Review, Arista™ AH Absorbable Hemostat. FDA PMA Response Letter [Online] Available: http://www.accessdata.fda.gov/cdrh_docs/pdf5/p050038a.pdf, 2006.
[36] R.M. Hakim, D.T. Fearon, J.M. Lazarus, Biocompatibility of dialysis membranes: effects of chronic complement activation, Kidney Int. 26 (2) (1984) 194–200.
[37] M. Kurisawa, J.E. Chung, Y.Y. Yang, S.J. Gao, H. Uyama, Injectable biodegradable hydrogels composed of hyaluronic acid-tyramine conjugates for drug delivery and tissue engineering, Chem. Commun. (Camb) (34) (2005) 4312–4314.
[38] A. Fakhari, C. Berkland, Applications and emerging trends of hyaluronic acid in tissue engineering, as a dermal filler and in osteoarthritis treatment, Acta Biomater. 9 (7) (2013) 7081–7092.
[39] Center for Devices and Radiological Health, Soft Tissue Fillers (Dermal Fillers) – Soft Tissue Fillers Approved by the Center for Devices and Radiological Health [Online]. Available: http://www.fda.gov/MedicalDevices/ProductsandMedicalProcedures/CosmeticDevices/WrinkleFillers/ucm227749.htm (accessed 02.06.15).
[40] S.R. Coleman, Cross-linked hyaluronic acid fillers, Plast. Reconstr. Surg. 117 (2) (2006) 661–665.
[41] H. Mojibian, M. Spector, N. Ni, D. Eliseo, J. Pollak, M. Tal, Initial clinical experience with a new heparin-coated chronic hemodialysis catheter, Hemodial. Int. 13 (3) (2009) 329–334.
[42] X. Ye, H. Wang, J. Zhou, H. Li, J. Liu, Z. Wang, et al., The effect of heparin-VEGF multilayer on the biocompatibility of decellularized aortic valve with platelet and endothelial progenitor cells, PLoS One 8 (1) (2013).
[43] S.M. Ghanaati, B.W. Thimm, R.E. Unger, C. Orth, T. Kohler, M. Barbeck, et al., Collagen-embedded hydroxylapatite-beta-tricalcium phosphate-silicon dioxide bone substitute granules assist rapid vascularization and promote cell growth, Biomed. Mater. 5 (2) (2010) 25004.
[44] X. Wang, R.A. Bank, J.M. TeKoppele, C. Mauli Agrawal, The role of collagen in determining bone mechanical properties, J. Orthop. Res. 19 (6) (2001) 1021–1026.

[45] B. Burton, A. Gaspar, D. Josey, J. Tupy, M.D. Grynpas, T.L. Willett, Bone embrittlement and collagen modifications due to high-dose gamma-irradiation sterilization, Bone 61 (2014) 71–81.
[46] ISO 10993-1:2009 Biological evaluation of medical devices Part 1: Evaluation and testing in the risk management process.
[47] FDA, Good Laboratory Practice Regulations (21 CFR Part 58). Code of Federal Regulations [Online]. Available: http://www.fda.gov/ohrms/dockets/98fr/980335s1.PDF.
[48] D.F. Williams, The Williams Dictionary of Biomaterials, vol. 5, Liverpool University Press, 1999.
[49] FDA Centre for Devices and Radiological Health, Use of International Standard ISO-10993, Biological Evaluation of Medical Devices Part 1: Evaluation and Testing, Draft Guidance Document (issued 23.04.13).
[50] F.J. Schoen, R.J. Levy, Tissue heart valves: current challenges and future research perspectives, J. Biomed. Mater. Res. 47 (4) (1999) 439–465.
[51] F.J. Schoen, R.J. Levy, Calcification of tissue heart valve substitutes: progress toward understanding and prevention, Ann. Thorac. Surg. 79 (3) (2005) 1072–1080.
[52] E. Rieder, M.T. Kasimir, G. Silberhumer, G. Seebacher, E. Wolner, P. Simon, et al., Decellularization protocols of porcine heart valves differ importantly in efficiency of cell removal and susceptibility of the matrix to recellularization with human vascular cells, J. Thorac. Cardiovasc. Surg. 127 (2) (2004) 399–405.
[53] E. Bell, B. Ivarsson, C. Merrill, Production of a tissue-like structure by contraction of collagen lattices by human fibroblasts of different proliferative potential in vitro, Proc. Natl. Acad. Sci. U.S.A. 76 (3) (1979) 1274–1278.
[54] R.A. Brown, In the beginning there were soft collagen-cell gels: towards better 3D connective tissue models, Exp. Cell Res. 319 (16) (2013) 2460–2469.
[55] M.L. Wong, L.G. Griffiths, Immunogenicity in xenogeneic scaffold generation: antigen removal vs. decellularization, Acta Biomater. 10 (5) (2014) 1806–1816.
[56] T. Fujita, Evolution of the lectin-complement pathway and its role in innate immunity, Nat. Rev. Immunol. 2 (5) (2002) 346–353.
[57] ISO 10993-10:2010 Biological evaluation of medical devices Part 10: Tests for irritation and delayed-type hypersensitivity.
[58] ISO 10993-20:2006 Biological evaluation of medical devices Part 20: Principles and methods for immunotoxicology testing of medical devices.
[59] P. Lucey, D.J. Goldberg, Complications of collagen fillers, Facial Plast. Surg. 30 (6) (December 2014) 615–622.
[60] J. Milland, M.S. Sandrin, ABO blood group and related antigens, natural antibodies and transplantation, Tissue Antigens 68 (6) (2006) 459–466.
[61] J. Geng, G. Mantovani, L. Tao, J. Nicolas, G. Chen, R. Wallis, et al., Site-directed conjugation of 'clicked' glycopolymers to form glycoprotein mimics: binding to mammalian lectin and induction of immunological function, J. Am. Chem. Soc. 129 (49) (2007) 15156–15163.
[62] J.C. Watts, S.B. Prusiner, Mouse models for studying the formation and propagation of prions, J. Biol. Chem. 289 (29) (2014) 19841–19849.
[63] P.E. Fraser, Prions and prion-like proteins, J. Biol. Chem. 289 (29) (2014) 19839–19840.
[64] FDA, "Medical Devices Containing Materials Derived from Animal Sources," FDA guidance documents [Online]. Available: http://www.fda.gov/downloads/MedicalDevices/DeviceRegulationandGuidance/GuidanceDocuments/UCM381491.pdf, 2014 (accessed 02.06.15).

Nondegradable synthetic polymers for medical devices and implants

2

P.A. Gunatillake, R. Adhikari
Commonwealth Scientific and Industrial Research Organisation (CSIRO) Manufacturing Flagship, Clayton, VIC, Australia

2.1 Introduction

The inert nature of many nondegradable synthetic polymers in biological environments and ease of processing have attracted researchers to explore their utility in biomedical applications. With the advancement of multitude of technologies over the second half of the twentieth century, many medical devices and implants have been developed from synthetic polymers and successfully used to help millions of patients worldwide. Today the biomaterial and medical device industry has developed to an estimated US$150 billion worldwide industry saving lives of millions and improving the quality of life for many millions more (Liu et al., 2012). Nondegradable synthetic polymers have played an important role in these products, often as inert materials, by contributing to the efficient functioning of the devices as well as providing mechanical support in many orthopaedic implants. For example, components in orthopaedic implants such as articulating surfaces, and scaffolds, or as protective coatings on electrically stimulating devices such as cardiac pacemakers. Among the synthetic polymers, the early materials explored for medical applications include silicone rubber, high density polyethylene, and polyesters such as Dacron. Since then, a wide spectrum of devices and implants comprised of inert synthetic polymer components have been developed and successfully used in numerous clinical applications. These applications include coatings on implants to improve blood compatibility, cardiovascular devices such as pacemakers, heart valves, and orthopaedic fixation devices such as knee and hip implants. Other applications include catheters and dialysis tubing, vascular grafts, implantable drug delivery systems such as drug eluting coatings on vascular stents. Since the early introduction of synthetic materials, significant advances have been made in polymer formulations and processing techniques to help optimise the performance and stability of these materials in the biological environment. With the realisation that inert materials may not always be the best in some of these applications, researchers have focused on improving the biological interaction of these materials through various surface modifications techniques and incorporating additives to help improve tissue integration with these materials.

With the emergence of tissue engineering and regenerative medicine as the next frontier technology to repair damaged tissues or organs to restore normal biological

Biosynthetic Polymers for Medical Applications. http://dx.doi.org/10.1016/B978-1-78242-105-4.00002-X

functions, many research groups worldwide have focused their attention to develop suitable biodegradable polymers to provide the material needs to further advance these technologies for clinical applications. Over the last two decades many reviews and research publications have appeared in the literature on new biodegradable materials and formulations. It is anticipated that these advancements will translate to clinically useful products and therapies in the near future. However, the use of nondegradable polymers in medical implants will continue to play a major role in many of the existing devices and next generation medical implants.

The aim of this chapter is to provide the readers with a review of the current nondegradable polymers used in biomedical applications, particularly covering the advancements over the past decade and to assess their biological performance based on long-term use in humans. A brief introduction to the chemistry, physical properties, biocompatibility and biostability of seven major classes of synthetic polymers will be provided. The term 'nondegradable' is used to imply that the polymers are resistant to degradation by hydrolytic and other mechanisms operating in the biological environments. This chapter will not cover biodegradable polymers and readers are referred to many excellent reviews (Martina and Hutmacher, 2007; Nair and Laurencin, 2007; Ulery et al., 2011; Place et al., 2009; Hazer et al., 2012).

2.1.1 Introduction to various classes of synthetic polymers

Synthetic polymers with chemical linkages resistant to hydrolytic, oxidative, and other degradation mechanisms operating in biological environments have been evaluated extensively for biomedical applications; however, only a few have made it to devices or implants in clinical use. A major attraction to use synthetic nondegradable polymers in biomedical applications stems from the ability to tailor mechanical properties and biological inertness, as well as a variety of available processing options. The main classes of nondegradable synthetic polymers used in biomedical applications include poly(olefins), poly(urethanes), poly(carbonates), poly(siloxanes), poly(amides), poly(ethers), poly(sulphones) and certain types of poly(esters). Table 2.1 lists representative chemical structures, general material properties and main biomedical applications of nondegradable synthetic polymers. The following sections outline the general chemistry, synthesis, properties and their suitability for biomedical applications based on numerous in vitro and in vivo evaluations.

2.2 Ultra-high molecular weight poly(ethylene) (UHMWPE)

Poly(ethylene) (PE) is one of the most commonly used synthetic polymers for industrial and commercial products with millions of metric tons produced annually. Polymerisations using Ziegler Natta or metallocene-based catalysts are the most widely used method for production of many different grades of PE for commercial applications. PE is classified into different grades based on its density and branching; ultra-high molecular weight PE (UHMWPE), high density PE (HDPE) and ultra-low molecular weight PE (ULMWPE) are examples. UHMWPE is a very tough material and has outstanding toughness and resistance to cut, wear and chemicals as well as very low moisture permeability and very low coefficient of friction. For these reasons UHMWPE has been used for the construction of articulating portions of implants used in hip and knee replacements (Kurtz, 2004) and has a history of over four decades of use in bearing surfaces of total joint replacements (Sobieraj and Rimnac, 2009). Table 2.2 lists some of the key properties of UHMWPE and its mechanical properties are dependent on its molecular weight, degree of crosslinking and the relative amounts of crystalline and amorphous phases.

2.2.1 Biomedical applications of UHMWPE

Since the first introduction of UHMWPE in hip replacements in 1962, the material is currently used in over 1.4 million patients around the world annually for implants in hip, knee, upper extremities and spine surgery (Kurtz et al., 1999b, Kurtz, 2004). This success is largely due to superior wear resistance of the polymer along with high fracture toughness and biocompatibility compared to other polymers. However, the long-term performance of these implants is less than optimal and in some cases revision surgery is required due to poor material performance. The failure of UHMWPE in joint replacement devices is primarily due to oxidative degradation, resulting in loss of mechanical properties (Kurtz et al., 1999a; Besong et al., 1998; del Prever et al., 2009). Over the last few decades many research groups have investigated the factors responsible for the material failure and have developed PE materials with improved performance. The major approaches investigated include minimisation of processing requirements during fabrication of the implants. These include sterilisation effects, crosslinking of the polymer using high energy radiation, blending with other materials and improvement of the surface properties.

Due to the extremely high molecular weight of UHMWPE, the molten polymer produced from granules does not flow like its low molecular weight counterparts; as such the conventional thermoplastic processing equipment cannot be used for its processing. The material must be consolidated using controlled pressure, temperature and time to produce moulded or extruded parts. The consolidation process is diffusion controlled and UHMWPE requires sufficient time at elevated temperature and pressure for the molecular chains to migrate across grain boundaries (Kurtz, 2009). Specially designed and modified techniques of extrusion, compression moulding, direct compression moulding, ram extrusion and hot isotactic pressing allow the polymer to be extruded for the production of medical grade products.

2.2.2 Biocompatibility and stability of UHMWPE

It is well known that UHMWPE is susceptible to oxidative degradation following radiation-induced sterilisation, leading to loss of mechanical properties affecting the long-term performance of implants with components fabricated from it. Many studies have investigated the effect of gamma irradiation on mechanical properties and wear

Table 2.1 The chemical structure, general properties and major biomedical applications of nondegradable synthetic polymers

Polymer	Chemical structure	Key properties	Major biomedical applications
Poly(ethylene)	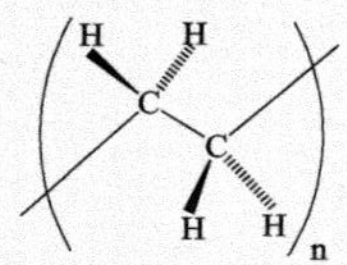	Linear thermoplastic Low and high-density grades Excellent chemical resistance	Total hip, knee and spine implants
Poly(propylene)	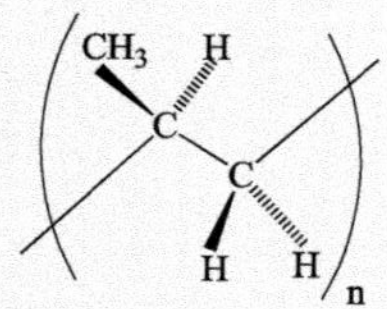	Linear thermoplastic Tough, flexible with good fatigue resistance	Nonabsorbable suture, medical pouches and hernia mesh
Poly(methyl methacrylate)	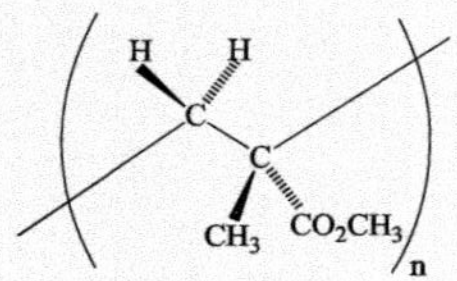	Lightweight transparent thermoplastic, good impact strength, poor resistance to chemicals	Orthopaedic prosthesis, dental, encapsulation device for cells, slow release of peptide and protein drug

Poly(dimethyl siloxane)	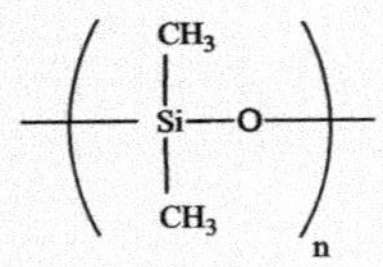	Transparent, elastic solid, nontoxic, inert, nonflammable, excellent viscoelastic properties	Breast implant, contact lens, prosthesis
Poly(ether ether ketone)	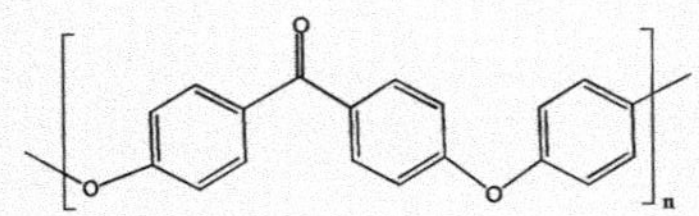	Semicrystalline thermoplastic with excellent mechanical properties and chemical resistance	Spinal fusion, disc arthroplasty, pedicle-based rod systems for nonfusion, interspinous spacers, minimally invasive fusion surgery, motion preservation and dynamic stabilisation
Polyurethane	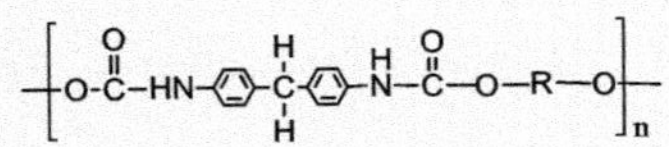	Linear thermoplastic or cross-linked thermoset can be formulated as soft elastomers or rigid materials to have either biostable or biodegradable properties	Pacemaker lead insulators, vascular grafts, catheters

Table 2.2 Properties of nondegradable synthetic polymers

Polymer	Melting temp °C	Ultimate tensile strength (MPa)	Ultimate tensile elongation (%)	T_g °C	References
Ultra-high molecular weight poly(ethylene) (UHMWPE) Extruded GUR 1020	135	54	452 + 19	−110	Kurtz (2009)
Poly(propylene) (PP)	120−176	26−32	10−140	−8	Handbook of Polymers (2012)
Poly(methyl methacrylate) (PMMA)	160	48−76	2−10	105	Livermore and Voldman (2013)
Poly(urethane) (PU) Elast-Eon™	180−185	23	>500	45	Gunatillake et al. (2003)
Poly(siloxane)	NA	4−12	>500	−127	Mata et al. (2005)
Poly(ether ether ketone) PEEK	343	90−100	1.5−40	143	Kurtz and Devine (2007)

performance of UHMWPE-based components used in hip, knee and other implants (Adrian et al., 2008; Berry et al., 2012; Affatato et al., 2002; Bracco et al., 2006; Carpentieri et al., 2011; Coote et al., 2000; Costa et al., 1998; Kaneeda et al., 1999; Sugano et al., 2004; Xiong et al., 2007; Xiong and Xiong, 2012). The free radicals generated during radiation sterilisation are responsible for initiating the chemical events leading to polymer degradation and subsequent deterioration of mechanical properties. The free radicals can react with the oxygen present forming hydroperoxides as the first product, which upon decomposition regenerate free radicals (Bracco et al., 2006; Costa et al., 2002, 2008). This autocatalytic process causes polymer main chain degradation leading to fragments with ketone, carboxyl and alcohol functional groups. The degradation process can continue as long as oxygen is available and it can continue without further irradiation (Bracco et al., 2006). This postirradiation ageing process leads to a reduction in the following properties: polymer elongation, modulus, ultimate tensile strength, fracture toughness, crack propagation and overall wear performance.

Many studies have focused on the effect of the radiation dose and conditions on the postirradiation ageing process (Adrian et al., 2008; Bracco et al., 2006; Coote et al., 2000; Kaneeda et al., 1999; Carpentieri et al., 2011). Irradiation in an inert atmosphere or in vacuum packaging to eliminate oxygen can reduce or retard the ageing process (Kurtz et al., 1999a) but cannot be completely eliminated. While these approaches help reduce the onset of degradation during storage, the oxidation can still occur once implanted due to available oxygen in vivo. The free radicals produced during sterilisation are considered to have different resident times depending on whether they are residing in the amorphous or the crystalline phase (Carpentieri et al., 2011), with those in the amorphous phase decaying fastest. A similar in vivo oxidation response has been shown for implants sterilised under inert atmospheric conditions (Berry et al., 2012; Sugano et al., 2004; Kaneeda et al., 1999; Kumakura et al., 2009).

The design of the components in implants has an influence on the extent and the location of degradation leading to gross fracture and cracking of the UHMWPE components. For example, cracks and gross fracture have occurred in acetabular rims (Berry et al., 2012; Sugano et al., 2004), the stabilising posts in noncruciate sparring tibial components (Hendel et al., 2003; Mariconda et al., 2000), and along rims of total spinal disc replacements (Kurtz et al., 2006a,b). The regions of these components where built-in stress is concentrated due to fabrication technique or the component design are more susceptible to fracture resulting from oxidation.

Crosslinking of UHMWPE using ionising radiation (gamma rays or electron beams) has been one of the main approaches employed to improve the wear properties. Typically radiation doses ranging from 50 to 100 kGy (Kurtz, 2004) are used. The irradiation is followed by thermal treatment to destroy any residual free radicals to minimise oxidative degradation. This annealing process is typically conducted by heating the material first below T_m followed by melting above T_m (Kurtz et al., 1999b). However, the residual free radical within crystalline domains may not be completely destroyed by this annealing process (McKellop et al., 2000). Both of these thermal treatments can influence the degree of crystallinity in the polymer. Annealing typically increases crystallinity (Medel et al., 2005) whereas remelting causes an irreversible

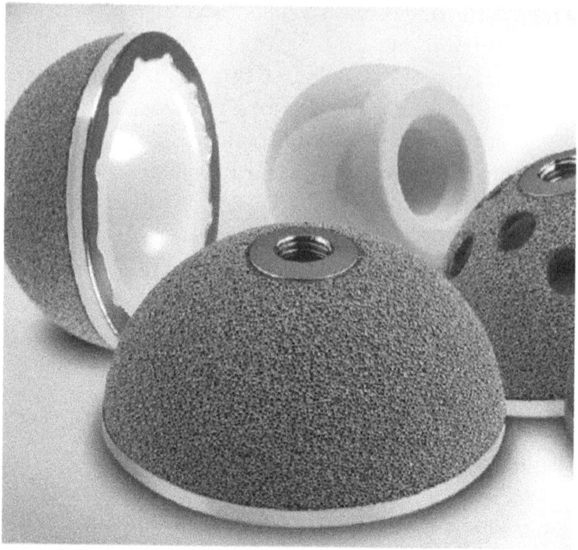

Figure 2.1 Vivacit-E® highly crosslinked polyethylene liner (containing vitamin E) for use with the Continuum Acetabular System.
Courtesy of Zimmer.

decrease in crystallinity (McKellop et al., 2000). The crosslinking process can produce the desired improvement in wear resistance but with a compromise on other mechanical properties. A reduction in both ultimate stress and strain has been observed for highly crosslinked UHMWPE (Lewis, 2001; Pruitt, 2005; Sobieraj and Rimnac, 2009). The reduction in these properties is relatively larger for gamma-irradiated materials compared to those irradiated with e-beam.

The incorporation of radical scavengers has been another approach to mitigate the effect of residual-free radicals in irradiated UHMWPE. Vitamin E (α-tocopherol) is arguably the most widely investigated radical scavenger (Affatato et al., 2012; Bracco and Oral, 2011; Mehmood et al., 2012; Wolf et al., 2006). Two methods have been employed to incorporate vitamin E: the first before irradiation and the second to allow it to diffuse into the polymer after irradiation (Shibata and Tomita, 2005).

These improvements to UHMWPE have shown promise in improving its performance in orthopaedic implants (see Figure 2.1) (Zimmer, 2012); however, there is little information available to-date for their clinical performance.

2.3 Polypropylene (PP)

Polypropylene (PP) is a thermoplastic polymer with a wide variety of industrial applications. The major industrial applications include packaging and labelling, carpets, reusable containers, laboratory equipment, automotive components, and bank notes.

Due to the unsymmetrical nature of the monomer propylene, the polymer produced can has three different chain conformations: isotactic, syndiotactic and atactic, depending on the special orientation of the methyl group on each monomer unit within the polymer chain. The most widely used commercial PP is isotactic and has intermediate crystallinity with a melting point in the range 160–166 °C, whereas the syndiotactic form has a melting point of 130 °C with a crystallinity of 30%. PP is hydrophobic and has good resistance to many chemical solvents and acids. PP is commercially produced using Ziegler–Natta and certain types of soluble metallocene catalysts. PP can be easily fabricated to various components using a variety of processing techniques, including compression, injection and blow moulding, and extrusion. The properties of PP are listed in Table 2.2.

2.3.1 Biomedical applications of PP

In addition to a wide variety of industrial applications, PP has found applications in medically related products. PP is the material of choice for medical supplies such as syringes, catheters, vials, blood transfusion bags, dialysers for blood purification, and for tubing and membranes used in diagnosis and treatment instruments. PP is also used in soft tissue applications and two of the most common applications are nonabsorbable sutures (e.g. Prolene™, manufactured by Ethicon Inc.) and PP meshes for hernia and pelvic organ repair. The understanding of the long-term biological performance of PP-based implants is largely from its use in these applications.

PP is liable to chain degradation, particularly when exposed to heat and UV radiation and the degradation is triggered by the free radicals formed on the tertiary carbon atom found in every repeat unit of the polymer; further reaction of the radical with oxygen can produce aldehydes and carboxylic acids leading to chain scission.

It is estimated that over 20 million hernia operations are performed globally every year (Sanders and Kingsnorth, 2012). Since its introduction in hernia surgery in 1962, PP has become the most widely used polymer for inguinal hernia repair (67.6%) and incisional hernia repair (44.4%). This is largely due to a few favourable properties of PP including high burst strength and good mechanical properties.

In hernia surgery, PP is used as a woven mesh to provide biomechanical strength to prevent the hernia from recurring by reinforcing the abdominal wall. The biological response to the foreign material is critical in the events after surgery leading to the completion of the wound healing process which can take up to 12 weeks (Majercik et al., 2006). The absorption of proteins on the surface of the implanted material occurs almost instantaneously upon implantation and is believed to be the first step in a series of biological events as part of the foreign-body reaction to the material. The material surface properties as well as the extent and the nature of these events influence the magnitude of the inflammatory response (Meintjes et al., 2011). While PP provides good mechanical support, one of the main disadvantages is the intensity of the foreign-body reaction, leading to less compliance and increased pain (Sanders and Kingsnorth, 2012).

The design of the mesh (Bellon, 2009; Klosterhalfen et al., 2005) and fabrication methods can significantly improve its long-term performance of hernia repair

(Nayak et al., 2012). Many research groups have investigated surface modification approaches to improve the overall biocompatibility of PP for implant applications. Low pressure nitrogen plasma surface modification (Gomathi et al., 2012), plasma-induced graft polymerisation of acrylic acid (Gupta et al., 2008), graft polymerisation with other hydrophilic monomers such as *N*-isopropyl acrylamide (NiPAm) (Desai et al., 2003), conjugation of gold nanoparticles (Grant et al., 2011), surface modification with glycopolymer (Yang et al., 2005), and zwitterionic polymers (Zhao et al., 2011, 2012) are among the main approaches reported to improve PP surface properties in implant applications.

The plasma surface modification is one of the main approaches used to surface modify PP as this can be carried out with fibres without modifying its mechanical performance. The approaches range from plasma modification with inert gases such as nitrogen (Gomathi et al., 2012) to plasma-induced polymerisation in the presence of hydrophilic monomers such as acrylic acid (Gupta et al., 2008), NiPAm (Contreras-Garcia et al., 2011; Desai et al., 2003), and acrylonitrile (Gupta et al., 2008). Surface modification with nitrogen plasma introduces nitrogen and oxygen containing functional groups (NH_2, NH and CO) onto PP surfaces improving cell compatibility and haemocompatibility (Gomathi et al., 2012). Plasma-induced graft polymerisation of acrylic acid followed by chitosan binding helps to improve antimicrobial properties of PP (Gupta et al., 2008; Saxena et al., 2011). A number of other hydrophilic monomers such as vinylimidazole, NiPAm (Contreras-Garcia et al., 2011), 2-acrylamido-2-methylpropane sulphonic acid (Song et al., 2011), D-gluconamidoethyl methacrylate (Yang et al., 2005), and zwitterionic monomers such as 2-methacryloyloxyethyl phosphocholine (Zhao et al., 2011, 2012) have also been reported. Overall, these surface chemical modifications have improved the wettability of PP and cell compatibility and growth. However, long-term in vivo data are needed to fully assess the impact of these modifications to improve the functional performance of membranes used in patients.

2.4 Poly(methyl methacrylate) (PMMA)

Poly(methyl methacrylate) is a transparent thermoplastic polymer produced by polymerisation of methyl methacrylate (Table 2.1). The polymer was developed in 1928 in various laboratories and was first brought to the market by Rohm and Hass Company under the trade name Plexiglass. Since then it has been sold under several different names such as Lucite and Perspex. PMMA is currently produced by emulsion, solution and bulk polymerisation methods. Generally, the polymerisation is carried out by free radical polymerisation methods including controlled radical polymerisation methods as well as anionic polymerisation. All commercial PMMA is produced by radical polymerisation and is atactic and completely amorphous.

The glass transition temperature of atactic PMMA is 105 °C but most commercial PMMA has T_g in a wide temperature range (85–165 °C) due to various commercial compositions incorporating comonomers to modify properties (Table 2.2). All common processing techniques such as injection moulding, compression moulding and extrusion used for thermoplastic polymers can be used to process PMMA. PMMA is a strong lightweight material with good impact strength and is transparent, transmitting up to 92% of visible light. PMMA swells and dissolves in many organic solvents and has poor resistance to many other chemicals. The PMMA homopolymer is versatile with many of its uses in a wide range of fields and applications but for most commercial applications the polymer is modified mostly by copolymerising with varying amounts of other monomers. It is widely used as a transparent glass substitute, for artistic and aesthetic uses, and for daylight redirection panels. PMMA has found many applications in medical technologies and implants as well. The major application areas include orthopaedic, cranial and facial reconstruction, ocular lenses, drug delivery and dentistry.

2.4.1 Biomedical applications of PMMA

Since the first use of acrylic bone cements in the 1960s (Charnley, 1960), PMMA bone cement has been used in many load-bearing orthopaedic fixation procedures, including anchoring total joint replacement, vertebral body augmentation procedures and in balloon Kyphoplasty (Kenny and Buggy, 2003). The commercial PMMA bone cement is supplied as a two-part system for mixing and delivery at the point of use. One component is a liquid consisting primarily methyl methacrylate monomer and a small amount of an accelerator (*N,N*-dimethyl-*p*-toluidine) with traces of hydroquinone whereas the other component is PMMA powder with components like radio-opaque compounds (e.g. barium sulphate or zirconium oxide) as well as the free radical initiator (benzoyl peroxide). The use of prepolymerised PMMA powder in the formulation reduces the volume shrinkage during polymerisation while helping to manage the temperature rise during polymerisation. The formulation details and properties of many commercial PMMA bone cements can be found in review articles (Jaeblon, 2010; Kenny and Buggy, 2003; DiMaio, 2002; Lewis, 2011) and in books (Kuhn, 2000). The two components when mixed form a clear and uniform mixture and the polymerisation of the monomer is initiated generating heat from the reaction exotherm. The peak temperature can reach 113 °C and the consistency of the reaction mixture changes from a low viscous sticky phase to a workable putty like consistency (dough) and finally to a hardening phase leading to a high strength solid mass. The mixture has to be delivered during the working phase to the implant site and for most commercial formulations the hardening occurs within 10–20 min.

In most implant applications PMMA cement serves as space filler or as an interphase between the implant and the host bone providing stability to the implant. The PMMA layer helps transfer the mechanical forces from the implant to the bone due to comparable mechanical properties of PMMA to bone. The long-term performance of the implants is dependent on the quality of the apposition of the implant-cement and cement-bone. The surgical technique, loading characteristics, as well as the properties of cement, bone and implant can have a significant influence on the long-term performance of the cement (Jaeblon, 2010).

PMMA bone cement is also used in the treatment of vertebral defects (Laredo and Hamze, 2004) using a procedure termed vertebroplasty. This procedure consists of percutaneous injection of PMMA into vertebral collapse in order to obtain pain relief and mechanical strengthening of the vertebral body. Kyphoplasty is a variant of vertebroplasty used to help restore the height of vertebral compression fractures (Lieberman et al., 2002). Although the procedure is used extensively, it is not free of complications and the leakage of PMMA during the procedure is the main source of complications.

2.4.2 Biocompatibility and stability of PMMA

Despite the success of PMMA bone cement in orthopaedic procedures, several problems have been identified associated with its use. Some of these problems are procedure related and the others are attributed to material properties and the polymerisation reaction employed to set the cement. For example, in the vertebroplasty procedure the leakage of the PMMA cement to spinal canal is very frequent, leading to associated complications. The technical refinements to reduce the risk of PMMA leakage are reviewed by Laredo (Laredo and Hamze, 2004) and readers are referred to this review article for further information.

Numerous in vitro studies have reported on the cytotoxicity issues related to the use of PMMA resins in a range of medical implant applications. A review summarised the biocompatibility of PMMA resins used in dentistry (Gautam et al., 2012). PMMA resins used in dentistry are considered cytotoxic on account of leaching of various potential toxic substances such as unreacted monomer and other additives present in various formulations which may include initiator residues, activators, and monomer degradation products and crosslinking agents. The amount of residual monomer can vary depending on the type of polymerisation with the autopolymerised resins exhibiting a higher level compared to heat-polymerised resin activated with benzoyl peroxide (Vallittu et al., 1998). Irritation of the oral mucosa is the main cytotoxic effect of MMA and the systemic toxicity is considered very low consistent with high oral LD_{50} of MMA in rats (9 g/kg) (Gautam et al., 2012). Although many in vitro studies have investigated the cytotoxicity issues of PMMA leachables, only few in vivo studies have been reported.

The heat generated during the polymerisation in PMMA bone cements has also been a concern as this could lead to cell necrosis in tissues closer to cement. It is reported that although the peak temperature during cure can reach about 113 °C, in vivo, it is much lower between 40 °C and 56 °C (Kuehn et al., 2005), largely due to rapid heat dissipation through blood flow around the area as well as heat conduction throughout the implant material.

2.5 Polyurethane (PU)

PUs represent an important class of synthetic polymers used in the manufacture of rigid and flexible foams, adhesives, surface coatings, sealants, and fibres covering a broad range of industrial applications (Ortel, 1994). Polyurethanes were first evaluated for biomedical applications in 1960 and since then numerous studies have explored their applications for a range of medical implants. The current major application is for insulating cardiac pacemakers. Polyurethanes have excellent mechanical properties and are easily formulated to have broad range of mechanical properties for applications as soft elastomers or high strength rigid materials. Polyurethanes are well tolerated in the body and exhibit good compatibility with cells and soft tissues (Lamba et al., 1998).

2.5.1 Synthesis and properties of PU

The chemical reaction between an isocyanate group and a hydroxyl or amine group generates urethanes (carbamates) and urea groups, respectively. This reaction has been employed to synthesise a range of thermoplastic polyurethanes (TPU) and thermoset polyurethanes (TS). TPUs are prepared by reacting a diisocyanate, a difunctional polyol (macrodiol) and a dihydroxy or diamine chain extender, whereas TSs are synthesised using the same reagents, except at least one of those reagents has to be tri or higher functional to produce branched or crosslinked polymers. A vast number of potential combinations of the three reagents have been explored to synthesise polyurethanes with a broad range of mechanical properties (Ortel, 1994). However, only a relatively few have been used in medical applications, primarily due to toxicity, stability and mechanical properties. Due to ease of handling, symmetrical structure and high reactivity, 4,4′-methylenediphenyl diisocyante is the most frequently used diisocyanate in formulating biostable polyurethanes for biomedical applications. The chain extender is usually a low molecular weight diol such as 1,4-butanediol, although low molecular weight diamines, such as ethylene diamine may be used. The macrodiol is a diol of higher molecular weight (600–2000 Da) and poly(tetramethylene oxide) (PTMO) is one of the common macrodiols used in polyurethanes such as Pellethane™ used in medical implants such as cardiac pacemakers (Szycher et al., 1996).

Polyurethanes can be prepared by one- or two-step batch procedures or by semicontinuous processes such as reactive extrusion (Ortel, 1994). One-step batch synthesis for thermoplastic polyurethanes involves reacting a mixture of the predried macrodiol and the chain extender with the diisocyanate. The reaction is generally catalysed with dibutyltin dilaurate, stannous octoate or amines and is exothermic. The 'one-step' process can also be carried out in special continuous mixing machines, or reactive extruders, or in continuous injection moulding machines. The reactive extrusion offers significant advantages in polyurethane synthesis for biomedical applications due to better control of reaction conditions as well as the ability to produce articles or components in one step, avoiding post synthesis processing steps.

Compared with the one-step procedure, the two-step procedure gives good control of polymer architecture and can be carried out in bulk or in solvents such as rigorously dried *N,N*-dimethylformamide or *N,N*-dimethylacetamide. This procedure is mostly used for laboratory-scale preparations and is less attractive in industry-scale synthesis. The two-step batch procedure involves the synthesis of a prepolymer in the first step by end-capping the polyol with diisocyanate, and chain extending in the second step by reacting with the chain extender.

2.5.2 Biostability and applications of PU

The attractive mechanical properties such as high strength, elongation, tear and abrasion resistance of polyurethanes are attributed to the micro-phase separated morphology brought about by the partial mutual insolubility of the different chemical segments in the block copolymers. One microphase is derived from the macrodiol and is generally referred to as 'soft' segment which imparts material softness and extensibility. The other segment referred to as the 'hard' segment which is derived from the diisocyanate and the chain extender imparts cohesive strength to the polymer matrix.

The chemical structures of 'soft' and 'hard' segments as well as their relative proportions within a polymer chain affect the stability of the polyurethane in the biological environment. It was recognised early that soft segments based on polyester macrodiols are susceptible to hydrolytic degradation and are not suitable for stable biomedical applications (Lamba et al., 1998; Stokes and McVennes, 1995). Accordingly, the polyurethane investigated for biomedical applications were based on polyether macrodiols such as PTMO. For example, Pellethane-80A used in pacemaker insulations was based on PTMO with a molecular weight of 1000. However, it was later realised that PTMO-based polyurethanes are susceptible to oxidative degradation (Szycher et al., 1996).

The mechanism of biologically induced degradation of polyurethanes has been the subject of much investigation. The results have been summarised in a number of review articles (Szycher et al., 1996; Santerre et al., 2005; Anderson et al., 2008; Ward et al., 2006b; Christenson et al., 2007). Although the exact mechanisms are not fully understood, it is widely held that oxidative pathways involving the polyether 'soft' segment leading to environmental stress cracking as one of the main mechanisms. This form of degradation is found to be concentrated in areas where residual polymer surface stresses are present due to device fabrication and not sufficiently reduced by annealing. Hydrolytic enzymes have also been implicated in polyurethane biodegradation (Santerre et al., 1995).

The polyurethanes investigated earlier for biomedical applications were not specifically designed for such applications and as such the understanding of the degradation mechanisms has led to commercial withdrawal of polyurethanes in the 1990s for chronic implants. This provided a stimulus to design more stable polyurethanes for medical applications. The design approaches were focused on the chemical structure of 'soft' segment forming macrodiols which are not susceptible to oxidative and hydrolytic degradation. The macrodiols investigated to date can be classified into four main groups based on the type of backbone functional groups. These are hydrocarbon, ether, siloxane and carbonate. In this field, the leading research groups are, Coury et al. (Takahara et al., 1991), Pinchuk (1995), Ward et al. (2006a), Szycher et al. (1996) and Gunatillake et al. (2003).

Hydrocarbon backbone macrodiols such as hydrogenated polybutadine diol and poly(isobutylene) results in PUs with significantly improved resistance to thermal, hydrolytic and UV degradation compared to polyether or polyester polyurethanes (Speckhard et al., 1983; Ojha et al., 2009). However, the mechanical properties are inferior to their polyether counterparts and their synthesis is more difficult, making them less attractive for biomedical applications. In another approach C-18 fatty acids were dimerised to form polyols with predominantly hydrocarbon backbone soft segments. The biostability of the resultant PU's improved but these materials were too stiff for most implant applications. Polyether macrodiols prepared from 1,6-hexanediol, 1,8-octanediol and 1,10 decanediol have shown significantly improved in vivo biostability compared with PTMO-based polyurethanes (Gunatillake et al., 2003); however, the polyurethanes exhibited higher modulus and stiffness as the number of ether linkages was reduced. Polycarbonate-based macrodiols yielded polyurethane with good mechanical properties and improved resistance to degradation in vivo compared to PTMO-based polyurethanes; however, in the longer term carbonate linkages were susceptible to degradation (Christenson et al., 2004).

The incorporation of PDMS into the polyurethane structure has the advantage of imparting good haemocompatibility, flexibility, excellent hydrolytic and oxidative stability to polyurethanes. One approach has been to incorporate PDMS segments as polyurethane chain end groups to improve the surface properties of PUs and to reduce oxidative degradation. Another approach was to incorporate PDMS segments to both 'soft' and 'hard' segments of polyurethane by using appropriate siloxane macrodiols and chain extenders. This second approach has been the most successful in developing polyurethanes with vastly improved biostability, over conventional and other polyurethanes developed in recent times (Figure 2.2).

The incorporation of siloxane segments as part of polyurethane structure is not straightforward due to the incompatibility between highly nonpolar siloxane segments with polar urethane segments. This incompatibility results in a high degree of phase separation yielding highly phase separated polyurethanes. This problem has been overcome by incorporating a small amount of a second macrodiol to improve compatibility as well as incorporating short siloxane chain extender segments to the 'hard' segment. By appropriate choice of catalysts both one and two-step methods have been adopted to prepare siloxane polyurethanes exhibiting good mechanical properties and processability. This new family (Elast-Eon™) (Table 2.2) of siloxane polyurethanes has been tested for biostability using both in vitro (Choi et al., 2009; Simmons et al., 2006) and in vivo tests and shown to have superior biostability. The in vitro oxidative stability of these polyurethanes is closely related to the morphology resulting from unlike segment demixing (Choi et al., 2009). Elast-Eon™ polyurethanes are currently used in cardiac pacemakers marketed by St. Jude Medical, USA as Optim™ (Figure 2.3). The biostability of Elast-Eon™ polyurethanes has been evaluated under both in vitro and in vivo conditions by a number of research groups. In a study (Wheatley et al., 2000, 2001) to evaluate the suitability of Elast-Eon™ polyurethane for tri-leaflet heart valves, bileaflet mechanical, Carpentier-Edwards porcine (bioprosthetic) and polyurethane heart valves (Figure 2.4) were implanted in juvenile sheep for six months. The study concluded that in the absence of valve-related deaths, and retention of good haemodynamic function, the PU valve was superior to bioprosthetic.

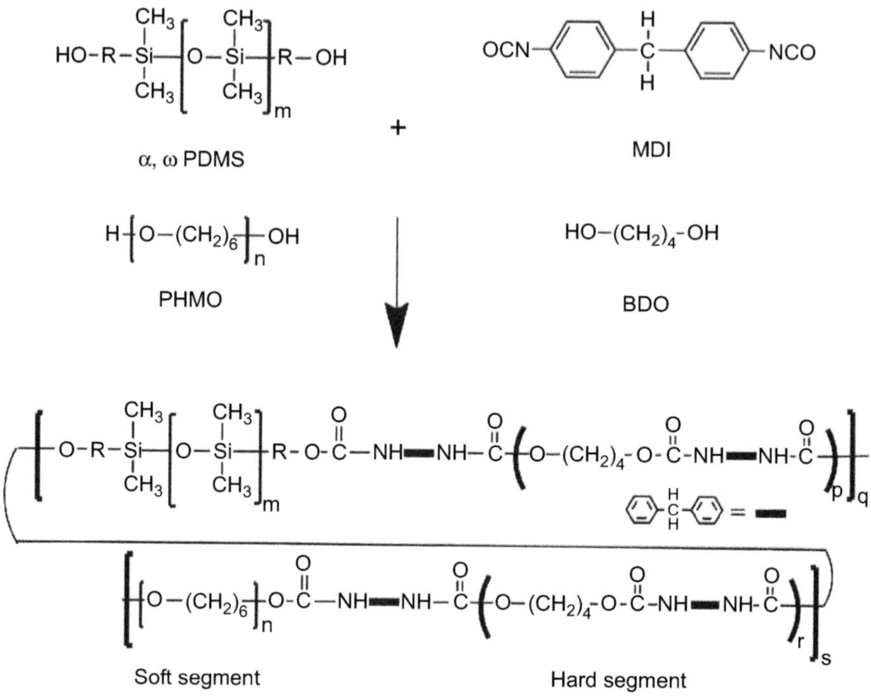

Figure 2.2 Chemical structure of Elast-Eon™ polyurethane.
Courtesy of Gunatillake P and Adhikari R with permission from AorTech Biomaterials Pty Ltd.

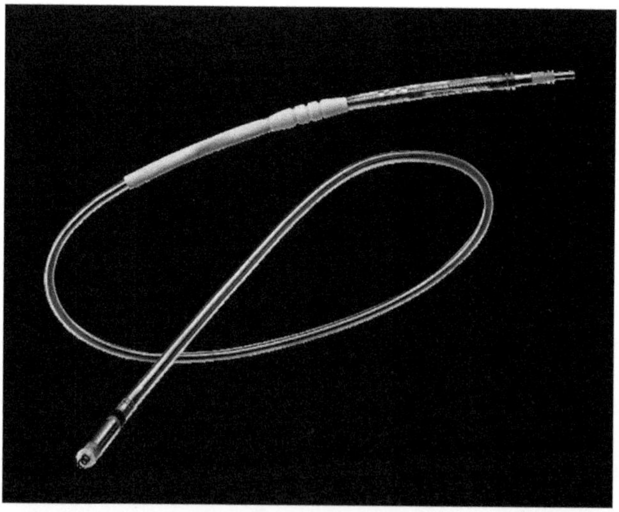

Figure 2.3 Elast-Eon™ polyurethane lead used for cardiac pacing applications.
Courtesy of Dr Ajay Padsalgikar with permission from AorTech Biomaterials Pty Ltd.

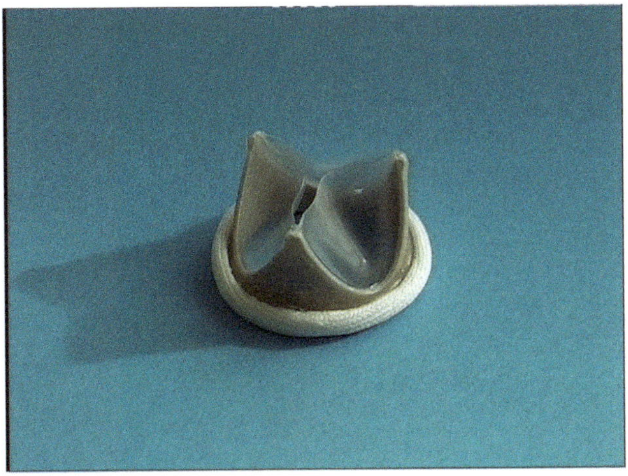

Figure 2.4 Prototype tri-leaflet heart valve.
Courtesy of Dr Robert Kerton with permission from CSIRO Publishing.

2.6 Poly(dimethyl siloxane) (PDMS)

Polysiloxanes are characterised by the presence of -Si-O-Si- linkage in the backbone and the most common polysiloxane is poly(dimethyl siloxane) (PDMS). The polymer in its pure form has very poor mechanical properties; PDMS with very high molecular weight tends to clod flow. For most applications, PDMS has to be crosslinked or reinforced with fillers to improve mechanical properties and is generally referred to as silicone rubber. Silicone rubber is nonreactive, stable and resistant to extreme environments and retains useful properties for applications in temperatures between −55 °C and +300 °C (Table 2.2). Silicone rubber has also favourable properties for biomedical applications because of its good biocompatibility. Due to these properties silicone rubber is used in a wide range of products, including automotive applications, cooking, baking and apparel such as undergarments, sportswear, footwear, electronics, medical devices and implants. The term 'silicone' is used to denote polymerised siloxanes or poly(siloxanes) with the chemical formula $[R_2SiO]_n$ where R is an organic group such as methyl, ethyl or phenyl present as side groups on Si along the -Si-O-Si-O- backbone. Silicones with a wide variety of properties and compositions can be prepared by varying the length of the backbone, the nature of the side groups or by crosslinking. The substitution of methyl groups along the chain with other groups such as phenyl, vinyl, trifluromethyl leads to silicones with unique properties. The polymers can vary from liquid to gel or to rubber and hard plastic.

2.6.1 Chemistry and synthesis of PDMS

PDMS is prepared from dimethyldichlorosilane which reacts with water to produce the linear polymer with either hydroxyl or chloride end groups and under different

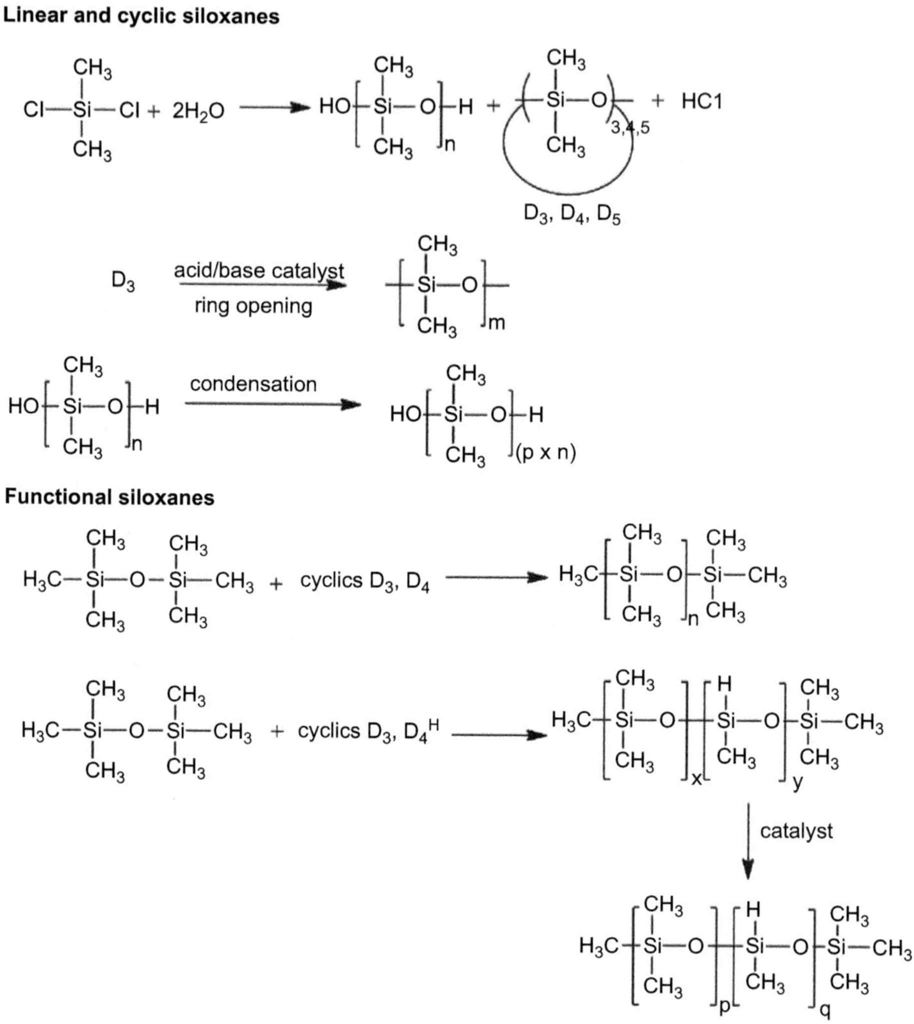

Figure 2.5 Principal chemical reactions in the synthesis of silicone polymers and functionalised silicones.

conditions, the polymer formed is cyclic (Figure 2.5). The cyclic monomers hexamethylcyclotrisiloxane (D3) and octamethylcyclotetrasiloxane (D4) can also be used to prepare PDMS using basic or acidic catalysts. Commonly used basic catalysts include potassium, sodium or tetramethylammonium silanolate. The reaction mixture typically consists of a monomer and an end-capper which is used to control molecular weight and stability. The mixture is heated under moderate temperature (60–150 °C) conditions to affect the polymerisation. Hexamethyldisiloxane is a common end-capper producing PDMS with trimethylsiloxy end groups which help stabilise the polymer from changes in viscosity and other properties for most fluid applications. The methyl groups on Si are not reactive and prevent further condensation. However, functional groups such as OH (silanols) or H (silanes) are reactive, for example, Si-OH groups are susceptible to condensation under acid or mild base conditions and they are intermediates for room temperature vulcanisable silicone formulations (Noll, 1968).

2.6.2 Biomedical applications of PDMS

The unique material properties of silicones and excellent biocompatibility make them well suited for a range of health care products covering numerous personalcare, pharmaceutical and medical device applications. The realisation in the mid-1940s that silicon coatings on glassware and needles prevents blood clotting for hours led to the use of silicon coatings on syringes, needles and blood collecting vials. Subsequently, silicone was used in fabricating implants for bile duct repair and artificial urethra demonstrating that there was no abnormal reaction by the body to silicone and the devices performed well. Perhaps, the most notable first application of silicone in the body is the hydrocephalus shunt in 1957 (Lafay, 1957). The interest of silicone for health care application continued in the 1960 with General Electric and Dow Corning supplying the materials for physicians and researchers, and by the end of the decade silicone was used or investigated in numerous applications, including orthopaedics, catheters, drains and shunts, blood oxygenators, heart-bypass machines, heart valves and aesthetic implants (Curtis and Colas, 2004b; McMillin, 2006).

For over 40 years, silicones have been used extensively in aesthetic and reconstructive surgery and despite the numerous allegations in the 1990s with regard to the safety of silicone breast implants, the use of silicones continues. Following the first implantation of a pair of silicone gel-filled breast implants (see Figure 2.6) (Friedman, 2010) in 1962, the popularity of silicone gel for breast reconstruction increased. The litigation related to breast implant safety raised controversial issues such as risk of breast cancer, autoimmune connective tissue disease as well as local or surgical complications such as rupture, infection, or capsular contraction. Many subsequent studies have found that these allegations are without sound scientific evidence and epidemiology studies have found that there was no association between breast implants and breast cancer. Many reports, papers and monographs have been published on this subject and the readers are referred to these excellent reviews for detailed information (Curtis et al., 2000; Brandon et al., 2003; Friedman, 2010; Brook, 2006).

2.6.3 Biocompatibility and stability of PDMS

Among the synthetic polymers, silicone can be considered as the material with the longest history in medical implant applications (De Nicola, 1950). Numerous in vitro and in vivo studies have provided evidence to claim that silicone materials are 'biocompatible' (Curtis and Colas, 2004a). However, such claims and the data supporting those claims should be carefully considered in view of the modern definition of biocompatibility, which was the subject of much discussion. The modern definition 'the ability of a material to perform with an appropriate host in specific

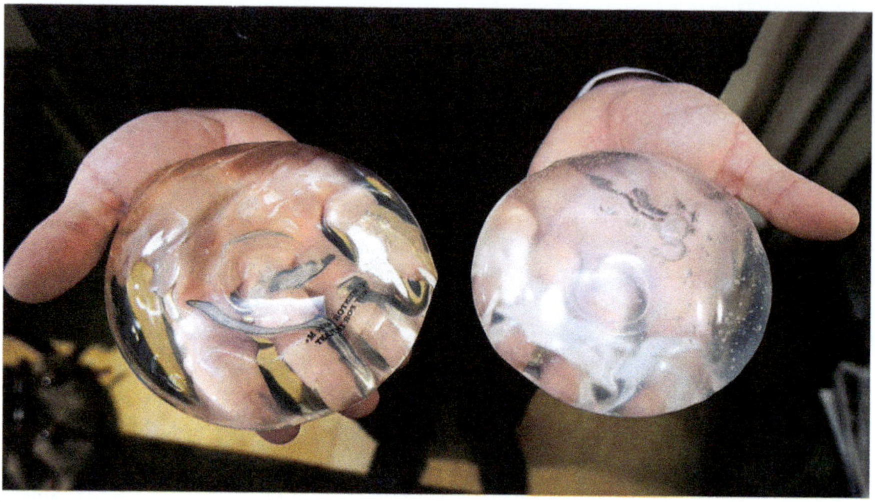

Figure 2.6 Silicon breast implant gels.
Courtesy of Richard Szabo with permission from Get Media, Leadewrs in Niche Digital Publishing.

situation' (Williams, 2003) warrants careful review of the type of biological fluids/ tissues that the material comes into contact with before making such claims. Silicone materials in various forms such as liquids, gels and elastomers have been used as implants in contact with biological tissues and fluids in different parts of the body. While the bulk polymer may not induce adverse reaction from the body, with synthetic materials it is often the impurities present in the material that causes biocompatibility issues. Silicones are no exception as catalysts are used in the polymerisation and subsequent crosslinking reactions to manufacture the silicone for various applications. However, in addition to the wealth of information from in vitro test results for various silicone formulations and applications, results of long-term in vivo studies as well as explant analysis results substantiate the claim that silicone biocompatibility is excellent.

Among the many studies to evaluate the biodurability of silicone elastomers and implants, the following can be cited as major studies to confirm long-term durability of silicon. In a comprehensive study to evaluate 42 silicone breast explants including human implantation duration of up to 32 years, Branden et al. (Brandon et al., 2003) reported that there was little or no degradation of the base polydimethylsiloxane during in vivo ageing of the explants they examined. In another study (Curtis et al., 2000) silicone breast implants were surgically excised and examined after 13.8–19.3 years. Only minor changes in the tensile strength of the shell were observed and the gel extract molecular weight remains unchanged.

Despite its excellent biocompatibility, the relatively poor mechanical properties limit applications of silicones in medical implants. In particular, poor tensile strength, abrasion and tear strength limit the application to less load-bearing capacity.

2.7 Polyether ether ketone (PEEK)

PEEK is a semicrystalline thermoplastic with excellent mechanical and chemical resistance properties which are retained at high temperatures. The polymer is very rigid with a Young's modulus of 3.6 GPa and tensile strength in the range 90–100 MPa. The glass transition temperature is around 143 °C (Table 2.2). The polymer is highly resistant to thermal degradation as well as degradation from organic and aqueous environments. The polymer can be dissolved in concentrated sulphuric acid. PEEK is the leading polymer candidate used in orthopaedic applications from a family of polymers generally referred to as polyaryl ether ketones (Kurtz and Devine, 2007).

2.7.1 Synthesis and properties of PEEK

PEEK polymers are synthesised by the dialkylation of the bisphenolate salts using step-growth polymerisation method. In a typical polymerisation procedure, 4,4′-difluorobenzophenone is reacted with disodium salt of hydroquinone and the reaction is carried out in polar aprotic solvents such as diphenylsulphone at approximately 300 °C to complete the nucleophilic substitution reaction (Figure 2.7).

PEEK can be processed using a range of commercial processing techniques, including injection moulding, extrusion and compression moulding at temperatures between 390 and 420 °C, which are significantly higher compared to that used for conventional thermoplastic polymers. The physical properties of PEEK are shown in Table 2.2.

The extremely high thermal and chemical resistance is attributed to its resonance stabilised chemical structure of PEEK. Its outstanding chemical resistance is also reflected in its resistance to postirradiation degradation, allowing PEEK to be sterilised by gamma and electron beam irradiation. Although free radicals may be formed during irradiation, unlike in polymers like UHMWPE the free radicals formed are believed to decay rapidly due to their mobility along the polymer chain. In a study by Li et al. (1999), no evidence of residual free radicals were observed in PEEK exposed to

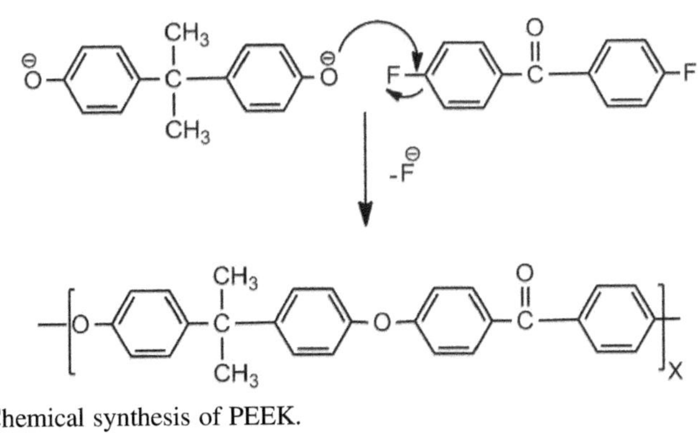

Figure 2.7 Chemical synthesis of PEEK.

gamma irradiation of up to 600 kGy, indicating that the life time of the free radical is less than 20 minutes. In another study (Kwarteng and Starck, 1990), repeated sterilisation doses up to four 25–40 kGy of gamma radiation in air confirmed that no significant changes in mechanical properties of PEEK resulted. As such, postirradiation degradation is not expected to be a clinically relevant concern with PEEK-based medical implants as it has been the case with UHMWPE.

Unmodified PEEK has considerable ductility and can accommodate large deformation plastic flow under both uniaxial tension and compression. Detailed studies of the true stress–strain behaviour of PEEK are reported in the literature (Rae et al., 2007; Hamdan and Swallowe, 1996). At room temperature and under very low strain (0.03) PEEK displays a linear relationship between stress and strain in both tension and compression. As the strain is increased the material exhibits a clear yield transition in the stress–strain curve. For industrial engineering applications, the mechanical properties of PEEK generally decreases with elevated temperatures up to 250 °C, with a significant decrease above 150 °C, which is slightly above the glass transition temperature (Rae et al., 2007). However, for biomedical applications where the application temperature is body temperature, PEEK elastic properties are relatively insensitive to temperature. For implant applications that involve heat generation, particularly load-bearing applications such as joint replacement require more detailed characterisation of PEEK with respect to plastic flow, and fracture behaviour is required (Kurtz and Devine, 2007). PEEK is gaining acceptance as a suitable material for fabrication of components for certain orthopaedic procedures, for example, in cranioplasty (Figure 2.8).

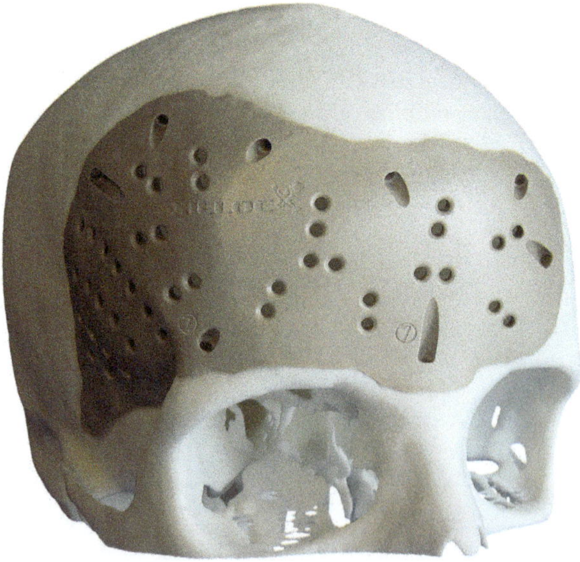

Figure 2.8 Custom skull implant fabricated from PEEK for use in cranioplasty. Courtesy of Xilloc, the Netherlands.

2.7.2 Biocompatibility and implant applications of PEEK

Numerous studies on the systemic and intracutaneous toxicity and intramuscular implantation have shown that PEEK and its composites do not illicit adverse tissue reactions (Williams et al., 1987; Petillo et al., 1994). The first (Williams et al., 1987; Toth, 2012) in vivo study in mice reported that PEEK elicited no adverse tissue reaction. A subsequent in vitro study using mouse fibroblasts by Wenz et al. (1990) showed that the cell cultures were healthy with no difference to negative controls. Numerous other in vitro studies using different cell types including human-derived osteoblasts, fibroblasts (Wenz et al., 1990; Hunter et al., 1995), murine macrophages (Scotchford et al., 2003) have confirmed the noncyctotoxicity of PEEK. The early investigations of PEEK polymers for orthopaedic implants occurred in the mid-to-late 1980s (Skinner, 1988; Brown et al., 1990) but it was only in the 1990s that PEEK received consideration in the field of spine implants. A book (Kurtz, 2012) titled 'PEEK Biomaterials Handbook' provides a comprehensive account of the development of PEEK as a biomaterial.

2.8 Future directions

For many decades nondegradable synthetic polymers have found applications in a variety of medical implants. The acceptance of these polymers for a wide variety of implants is based on the consideration of the mechanical properties, relative inertness of the polymers in their respective biological environments, and their ability to retain a required mechanical strength under dynamic environments for a long period of time. Since the first introduction of the synthetic polymers in implants in clinical use and subsequent findings from clinical experience about the material deficiencies, many research groups have investigated various approaches to improve their performance. In particular, the focus since the mid-1990s was to explore methods to minimise processing-related factors, imperfections at a molecular level and material surface properties to enhance biological tissue compatibility. Similar research is expected to continue as most of these polymers continue to play a major role in many of the existing and emerging implants. The adaption of techniques such as additive manufacturing will play a major role in minimising process-related defects in fabrication of implants and components based on synthetic polymers. And the incorporation of additives to control infections, improve biocompatibility and to deliver therapeutic agents will continue to be areas for further research.

The wear performance of crosslinked UHMWPEs has significantly improved over that of conventional UHMWPE based on short-term clinical studies. One of the main improvements is post processing following radiation-induced crosslinking to eliminate residual radicals which has helped the long-term stability of UHMWPE implants. The incorporation of radical scavengers such as vitamin E may also help to reduce polymer degradation. These developments are encouraging and can expect to extend the functional life of UHMWPE-based implants. However, long-term clinical data is still required to understand and assess the performance enhancements associated with these improvements. Further research into understanding the molecular-level changes resulting from these modifications and effects on mechanical performance needs to be conducted.

PMMA bone cement formulations have also been improved, enabling better curing characteristics (Copal®, Osteopal®) and bioactive loading capabilities (Palamed®, Refobacin®-Palacos®). Improvements are still needed as the toxicity associated with long-term exposure to unreacted methacrylate monomer will continue to be an issue of concern.

Silicone materials remain as a class of synthetic polymers thoroughly tested for a range of important medical implants due to their biocompatibility and biodurability. The limitation of the use of silicone materials in a wide range of medical implants is the relatively poor mechanical properties. Some of the recent advances in incorporating silicone segments to other high strength materials such as polyurethanes have resulted in materials with improved mechanical properties, expanding the range of applications. Further efforts in this area should lead to development of materials that can fulfil the materials needs for next generation medical implants, particularly in neural and vascular environments.

Based on recent developments, PEEK has been recognised as a next generation high strength biomaterial, particularly for spine implants. The attractiveness of PEEK stems from the fact that it is biocompatible, inert, radiolucent and inherently strong. The use of PEEK in more advanced fields such as total joint replacement and fracture fixation may take many more years as the introduction of new materials in the biomedical field is slow requiring extensive testing. However, as new implant designs progress PEEK may be considered as a material that can offer a number of advantages over the more conventional synthetic polymers used in orthopaedic implants. The on-going development in PEEK composites, particularly those incorporating additive such as hydroxyapatite may provide novel materials to improve the functional performance of orthopaedic implants.

Silicone-based polyurethanes such as Elast-Eon™ have shown to be significantly more biostable than conventional polyether polyurethanes and have shown excellent performance in devices such as cardiac pacemakers. With the expansion of the range of implants based on silicone polyurethanes, better understanding of the long-term biostability will emerge. These results will provide the researchers valuable information to broaden the application range as well as to address any materials deficiencies in specific applications.

References

Adrian, M., Zaharescu, T., Jipa, S., Silva, L.E., Oros, C., 2008. The assessment of thermal and radiation stability of UHMWPE. J. Optoelectron. Adv. Mater. 10, 826–829.

Affatato, S., Bordini, B., Fagnano, C., Taddei, P., Tinti, A., Toni, A., 2002. Effects of the sterilisation method on the wear of UHMWPE acetabular cups tested in a hip joint simulator. Biomaterials 23, 1439–1446.

Affatato, S., Bracco, P., Costa, L., Villa, T., Quaglini, V., Toni, A., 2012. In vitro wear performance of standard, crosslinked, and vitamin-E-blended UHMWPE. J. Biomed. Mater. Res. Part A 100A, 554–560.
Anderson, J.M., Rodriguez, A., Chang, D.T., 2008. Foreign body reaction to biomaterials. Semin. Immunol. 20, 86–100.
Bellon, J.M., 2009. Role of the new lightweight prostheses in improving hernia repair. Cir. Esp. 85, 268–273.
Berry, D.J., Currier, B.H., Mayor, M.B., Collier, J.P., 2012. Gamma-irradiation sterilization in an inert environment: a partial solution. Clin. Orthop. Relat. Res. 470, 1805–1813.
Besong, A.A., Tipper, J.L., Ingham, E., Al, E., 1998. Quantitative comparison of wear debries from UHMWPE that has and has not been sterilized by gamma irradiation. J. Bone Jt. Surg. 80, 340–344.
Bracco, P., Del Prever, E.M.B., Cannas, M., Luda, M.P., Costa, L., 2006. Oxidation behaviour in prosthetic UHMWPE components sterilised with high energy radiation in a low-oxygen environment. Polym. Degrad. Stab. 91, 2030–2038.
Bracco, P., Oral, E., 2011. Vitamin E-stabilized UHMWPE for total joint implants: a review. Clin. Orthop. Relat. Res. 469, 2286–2293.
Brandon, H.J., Jerina, K.L., Wolf, C.J., Young, V.L., 2003. Biodurability of retrieved silicone get breast implants. Plast. Reconstr. Surg. 11.
Brook, M.A., 2006. Platinum in silicone breast implants. Biomaterials 27, 3274–3286.
Brown, S.A., Hastings, R.S., Mason, J.J., Moet, A., 1990. Characterisation of short-fibre reinforced thermoplastics for fracture fixation devices. Biomaterials 11, 541–547.
Carpentieri, I., Brunella, V., Bracco, P., Paganini, M.C., Del Prever, E.M.B., Luda, M.P., Bonomi, S., Costa, L., 2011. Post-irradiation oxidation of different polyethylenes. Polym. Degrad. Stab. 96, 624–629.
Charnley, J., 1960. Bone cements and fillers: a review. J. Bone Jt. Surg. 42-B, 28.
Choi, T., Weksler, J., Padsalgikar, A., Hernandez, R., Runt, J., 2009. Polydimethylsiloxane-based polyurethanes: phase-separated morphology and in vitro oxidative biostability. Aust. J. Chem. 62, 794–798.
Christenson, E.M., Anderson, J.M., Hittner, A., 2007. Biodegradation mechanisms of polyurethane elastomers. Corros. Eng. Sci. Technol. 42, 312–323.
Christenson, E.M., Dadsetan, M., Wiggins, M., Anderson, J.M., Hiltner, A., 2004. Poly(carbonate urethane) and poly(ether urethane) biodegradation: in vivo studies. J. Biomed. Mater. Res. Part A 69A, 407–416.
Contreras-Garcia, A., Bucio, E., Concheiro, A., Alvarez-Lorenzo, C., 2011. Surface functionalization of polypropylene devices with hemocompatible DMAAm and NIPAAm grafts for norfloxacin sustained release. J. Bioact. Compat. Polym. 26, 405–419.
Coote, C.F., Hamilton, J.V., Mcgimpsey, W.G., Thompson, R.W., 2000. Oxidation of gamma-irradiated ultrahigh molecular weight polyethylene. J. Appl. Polym. Sci. 77, 2525–2542.
Costa, L., Bracco, P., Brach, E.M., Luda, M.P., 2002. Oxidation in prosthetic UHMWPE. Abstr. Pap. Am. Chem. Soc. 224, U507.
Costa, L., Carpentieri, I., Bracco, P., 2008. Post electron-beam irradiation oxidation of orthopaedic UHMWPE. Polym. Degrad. Stab. 93, 1695–1703.
Costa, L., Luda, M.P., Trossarelli, L., Del Prever, E.M.B., Crova, M., Gallinaro, P., 1998. Oxidation in orthopaedic UHMWPE sterilized by gamma-radiation and ethylene oxide. Biomaterials 19, 659–668.
Curtis, J., Colas, A., 2004a. Medical Applications of Silicones. Academic Press.
Curtis, J., Colas, A., 2004b. Silicone Biomaterials: History and Chemistry & Medical Applications of Silicones. Academic Press.

Curtis, J.M., Peters, Y.A., Swarthout, D.E., Kennan, J.J., Vandyke, M.E., 2000. Mechanical and chemical analysis of retrieved breast implants demonstrate material durability. In: Transactions of the Sixth World Biomaterials Congress.

Del Prever, E.M.B., Bistolfi, A., Bracco, P., Costa, L., 2009. UHMWPE for arthroplasty: past or future. J. Orthop. Traumatol. 10, 1–8.

De Nicola, R.R., 1950. Permanent artificial (silicone) urethra. J. Urol. 63, 168–172.

Desai, S.M., Solanky, S.S., Mandale, A.B., Rathore, K., Singh, R.P., 2003. Controlled grafting of N-isopropyl acrylamide brushes onto self-standing isotactic polypropylene thin films: surface initiated atom transfer radical polymerization. Polymer 44, 7645–7649.

DiMaio, F.R., 2002. The science of bone cement: a historical review. Orthopedics 25, 1399–1407.

Friedman, R.M., 2010. Silicon Breast Implants [Online]. Available: http://www.plasticsurgerydallas.com/blog/which-should-i-choose-saline-breast-implants-or-silicone-gel-breast-implants/.

Gautam, R., Singh, R.D., Sharma, V.P., Siddhartha, R., Chand, P., Kumar, R., 2012. Biocompatibility of polymethylmethacrylate resins used in dentistry. J. Biomed. Mater. Res. Part B Appl. Biomater. 100B, 1444–1450.

Gomathi, N., Rajasekar, R., Babu, R.R., Mishra, D., Neogi, S., 2012. Development of bio/blood compatible polypropylene through low pressure nitrogen plasma surface modification. Mater. Sci. Eng. C Mater. Biol. Appl. 32, 1767–1778.

Grant, D.N., Benson, J., Cozad, M.J., Whelove, O.E., Bachman, S.L., Ramshaw, B.J., Grant, D.A., Grant, S.A., 2011. Conjugation of gold nanoparticles to polypropylene mesh for enhanced biocompatibility. J. Mater. Sci. Mater. Med. 22, 2803–2812.

Gunatillake, P.A., Martin, D.J., Meijs, G.F., Mccarthy, S.J., Adhikari, R., 2003. Designing biostable polyurethane elastomers for biomedical implants. Aust. J. Chem. 56, 545–557.

Gupta, B., Saxena, S., Ray, A., 2008. Plasma induced graft polymerization of acrylic acid onto polypropylene monofilament. J. Appl. Polym. Sci. 107, 324–330.

Hamdan, S., Swallowe, G.M., 1996. Strain rate and temperature dependence of the mechanical properties of polyetherketone polyetheretherketone. J. Mater. Sci. 31, 1415–1423.

Handbook of Polymer, Copyright, 2012. ChemTec Publishing, p. 482.

Hazer, D.B., Kilicay, E., Hazer, B., 2012. Poly(3-hydroxyalkanoate)s: diversification and biomedical applications. A state of the art review. Mater. Sci. Eng. C Mater. Biol. Appl. 32, 637–647.

Hendel, G., Garti, A., Al, E., 2003. Fracture of the central polyethylene tibial spine in posterior stabilized total knee arthroplasty. J. Arthroplasty 15, 672–674.

Hunter, A., Archer, C.W., Walker, P.S., Blunn, G.W., 1995. Attachment and proliferation of osteoblasts and fibroblasts on biomaterials for orthopedic use. Biomaterials 16, 635–646.

Jaeblon, T., 2010. Polymethylmethacrylate: properties and contemporary uses in orthopaedics. J. Am. Acad. Orthop. Surg. 18, 297–305.

Kaneeda, T., Utsumi, M., Watanabe, E., Aspe, 1999. Effects of gamma irradiation and accelerated aging on wear properties of UHMWPE artificial joint. In: Proceedings of the Fourteenth Annual Meeting of the American Society for Precision Engineering, pp. 167–170.

Kenny, S.M., Buggy, M., 2003. Bone cements and fillers: a review. J. Mater. Sci. Mater. Med. 14, 923–938.

Klosterhalfen, B., Junge, K., Klinge, U., 2005. The lightweight and large porous mesh concept for hernia repair. Expert Rev. Med. Devices 2, 103–117.

Kuehn, K.D., Ege, W., Gopp, U., 2005. Acrylic bone cements: composition and properties. Orthop. Clin. North Am. 36, 17–28.

Kuhn, K.-D., 2000. Bone Cements. Springer Valley, Heidelberg, Germany.

Kumakura, T., Puppulin, L., Yamamoto, K., Takahashi, Y., Pezzotti, G., 2009. In-depth oxidation and strain profiles in UHMWPE acetabular cups non-destructively studied by confocal Raman microprobe spectroscopy. J. Biomater. Sci. Polym. Ed. 20, 1809–1822.
Kurtz, S.M., 2004. Ultrahigh Molecular Weight Polyethylenes (UHMWPE). Academic Press, London.
Kurtz, S., Muratoglu, O., Mark, E., Al, E., 1999a. Advances in the processing, sterilization, and crosslinking of ultra-high molecular weight polyethylene for total joint arthroplasty. Biomaterials 20, 1659–1688.
Kurtz, S., Van Ooij, A., Al, E., 2006a. Polyethylene wear and rim fracture in total disc arthroplasty. Spine J. 7, 12–21.
Kurtz, S.M., 2009. UHDMWPE Biomaterials Handbook, Chapter2. Academic Press, London, UK, pp. 7–19.
Kurtz, S.M., 2012. PEEK Biomaterials Handbook. William Andrew Publication, Oxford, UK.
Kurtz, S.M., Devine, J.N., 2007. PEEK biomaterials in trauma, orthopedic, and spinal implants. Biomaterials 28, 4845–4869.
Kurtz, S.M., Hozack, W.J., Purtill, J.J., Marcolongo, M., Kraay, M.J., Goldberg, V.M., Sharkey, P.F., Parvizi, J., Rimnac, C.M., Edidin, A.A., 2006b. 2006 Otto Aufranc Award paper – significance of in vivo degradation for polyethylene in total hip arthroplasty. Clin. Orthop. Relat. Res. 47–57.
Kurtz, S.M., Muratoglu, O.K., Evans, M., Edidin, A.A., 1999b. Advances in the processing, sterilization, and crosslinking of ultra-high molecular weight polyethylene for total joint arthroplasty. Biomaterials 20, 1659–1688.
Kwarteng, K.B., Starck, C., 1990. Carbon fibre reinforced PEEK (APC-2/AS-4) composites for orthopaedic implants. SAMPE Q. 10–14.
Lafay, H., 1957. A father's last chance invention saves his son. Reader's Digest.
Lamba, K., Woodhouse, K., Coper, S.L., 1998. Polyurethanes in Biomedical Applications. CRC Press, New York.
Laredo, J.D., Hamze, B., 2004. Complications of percutaneous vertebroplasty and their prevention. Skeletal Radiol. 33, 493–505.
Lewis, G., 2001. Properties of crosslinked ultra-high-molecular-weight polyethylene. Biomaterials 22, 371–401.
Lewis, G., 2011. Viscoelastic properties of injectable bone cements for orthopaedic applications: state-of-the-art review. J. Biomed. Mater. Res. Part B Appl. Biomater. 98B, 171–191.
Li, H.M., Fouracre, R.A., Given, M.J., Banforn, H.M., Wysocki, S., Karolczak, S., 1999. Effects on polyetheretherketone and polyether sulfone of electron and gamma irradiation. Dielectr. Electr. Insul. IEEE Trans. 6, 295–303.
Lieberman, I., Dudeney, S., Reinhardt, M.-K., Bell, G., 2002. Initial outcome and efficacy of "kyphoplasty" in the treatment of painful osteoporotic vertebral compression fractures. Spine 26, 1631–1638.
Liu, Q.Y., Jiang, L., Shi, R., Zhang, L.Q., 2012. Synthesis, preparation, in vitro degradation, and application of novel degradable bioelastomers-a review. Prog. Polym. Sci. 37, 715–765.
Livermore, C., Voldman, J., 2004. Design and Fabrication of Microelectromechanical Devices Material Property Database, 2004 [cit 14.05.2013].
Majercik, S., Tsikitis, V., Iannitti, D.A., 2006. Strength and tissue attachment to mesh after ventral hernia repair with synthetic composite mesh in a porcine model. Surg. Endosc. 20, 1671–1674.
Mariconda, M., Lotti, G., Al, E., 2000. Fracture of posterior-stabilized tibial insert in a genesis knee prosthesis. J. Arthroplasty 15, 529–530.

Martina, M., Hutmacher, D.W., 2007. Biodegradable polymers applied in tissue engineering research: a review. Polym. Int. 56, 145–157.

Mata, A., Fleischman, A.J., Roy, S., 2005. Biomed. Microdevices 7, 281–293.

Mckellop, H., Shen, F.W., Lu, B., Campbell, P., Salovey, R., 2000. Effect of sterilization method and other modifications on the wear resistance of acetabular cups made of ultra-high molecular weight polyethylene – a hip-simulator study. J. Bone Jt. Surg. Am. Vol. 82A, 1708–1725.

Mcmillin, C.R., 2006. Biomedical applications of rubbers and elastomers. Rubber Chem. Technol. 79, 500–519.

Medel, F.J., Garcia-Alvarez, F., Gomez-Barrena, E., Puertolas, J.A., 2005. Microstructure changes of extruded ultra high molecular weight polyethylene after gamma irradiation and shelf-aging. Polym. Degrad. Stab. 88, 435–443.

Mehmood, M.S., Hafeez, U., Jahan, M.S., Mishra, S., Walters, B.M., Ikram, M., 2012. The effect of high dose of gamma-irradiation on residual radicals concentration in ultra-high molecular weight polyethylene (UHMWPE) in the presence of vitamin E. Polym. Sci. Ser. A 54, 343–348.

Meintjes, J., Yan, S., Zhou, L., Zheng, S.S., Zheng, M.H., 2011. Synthetic, biological and composite scaffolds for abdominal wall reconstruction. Expert Rev. Med. Devices 8, 275–288.

Nair, L.S., Laurencin, C.T., 2007. Biodegradable polymers as biomaterials. Prog. Polym. Sci. 32, 762–798.

Nayak, R., Kyratzis, I.L., Truong, Y.B., Padhye, R., Arnold, L., Peeters, G., Nichols, L., O'shea, M., 2012. Fabrication and characterisation of nanofibres by meltblowing and melt electrospinning. In: Chen, W.Z., Xu, X.P., Dai, P.Q., Chen, Y.L. (Eds.), Advanced Manufacturing Technology, Pts 1–4.

Noll, W., 1968. Chemistry and Technology of Silicones. New York.

Ojha, U., Kulkarni, P., Faust, R., 2009. Syntheses and characterization of novel biostable polyisobutylene based thermoplastic polyurethanes. Polymer 50, 3448–3457.

Ortel, G., 1994. Polyurethane Handbook. Hanser Gardner, Berlin.

Petillo, O., Peluso, G., Ambrosio, L., Nicolais, L., Kao, W.J., Anderson, J.M., 1994. In vivo induction of macrophage Ia antigen (MHC Class II) expression by biomedical polymers in the cage implant system. J. Biomed. Mater. Res. 28, 635–646.

Pinchuk, L., 1995. A review of the biostability and carcinogenicity of polyurethanes in medicine and the new generation of biostable polyurethanes. J. Biomater. Sci. Polym. Ed. 6, 225–267.

Place, E.S., George, J.H., Williams, C.K., Stevens, M.M., 2009. Synthetic polymer scaffolds for tissue engineering. Chem. Soc. Rev. 38, 1139–1151.

Pruitt, L.A., 2005. Deformation, yielding, fracture and fatigue behavior of conventional and highly cross-linked ultra high molecular weight polyethylene. Biomaterials 26, 905–915.

Rae, P.J., Brown, E.N., Orler, E.B., 2007. The mechanical properties of poly(ether-ether-ketone) (PEEK) with emphasis on the large compressive strain response. Polymer 48, 598–615.

Sanders, D.L., Kingsnorth, A.N., 2012. Prosthetic mesh materials used in hernia surgery. Expert Rev. Med. Devices 9, 159–179.

Santerre, J.P., Woodhouse, K., Laroche, G., Labow, R.S., 2005. Understanding the biodegradation of polyurethanes: from classical implants to tissue engineering materials. Biomaterials 26, 7457–7470.

Santerre, P., Duguay, D., Labow, R., Brash, J., 1995. Interaction of hydrolytic enzymes at an aqueous-polyurethane interface. Proteins at interfaces II. J. Am. Chem. Soc. 352–370.

Saxena, S., Ray, A.R., Kapil, A., Pavon-Djavid, G., Letourneur, D., Gupta, B., Meddahi-Pelle, A., 2011. Development of a new polypropylene-based suture: plasma grafting, surface treatment, characterization, and biocompatibility studies. Macromol. Biosci. 11, 373–382.
Scotchford, C.A., Garle, M.J., Batchelor, J., Bradley, J., Grant, D.M., 2003. Use of a novel carbon fibre composite material for the femoral stem component of a THR system: in vitro biological assessment. Biomaterials 24, 4871–4879.
Shibata, N., Tomita, N., 2005. The anti-oxidative properties of alpha-tocopherol in gamma-irradiated UHMWPE with respect to fatigue and oxidation resistance. Biomaterials 26, 5755–5762.
Simmons, A., Hyvarinen, J., Poole-Warren, L., 2006. The effect of sterilisation on a poly (dimethylsiloxane)/poly(hexamethylene oxide) mixed macrodiol-based polyurethane elastomer. Biomaterials 27, 4484–4497.
Skinner, H.B., 1988. Composite technology for total hip arthroplasty. Clin. Orthop. Relat. Res. 235, 224–236.
Sobieraj, M.C., Rimnac, C.M., 2009. Ultra high molecular weight polyethylene: mechanics, morphology, and clinical behavior. J. Mech. Behav. Biomed. Mater. 2, 433–443.
Song, L.J., Zhao, J., Yang, H.W., Jin, J., Li, X.M., Stagnaro, P., Yin, J.H., 2011. Biocompatibility of polypropylene non-woven fabric membrane via UV-induced graft polymerization of 2-acrylamido-2-methylpropane sulfonic acid. Appl. Surf. Sci. 258, 425–430.
Speckhard, T., Ver Strate, G., Gibson, P., Sl, C., 1983. Properties of polyisobutylene-polyurethane block copolymers: I. Macroglycols from ozonolysis of isobutylene copolymer. Polym. Eng. Sci. 23, 337–349.
Stokes, K., Mcvennes, R., 1995. Polyurethane elastomer biostability. J. Biomater. Appl. 9, 321–335.
Sugano, N., Saito, A., Yamamoto, T., Nishii, T., Yau, S.S., Wang, A., 2004. Analysis of a retrieved UHMWPE acetabular cup crosslinked in air with 1000 kGy of gamma radiation. J. Orthop. Res. 22, 828–831.
Szycher, M., Reed, A.M., Soc Plast Engineers, I.N.C., 1996. Medical-grade polyurethanes: a critical review. In: Antec '96: Plastics – Racing into the Future, Vols I-III: Vol I: Processing; Vol II: Materials; Vol III: Spacial Areas, 42, pp. 2758–2766.
Takahara, A., Coury, A., Hergenrother, R., Cooper, S., 1991. Effect of soft segment chemistry on the biostability of segmented polyurethanes. I. In vitro oxidation. J. Biomed. Mater. Res. 25, 341–356.
Toth, J.M., 2012. Biocompatibility of Polyaryletheretherketone Polymers. Elsevier Inc.
Ulery, B.D., Nair, L.S., Laurencin, C.T., 2011. Biomedical applications of biodegradable polymers. J. Polym. Sci. Part B Polym. Phys. 49, 832–864.
Vallittu, P.K., Ruyter, I.E., Buykuilmaz, S., 1998. Effect of polymerization temperature and time on the residual monomer content of denture base polymers. Eur. J. Oral Sci. 106, 588–593.
Ward, R., Anderson, J., Mcvenes, R., Stokes, K., 2006a. In vivo biostability of polysiloxane polyether polyurethanes: resistance to biologic oxidation and stress cracking. J. Biomed. Mater. Res. Part A 77A, 580–589.
Ward, R., Anderson, J., Mcvenes, R., Stokes, K., 2006b. In vivo biostability of shore 55D polyether polyurethanes with and without fluoropolymer surface modifying endgroups. J. Biomed. Mater. Res. Part A 79A, 836–845.
Wenz, L.M., Merritt, K., Brown, S.A., Moet, A., Steffe, A.D., 1990. In vitro biocompatibility of polyetheretherketone and polysulfone composites. J. Biomed. Mater. Res. 24, 207–215.
Wheatley, D.J., Bernacca, G.M., Tolland, M.M., O'connor, B., Fisher, J., Williams, D.F., 2001. Hydrodynamic function of a biostable polyurethane flexible heart valve after six months in sheep. Int. J. Artif. Organs 24, 95–101.

Wheatley, D.J., Raco, L., Bernacca, G.M., Sim, I., Belcher, P.R., Boyd, J.S., 2000. Polyurethane: material for the next generation of heart valve prostheses? Eur. J. Cardiothorac. Surg. 17, 440–447.

Williams, D.F., 2003. Revisiting the definition of biocompatibility. Med. Device Technol. 14, 10–13.

Williams, D.F., Mcnmara, A., Turner, R.M., 1987. Potential of polyetheretherketone (PEEK) and carbon-fibre-reinforced PEEK in medical applications. J. Mater. Sci. Lett. 6, 188–190.

Wolf, C., Maninger, J., Lederer, K., Fruhwirth-Smounig, H., Gamse, T., Marr, R., 2006. Stabilisation of crosslinked ultra-high molecular weight polyethylene (UHMW-PE)-acetabular components with alpha-tocopherol. J. Mater. Sci. Mater. Med. 17, 1323–1331.

Xiong, D., Ma, R., Lin, J., Wang, N., Jin, Z.M., 2007. Tribological properties and structure of ultra-high molecular weight polyethylene after gamma irradiation. Proc. Inst. Mech. Eng. Part J J. Eng. Tribol. 221, 315–320.

Xiong, L., Xiong, D.S., 2012. The influence of irradiation dose on mechanical properties and wear resistance of molded and extruded ultra high molecular weight polyethylene. J. Mech. Behav. Biomed. Mater. 9, 73–82.

Yang, Q., Xu, Z.K., Dai, Z.W., Wang, J.L., Ulbricht, M., 2005. Surface modification of polypropylene microporous membranes with a novel glycopolymer. Chem. Mater. 17, 3050–3058.

Zhao, J., Shi, Q., Luan, S.F., Song, L.J., Yang, H.W., Stagnaro, P., Yin, J.H., 2012. Polypropylene non-woven fabric membrane via surface modification with biomimetic phosphorylcholine in Ce(IV)/HNO3 redox system. Mater. Sci. Eng. C Mater. Biol. Appl. 32, 1785–1789.

Zhao, J., Shi, Q.A., Luan, S.F., Song, L.J., Yang, H.W., Shi, H.C., Jin, J., Li, X.L., Yin, J.H., Stagnaro, P., 2011. Improved biocompatibility and antifouling property of polypropylene non-woven fabric membrane by surface grafting zwitterionic polymer. J. Membr. Sci. 369, 5–12.

Zimmer, 2012. Vitamin E Containing UHMWPE in Continuum Acetabular Shell System (Vivacit). Zimmer, Inc. http://www.zimmer.com/content/pdf/en-US/zimmer_continuum_acetabular_system_with_vivacit-e_surgical_technique.pdf.

Biodegradable and bioerodible polymers for medical applications

3

K.E. Uhrich[1], *D. Abdelhamid*[2]
[1]Rutgers University, Piscataway, NJ, USA; [2]Minia University, Minia, Egypt

3.1 Introduction

Historically, early biomedical polymers were chosen for their stability in physiological conditions as well as meeting a medical need. For example, poly(methyl methacrylate) (PMMA) was one of the earliest synthetic polymers for medical applications; it was used as a corneal implant because of its optical transparency and biocompatibility, as demonstrated by PMMA shards tolerated in the eyes of fighter pilots (Davis, 2003). For many medical applications, particularly tissue-engineered constructs, it is desirable for the polymer to permanently remain in place. For example, Teflon-coated hip implants reduce friction, and this antifriction property is expected to persist throughout the lifetime of the device. Yet, many medical applications would benefit from a temporary polymer – a polymer that would "disappear" after the drug has been delivered or the tissue has properly healed. This chapter focuses on polymers that are temporary; they ultimately break down in physiological conditions (i.e. biodegrade) or solubilise (i.e. bioerode).

3.2 Concepts and terminology

3.2.1 *Biodegradable and bioerodible*

Several terms are often used interchangeably, we will use chemical and physical mechanisms to clarify and differentiate the terms (Uhrich et al., 1999). First, we define "biodegradation" as a biologically based process that leads to degradation. Biological processes encompass human enzymes, microbial enzymes and even hydrolysis – as water is the most abundant molecule in the human body. Degradation refers to bond cleavage and includes hydrolysis of ester bonds or ultraviolet-promoted cleavage of the C–C bonds. Typically, biodegradable polymers would include hydrolytically and/or enzymatically susceptible bonds such as polyesters, polyanhydrides, polycarbonates, polyamides and polyurethanes. Table 3.1 shows representative examples of biodegradable polymers, their chemical structures and applications. Second, we define "bioerodible" as using biological processes to mechanically erode a polymer. Just as water eroded rock to produce the Grand Canyon, water can erode a polymer via mechanical means (e.g. friction) and/or solubilise the polymer. In this sense, "bioresorbable" is a synonym of bioerodible; the implication is that the polymer is resorbed, or adsorbed,

Biosynthetic Polymers for Medical Applications. http://dx.doi.org/10.1016/B978-1-78242-105-4.00003-1

Table 3.1 Examples of biodegradable polymers, their chemical structures and applications

Polymer type	Polymer name	Chemical structure (of repeat unit)	Applications
Polyether	Poly(ethylene glycol) (PEG)	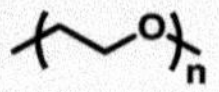	• Diffusion-controlled tablet formulation • Crosslinked hydrogels • Polymer–drug conjugates • Block copolymers
Polyester	Poly(glycolic acid) (PGA)	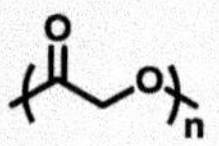	• Woven medical devices (e.g. sutures and meshes)
	Poly(lactic acid) (PLA)	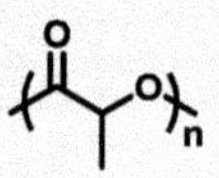	• Resorbable sutures • Block copolymers (PLGA)
	Poly(ε-caprolactone) (PCL)	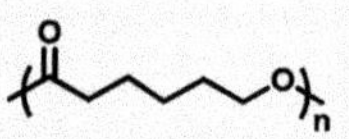	• Slow-degrading polymer • Sutures • Adhesion barrier
Polyanhydride	Poly(sebacic acid)	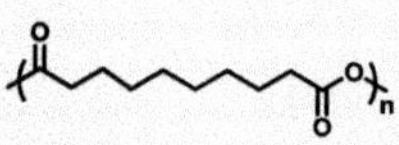	• Copolymer for admixed drug delivery systems
Poly(anhydride-ester)	Poly(salicylic acid)	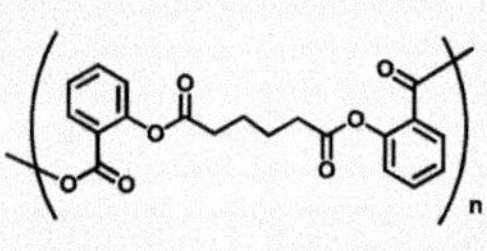	• Hydrolytically controlled release of anti-inflammatory drugs
Polyamides	Polylysine	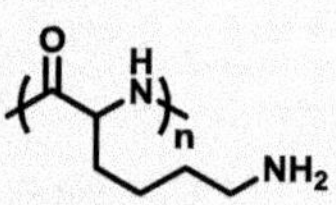	• Copolymer microspheres for deep lung delivery
Polyurethanes	Polyurethanes	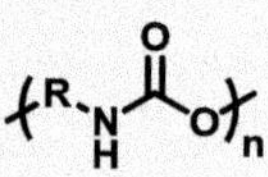	• Hard and soft-segments modified for temporal controlled release
Poly(ether-ester)	Azopolymer	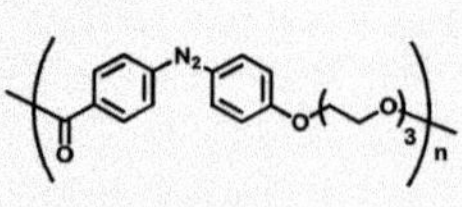	• Colon-specific delivery of chemotherapeutics
Polyphosphazene	Poly(bis [carboxylatophenoxy] phosphazene)	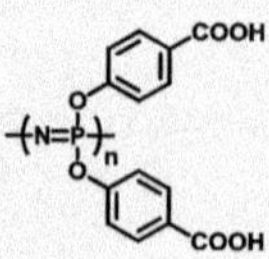	• Microspheres for temporal controlled release

into the surrounding tissue. Thus, the chemistry of the polymer is not fundamentally changed; rather, the physical state has changed from a solid structure to a solubilised polymer. An example of a bioresorbable polymer is poly(ethylene-glycol) (PEG); a ubiquitous polyether that is frequently used for biomedical applications because of its biocompatibility and water solubility.

Therapeutically viable polymers are often designed to be stable, biocompatible, soluble, and preferably, target-specific (Liu et al., 2009; Watson et al., 2001). Several medical conditions, however, would benefit from polymers that degrade in vivo. Nondegradable polymers require removal or further treatment after introduction into the body. Biodegradable polymers overcome these shortcomings as they are liable to hydrolysis under physiological conditions due to the presence of unstable functional groups (e.g. anhydride, ester, amide, bonds) (Uhrich et al., 1999). As described above, hydrolytic or enzymatic degradation may result in polymer backbone scission or cleavage of water-soluble side chains. The cleavage products can then be metabolised and excreted, resulting in complete removal. Biodegradability and bioerodibility are both considered desirable characteristics for controlled drug delivery; as such, devices do not require a second surgery for removal. As examples, biodegradable and/or bioerodible polymers can be used as sutures or adhesives in wound management, pins and rods in orthopedic devices, stents for treating cardiovascular diseases, guided tissue regeneration membranes, and void fillers after tooth extraction.

3.2.2 Natural and synthetic polymers

Biocompatibility and minimal side effects are critical factors for polymer therapeutic applicability. Natural polymers, often referred to as biopolymers due to inherent biocompatibility, are biomacromolecules that are used in therapeutics; examples include carbohydrates (e.g. cellulose, starch and chitosan) (Uhrich et al., 1999) and polysulfates (e.g. gelatin, fibrin, collagen and hyaluronan) (Duncan, 2003). These biomacromolecules are extracted from animals or plants, and often possess desirable bioactive properties (e.g. antiviral and antitumour) (Seymour, 1991). Despite their biocompatibility, the applicability of naturally occurring polymers is limited by their physicochemical properties which often can only be manipulated in the bulk material (Uhrich et al., 1999). One particular issue is polydispersity (PDI), which is defined as the ratio of weight−average molecular weight (Mw) and number−average molecular weight (Mn) (PDI = Mw/Mn). Polydispersity measures the presence of individual molecules of different chain lengths within the polymer sample. As examples, polysaccharides and chitosans are typically characterised by high Mw (>200,000 g/mole) and high PDI (>2) (Duncan, 2003) compared with smaller bioactives (i.e. drugs) that have relatively low Mw values with PDI values of 1.

Significant advances in organic synthesis and characterisation techniques have yielded synthetic polymers with well-defined, three-dimensional structures and with the potential to mimic biomacromolecules. These well-structured polymers include block copolymers (Pechar et al., 2000), branched polymers, graft polymers (Langer and Peppas, 1981), dendronized polymers (Kwon and Kataoka, 1995), multivalent polymers (Langer, 1995), and polymers with biomimetic features (Duncan, 2003).

Depending on the polymerisation method, synthetic polymers can have very narrow PDI values; an excellent example is PEG, which is commercially available with narrow PDI values (~1.01). As another example, many dendronized polymers or dendrimers can be produced as monodispersed polymers (Duncan, 2003). Furthermore, careful design of the polymer synthetic routes allows tailoring of the mechanical, physicochemical and degradation properties of the resulting polymers.

3.2.3 Controlled release

Different classes of drugs may require differences in delivery methods to improve their therapeutic efficiency, decrease side effects and/or reduce the frequency of administration. Examples of drug classes include chemotherapeutics (Walter et al., 1995; Dang et al., 1994), immunosuppressants (Katayama et al., 1995), antiinflammatory agents (Wagenaar and Muller, 1994; Conforti et al., 1996), antibiotics, (Schierholz et al., 1997) opioid antagonists, (Falk et al., 1997) steroids (Ye and Chien, 1996), hormones (Johnson et al., 1996), anesthetics (Park et al., 1998), and vaccines (McGee et al., 1994). Moreover, protein drugs and gene therapy can require specific and time-controlled delivery to target cells. Thus, controlled release systems were developed to improve the effectiveness of these drugs via either temporal or distribution release mechanisms (Uhrich et al., 1999).

3.2.3.1 Temporal control

In temporal control (Figure 3.1), the drug is delivered over an extended period or at a specific time point. The extended period may enable longer circulation time for drugs that are rapidly metabolised and eliminated in vivo. Temporally controlled systems delay the dissolution of the drug and inhibit its diffusion for a specific period of time to postpone reaching its target cells (Uhrich et al., 1999). This effect is usually achieved with a polymer coating that dissolves at a slower rate than the drug molecules, delaying exposure to the physiological aqueous environment.

3.2.3.2 Distribution control

In distribution control, the drug is delivered at a specific site in the body that can be beneficial in specific situations. When drug molecules are evenly distributed to many tissues, major side effects may occur and prevent further treatment. This example is often encountered in cancer chemotherapy, potentially causing treatment interruption due to the death of bone marrow cells. In another example, the drug cannot reach its target site via natural distribution, such as a drug that acts on brain receptors but cannot cross the blood–brain barrier. Thus, for distribution controlled delivery systems, a targeting mechanism is employed (Uhrich et al., 1999). Physically encapsulated drugs and polymer–drug conjugates are mostly applied in distribution control mechanisms. In these systems, targeting moieties are chemically incorporated into the polymeric structure. Examples of these moieties include immunoglobulins and carbohydrates. Some block copolymers such as Pluronics (composed of PEG and

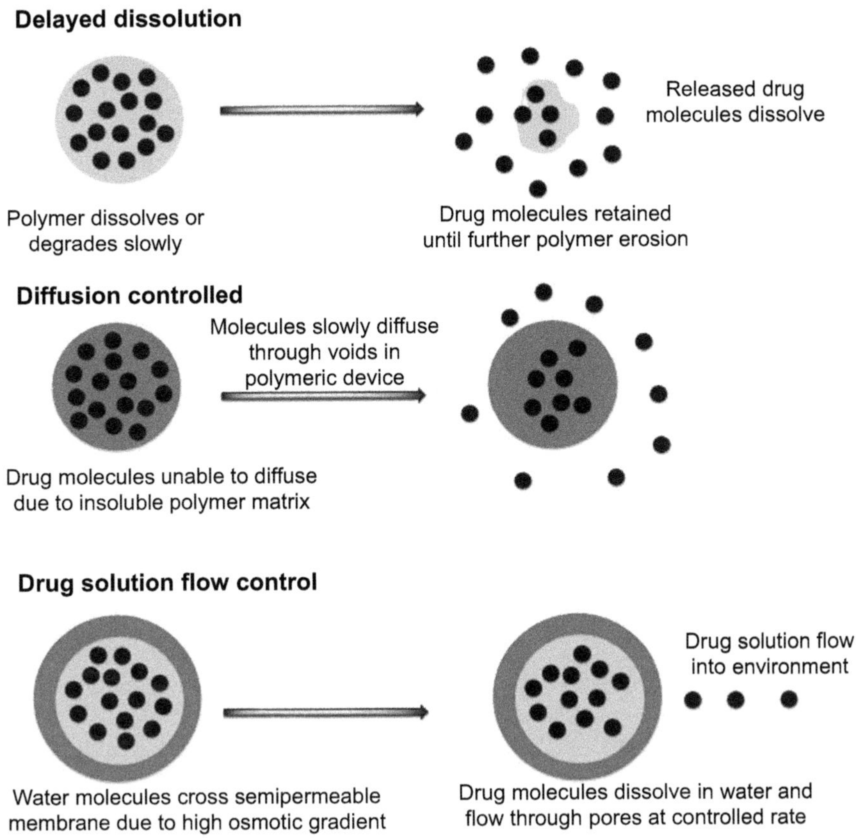

Figure 3.1 Examples of mechanisms of temporal controlled release: delayed dissolution, diffusion-controlled and membrane-controlled.

poly(propylene oxide) blocks) possess inherent distribution control due to their ability to minimise protein adsorption on the particle surface (Amiji and Park, 1992; Topchieva et al., 1995). Some polymer–drug conjugates possess site-specific cleavable linkages, such as colon-targeting delivery systems that are susceptible to gastrointestinal bacteria (Putnam et al., 1996).

3.2.4 Polymer–drug conjugates

The concept of a polymer–drug conjugate was introduced in the 1970s by Ringsdorf, who envisioned the attachment of an anticancer-drug to the polymer backbone through a linker molecule (Figure 3.2) (Haag and Kratz, 2006). Many other polymer–drug systems have since been developed (Khandare and Minko, 2006). Typically, the linkage between the polymer and the drug is designed with predetermined cleavable bonds that respond to changes in physiological conditions such as temperature, pH, and action of enzymes, which then release the drug at the target site. Additional solubilising groups

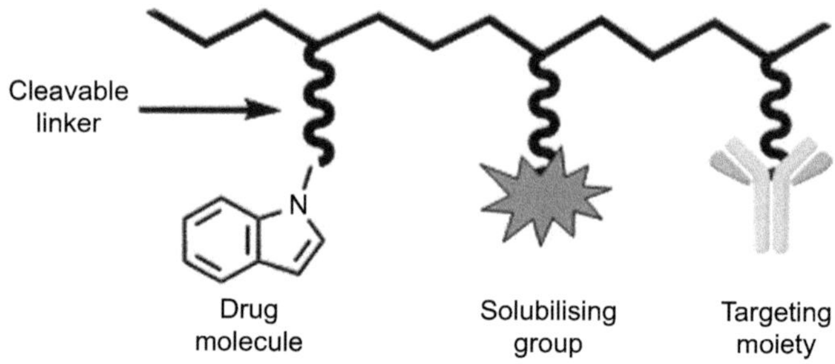

Figure 3.2 Ringsdorf model for polymer therapeutic – with drug, solubilising group and targeting moiety attached to the base polymer.

(e.g. PEG) and/or targeting moieties (e.g. antibodies) can be attached to improve drug solubility (Greenwald, 2001), bioavailability, targeting specificity and pharmacodynamic properties (Haag and Kratz, 2006). Ideally, the polymer should be water-soluble, biocompatible, nonimmunogenic, and most importantly, possess functional groups for attaching the drug (Godwin et al., 2001). Linear polymers (e.g. *N*-(2-hydroxypropyl) methacrylamide (HPMA)) were the first type to be investigated, followed by various polymer architectures (Rihova and Kubackova, 2003; Kopecek et al., 2000).

In addition to linkers that are physiologically triggered, polymer–drug conjugate designs can also address adequate drug loading capacity and targeting mechanism (de Duve et al., 1974). To date, the majority of research has focused on linkers that are stable during transport, yet allow sustained drug release at the appropriate site. Enzyme-sensitive peptide linkers were successfully applied after the popularisation of HPMA copolymer–Gly–Phe–Leu–Gly–doxorubicin conjugates (Rejmanova et al., 1985). This tetrapeptide is stable to blood circulation (Rejmanova et al., 1985) and cleaved by the lysosomal, thiol-dependent protease cathepsin B following endocytic uptake. pH-sensitive linkages such as hydrazone and acetal linkages have also been investigated (Duncan, 2003). In these cases, drug release is triggered by the acidic medium of endosomes or lysosomes following uptake. Similar to the tetrapeptide conjugate, a doxorubicin conjugate bound to an HPMA copolymer via hydrazone linkages has shown in vivo antitumour activity against lymphoma (Etrych et al., 2001).

3.2.5 Polymeric delivery systems

Polymer delivery vehicles are polymer-based systems in which the drug is physically entrapped (rather than chemically connected) to the polymer. Similar to the polymer–drug conjugates, polymeric delivery systems were developed to overcome the limitations of small drug molecule and macromolecule (e.g. DNA, RNA, proteins) delivery (Liu et al., 2009). These systems are mainly designed to protect drugs from physiological degradation or inactivation, yet allow drug release at a specific rate and/or site. To build upon a previous review article on polymers for drug delivery (Uhrich et al., 1999), this work describes only a few delivery systems – hydrogels, self-assemblies and complexes.

3.2.5.1 Hydrogels

Polymer matrices such as hydrogels (Figure 3.3) consist of multiple polymer chains which can physically entrap hydrophobic drugs (Liu et al., 2009). The drug is released via passive diffusion between polymer chains. In addition to swelling in the presence of water, the polymer matrix can be affected by changes in pH, temperature, or enzymatic action that lead to drug release. Natural and synthetic hydrogels have a long history of applications in drug delivery and repairing tissues and organs (Liu et al., 2009). Poly(hydroxyethylmethacrylic acid) hydrogels were introduced in the 1960s, and calcium alginate microcapsules in the 1980s (Liu et al., 2009; Kim et al., 2010; Lim and Sun, 1980). These hydrogels are biocompatible, biodegradable, withstand sterilisation and their chemical structures influence their mechanical and hydrophilic properties (Keys et al., 1998). Novel, superporous hydrogels based on poly(acrylic acid) (Chen et al., 1999) and disulphide-crosslinked (poly(oligo(ethyleneoxide) monomethyl ether methacrylate)) (POEOMA) nanogels have been developed using a uniquely sensitive linker. POEOMA nanogels degrade via the reducing action of glutathione that underlines their potential for specific target cell delivery (Oh et al., 2007).

3.2.5.2 Self-assembled systems

In aqueous media, amphiphilic molecules form core—shell aggregates such as micelles upon reaching a specific concentration (critical micelle concentration, CMC) (Gindy et al., 2008). Micelles and liposomes are types of physical aggregates that are used for drug delivery (Haag and Kratz, 2006). Drug molecules can be physically entrapped in these assemblies (Figure 3.4) via passive diffusion or in situ loading during formation (Hubbell, 2003). Micelles play a role in drug delivery as they provide high drug loading, control drug release, lengthen plasma circulation time and slow in vivo clearance. Despite these important properties, polymeric micelle stability can be compromised upon exposure to physiological conditions (Kim et al., 2010; Chen et al., 2008). The micelle size typically ranges between 20 and 50 nm with relatively narrow distribution, and can partially be controlled by the polymer chemical structure (Jones et al., 2003). These sizes are similar to those of viruses, lipoproteins and natural transporters (Kataoka et al., 2001), and therefore, are subject to nonspecific uptake by the reticuloendothelial system. Liposomes are also important in drug delivery, with many

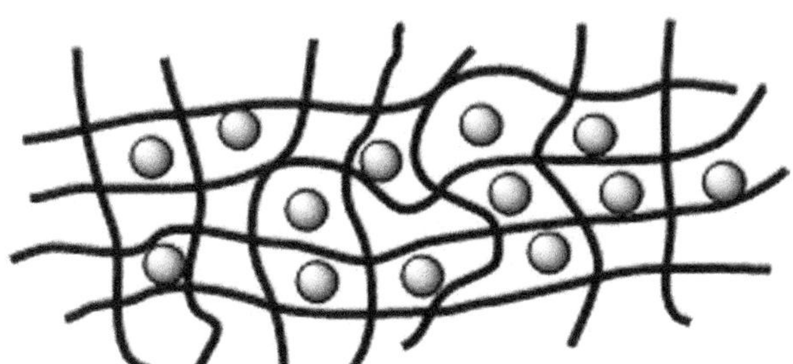

Figure 3.3 Drug molecules entrapped within the crosslinked polymer matrix.

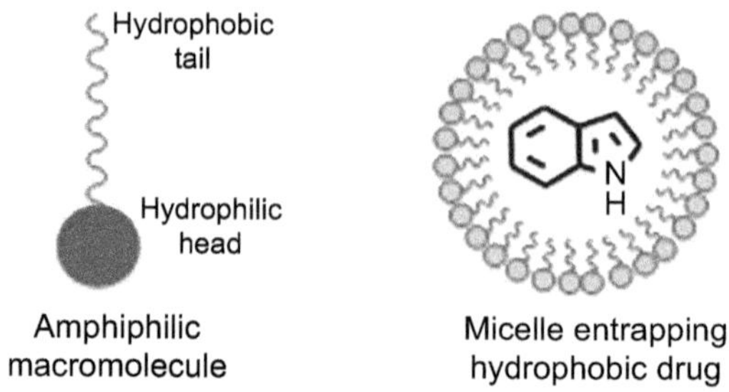

Figure 3.4 Drug molecules encapsulated within the micelle.

formulations in clinical use. Several excellent reviews on liposomes for drug delivery are recommended (Gregoriadis and Florence, 1993; Torchilin, 2012).

3.2.5.3 Complexes

As stated above, the biotechnology revolution has led to the development of sophisticated biomacromolecules such as recombinant nucleic acids (RNA and DNA) as viral vectors. Unfortunately, low selectivity, immunogenicity and liability to degradation upon cellular uptake are problems which limit their utility (Wolff, 2002). Cationic polymers or amphiphiles are being investigated as viral-protecting agents by forming electrostatic complexes with negatively charged DNA/RNA fragments (Figure 3.5). The most commonly used polymers for gene delivery are poly(ethylene imine) (PEI), poly(L-lysine), and chitosans. The polymers must form robust complexes that must transport through the cytoplasm, avoid degradation in the endosomes and lysosomes, and enter the nucleus (Figure 3.5). The physical and chemical properties of the complexes affect the rate and efficiency of gene delivery to cells, including the size, charge, hydrophobicity and buffering capacity of the complexes (Liu et al., 2009). Yet, some complexes are nonspecific, toxic and unstable in serum. Approaches to increase the efficiency of these delivery systems focus on polymers with variable primary and secondary amines such as PEI. Such polymers form complexes that bind with high affinity to DNA, and protect it from serum degradation (Srinivasachari et al., 2006, 2007). Generally, increasing the amine content increases the efficiency of DNA binding, cellular uptake and genetic expression. As another example, DNA polyplexes that contain PEG and heparin-binding proteins increase cell-surface adhesion and uptake, both are unique features favourable for nucleic acid delivery (Fichter et al., 2008). The therapeutic potential of these complexes for transgenic delivery relies on simple formulation and ability to transport large genes (Haensler and Szoka, 1993; Boussif et al., 1995; Kukowska-Latallo et al., 1996; Richardson et al., 1999; Joester et al., 2003; Murthy et al., 2003).

Small-interfering ribonucleic acid (siRNA) is considered a promising gene-based therapeutic approach for many diseases (Fire et al., 1998). However, due to the anionic nature of siRNA and the presence of RNases in the bloodstream, siRNA delivery is limited by inadequate cellular uptake and poor stability under physiological conditions (Gooding et al., 2012; Buyens et al., 2012; Dang and Leong, 2006). To overcome

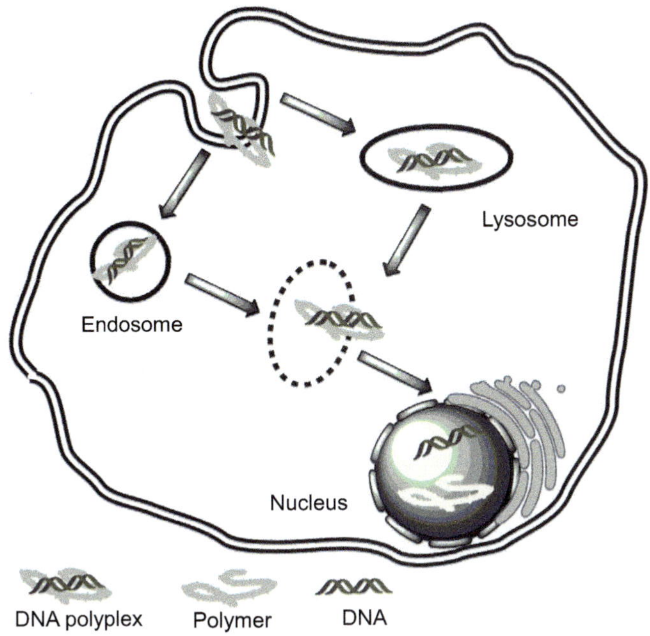

Figure 3.5 Cationic polymers complex with DNA and form DNA polyplex that protects genetic material.

this limitation, amphiphilic macromolecules (AMs) were synthesised with linear ethyleneimines to obtain cationic AMs capable of protecting and delivering siRNA (Sparks et al., 2011). Modest transfection efficiency with low cytotoxicity was shown when using AMs as the siRNA carrier. Further improvement of the transfection efficacy was attained using cationic AM–lipid complexes. In this case, the AMs stabilise liposomes and cationic lipid head groups provide enhanced siRNA protection (Gu et al., 2013).

3.3 Motivating factors for using polymer–drug conjugates

The main driving force for using synthetic polymers (vs naturally occurring polymers) is the ability to manipulate their properties by manipulating the chemical composition, which impacts solubility, tensile strength, biocompatibility, thermal stability and a myriad of other properties. Further, synthetic polymers provide unique advantages to overcome the limitations of small drug molecules as well as macromolecules (proteins, oligonucleotides and antibodies); their broad therapeutic applicability is based on their safety and tunable physicochemical properties (Fischbach and Mooney, 2007; Langer and Tirrell, 2004; Lutolf and Hubbell, 2005). Small molecules evenly diffuse throughout the body, which limits the effective drug concentration at the target site and can lead to side effects. By conjugating the drug molecules to a polymer, such as PEG, the polymer–drug conjugate's circulation time increases which improves the drug efficacy and provides the targeted drug delivery (Greenwald et al., 2003). Natural macromolecules, such as proteins, often suffer from immunogenicity and instability. These limitations can also be diminished by conjugation to hydrophilic polymers (e.g. PEG) that elongates their biological half-life and evades frequent administration (Knop et al., 2010).

Several biological factors and unmet medical needs have stimulated the fruitful research in the use of synthetic polymers in therapeutic applications. Several key concepts illustrating the use of polymers, specifically polymer–drug conjugates, are detailed below.

3.3.1 Passive accumulation: drug targeting via the EPR effect

Small molecules diffuse through endothelial cells of the capillary walls into normal and tumour tissues (Haag and Kratz, 2006). Macromolecules, however, can only diffuse through tumour tissues that have a leaky vasculature. Because of the defective lymphatic drainage system of tumours, macromolecules tend to passively accumulate in tumours. This phenomenon is called the "enhanced permeability and retention (EPR) effect" (Figure 3.6), which is due to the biochemical and physiological characteristics of malignant tissues (Maeda and Matsumura, 1989; Maeda et al., 2000). The EPR effect is observed for macromolecules within the molecular weight

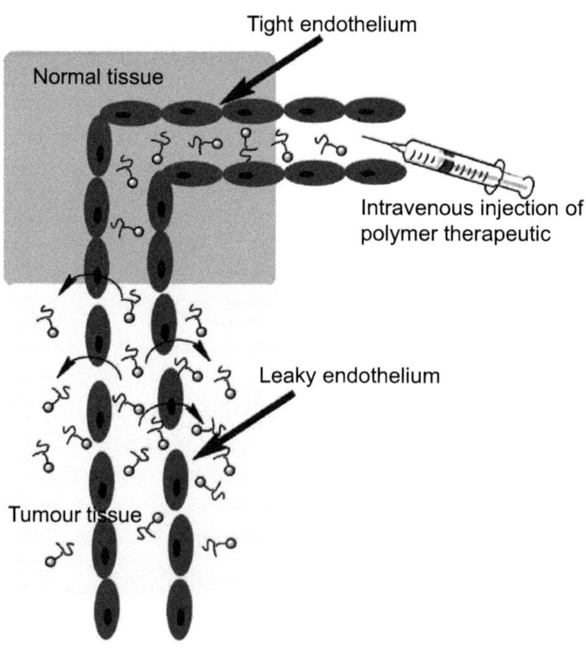

Figure 3.6 Tumour targeting by the EPR effect, relative to normal tissue.

range of 20–200 kDa (Haag and Kratz, 2006; Amiji and Park, 1992). Therefore, many polymers and related delivery systems were developed as tumour-targeted, drug delivery vehicles due to their selective retention in tumour tissues. Preclinical studies have shown that the physicochemical properties of polymers greatly influence their biodistribution and tumour accumulation (Greish et al., 2003; Maeda et al., 2001). These properties include molecular weight (Mw), overall charge, hydrophobicity, immunogenicity and conformation. Tumor size also influences the polymer uptake rate; polymers tend to accumulate more in small tumours (Satchi-Fainaro, 2002). This characteristic is useful for designing tumour-imaging agents to detect small tumours. Similarly, inflamed and infected tissues are characterised by leaky tissues, which can also lead to passive accumulation of polymers (Greish et al., 2003; Maeda et al., 2001).

3.3.2 Site-specific drug release

Small-molecule drugs tend to distribute uniformly throughout the body (i.e. systemic distribution), lowering the amount of drug that reaches the target site and elevates the probability of unwanted side effects. Site-specific drug release is accomplished through careful design of polymer–drug conjugates that are prone to biochemical or enzymatic hydrolysis. In cancer, site-specificity can be achieved with the overexpression of enzymes specifically associated with different tumours, as well as the hypoxic or acidic nature of other tumours (Shamis et al., 2004). This successful approach has provided higher drug concentration at target sites and ultimately increases drug efficacy (Greenwald et al., 2000). Cells take up polymers through receptor-mediated, adsorptive or fluid-phase endocytosis (Figure 3.7) (Mukherjee et al., 1997). Thus, the polymer is exposed to a significant pH drop from the physiological pH (~7.4) to an acidic pH (~5) in the endosomes or pH (~4) in the lysosomes. In addition to the pH change, polymers are exposed to the various enzymes in the vesicles (e.g. esterases, lipases, nucleases, phosphatases and proteases) (Haag and Kratz, 2006). When a polymer–drug conjugate with labile linkages encounters these conditions, the drug can be released by enzymatic or pH-dependent hydrolysis (Figure 3.7).

3.3.3 Improved stabilisation

The biotechnology revolution has provided an increasing number of protein-based therapeutic agents. Their application, however, can be limited by issues such as poor stability, immunogenicity, and short half-life. Research aimed at improving these shortcomings yielded "PEGylation," in which relevant proteins are conjugated to PEG (Harris and Chess, 2003). PEG is widely applied as a highly water-soluble pharmaceutical excipient that provides a protective hydrodynamic barrier against protein adsorption (Haag and Kratz, 2006). In general, PEGylation improves solubility and stability and reduces immunogenicity (Duncan, 2003). Moreover, PEGylation avoids rapid clearance of small molecular weight proteins and protein uptake by the reticuloendothelial system, which ultimately prolongs blood circulation time and improves efficacy. Consequently, longer duration reduces the frequency of administration and

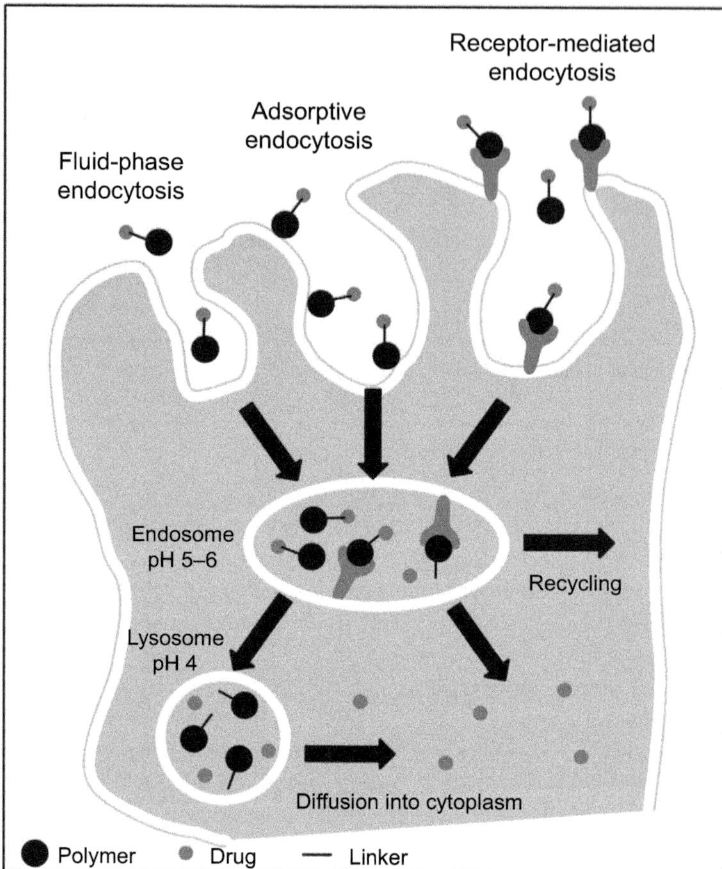

Figure 3.7 Cells uptake polymers through receptor-mediated, adsorptive or fluid-phase endocytosis.

encourages patient compliance. Table 3.2 provides examples of marketed PEGylated proteins and their clinical diseases.

Conjugation to polymers, including PEG as described above, provides many advantages to therapeutically relevant proteins (Caliceti and Veronese, 2003; Pedder, 2003). Given that several excellent review articles are available on the advantages of drug-PEG conjugates, we will not delve further on this particular class of polymer–drug conjugates.

3.3.4 Multivalent interactions

Multivalent polymer–drug conjugates consist of several drug molecules bridged together via spacers from a polymer backbone (Figure 3.8). This multivalent complex can provide a remarkably high binding constant as compared to individual drug molecules due to the high entropic gain when the multivalent complex is formed (Haag and Kratz, 2006).

Table 3.2 Polymer-protein conjugates on market or in clinical trials (Duncan, 2003)

Compound	Name	Indication	Year
PEG–adenosine deaminase	Adagen	SCID syndrome	1990
SMANCS	Zinostatin, Stimalmer	Hepatocellular carcinoma	1993 (Japan)
PEG-L-asparaginase	Oncaspar	Acute lymphoblastic leukemia	1994
PEG-α interferon 2b	PEG–INTRON™	Hepatitis C	2000
PEG-α–interferon 2b	PEG–INTRON™	Cancer, multiple sclerosis, HIV/AIDS	Various clinical trials
PEG-α–interferon 2a	PEGASYS	Hepatitis C	2002
PEG–HGR	Pegvisomant	Acromegaly	2002 (approved EU)
PEG–G–CSF	PEG–filgrastim	Prevention of neutropenia associated with cancer chemotherapy	2002
PEG–antiTNF Fab	CD870	Rheumatoid arthritis	Phase II

EU, European Union; G-CSF, granulocyte colony-stimulating factor; HGR, human growth hormone; HIV, human immunodeficiency virus; PEG, polyethylene glycol; SCID, severe combined immunodeficiency; SMANCS, styrene maleic anhydride; TNF, tumour necrosis factor.

Polymers are appropriate for creating multivalent polymer–drug complexes due to their ability to imitate biomacromolecules especially proteins (e.g. histones) and polysaccharides (e.g. heparin) (Haag and Kratz, 2006). Surface charges of polymers can imitate the biomacromolecules' surface charges: cationic polymers are useful for synthesis of DNA-binding agents and anionic polymers for anticoagulants, antiinflammatory drugs and anti-HIV agents (Haag and Kratz, 2006).

3.4 Current and future trends

As discussed above, a significant amount of research has focused on designing polymers to enhance the properties of small molecular and macromolecular drugs. An area of particular interest is designing polymer therapeutics and polymers with inherent

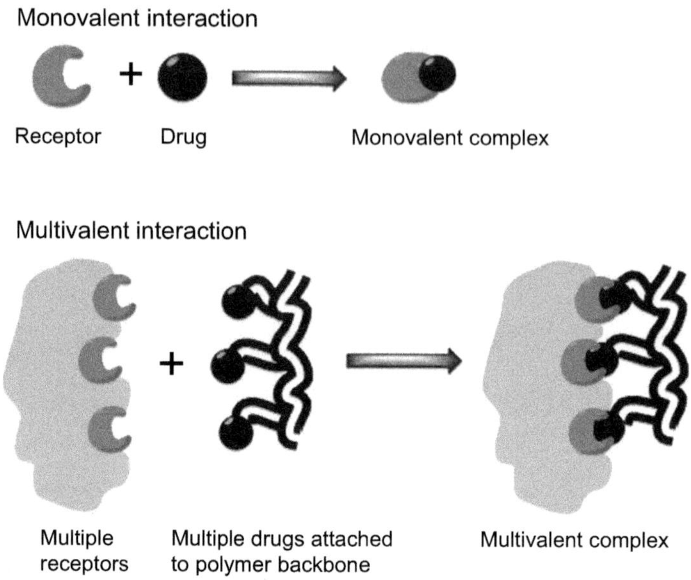

Figure 3.8 Monovalent (top) and multivalent drug interactions.

bioactivity (Kiick, 2007). With a primary focus on the nanoscale, Duncan published an excellent review of this field (Duncan, 2003; Duncan et al., 2006; Dhal et al., 2006). In this section, we provide two different types of polymer therapeutics; these are examples of bioactive and biodegradable polymers that represent some future trends.

3.4.1 Bioactive polymers

One example is AMs, which are similar to polymer micelles but lack the consistent, structural elements that strictly define a polymer (Figure 3.9). While investigating their ability to solubilise hydrophobic drugs (in effect, behaving as polymeric micelles), AMs were discovered to have a unique ability to intervene in atherosclerosis, an inflammatory disease that leads to arterial plaque development (Chnari et al., 2006a). The AMs competitively inhibit oxidised low density lipoprotein (oxLDL) uptake by macrophages (Iverson et al., 2010) through scavenger receptors to reduce cholesterol intake and consequent inflammatory cytokine release which leads to atherosclerotic plaques (Chnari et al., 2006b). From studies to date, anionic charge is essential for bioactivity, as is stereochemistry and hydrophobicity (Iverson et al., 2010).

Several other examples exist for bioactive polymers, particularly with the polymers designed as sequestrants – from cholesterol to iron. Dhal et al. (2009) authored an excellent, extensive review on polymers as therapeutic agents.

3.4.2 Polymers that degrade into bioactives

Many researchers have developed polymer–drug conjugates where the polymer serves no function once the drug is delivered/released. For example, nondegradable polymers

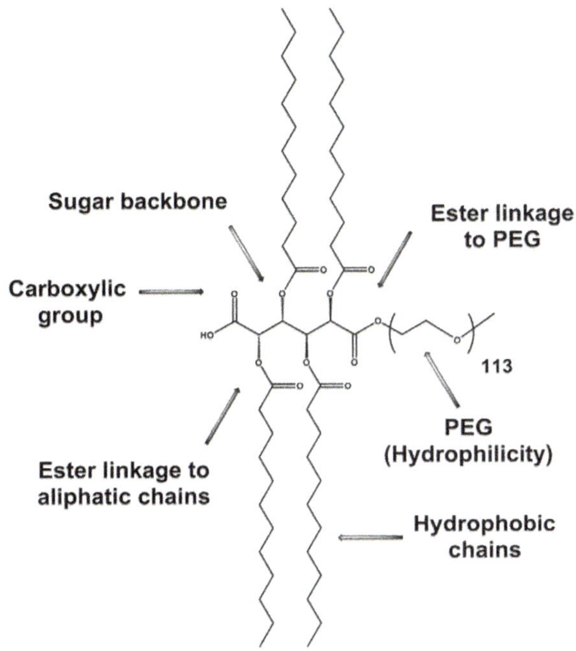

Figure 3.9 Key structural motifs of amphiphilic macromolecules (AMs).

such as PEG are excreted, whereas biodegradable polymers such as poly(lactide-glycolide) (PLGA) breakdown into lactic acid and glycolic acid that, depending on the conditions, are also excreted yet can cause localised inflammation.

For nearly two decades, we have synthesised polymers from bioactives that then ultimately breakdown into bioactives, which are also the starting materials. The first example was a poly(anhydride-ester) composed of salicylic acid and adipic acid (Figure 3.10); a unique feature is the high drug loading, nearly 70 wt% (Schmeltzer et al., 2003). Similarly, other nonsteroidal antiinflammatory drugs (NSAIDs), such as ibuprofen and naproxen, were chemically incorporated into polyester as pendant groups (Rosario-Melendez et al., 2013). Besides NSAIDs, other relevant bioactives have been incorporated into polymers, including antioxidants such as ferulic acid (Ouimet et al., 2013), antibiotics such as ampicillin (Prudencio and Uhrich, 2009),

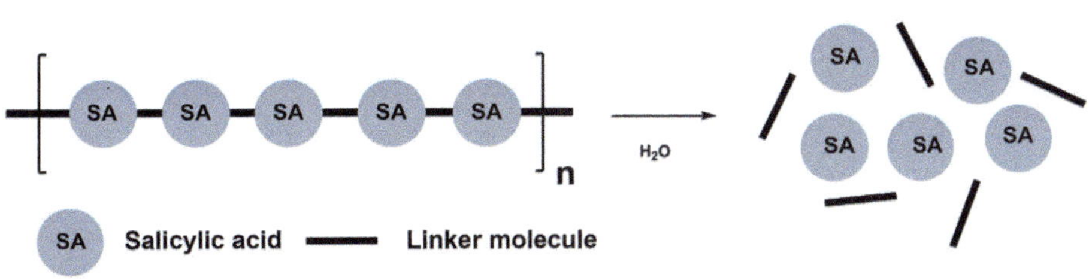

Figure 3.10 Generic structure of a salicylic acid-based polymer.

and a narcotic analgesic, morphine (Rosario-Meléndez et al., 2012). The potential to include a broad array of bioactives is enormous, yet only useful if the need for localised, sustained polymer-based delivery is appropriate.

Other general trends are advances made in a novel synthetic methodology and increasing focus on 'green chemistry'. While many researchers have spent decades developing polymers considered safe and nontoxic, another important trend is searching for 'greener' methods to reduce the potential toxicity of trace impurities and environmental/workplace hazards associated with synthesis, purification and/or large-scale production of biodegradable and/or bioerodible polymers.

Acknowledgments

Thank to National Institutes of Health and the National Science Foundation for support over the years.

References

Amiji, M., Park, K., 1992. Prevention of protein adsorption and platelet adhesion on surfaces by PEO/PPO/PEO triblock copolymers. Biomaterials 13, 682–692. http://dx.doi.org/10.1021/js960001i.

Boussif, O., Lezoualc'h, F., Zanta, M.A., Mergny, M.D., Scherman, D., Demeneix, B., Behr, J.P., 1995. A versatile vector for gene and oligonucleotide transfer into cells in culture and in vivo: polyethylenimine. Proc. Natl. Acad. Sci. U.S.A. 92, 7297–7301.

Buyens, K., De Smedt, S.C., Braeckmans, K., Demeester, J., Peeters, L., Van Grunsven, L.A., de Mollerat du Jeu, X., Sawant, R., Torchilin, V., Farkasova, K., Ogris, M., Sanders, N.N., 2012. Liposome based systems for systemic siRNA delivery: stability in blood sets the requirements for optimal carrier design. J. Control. Release 158, 362–370. http://dx.doi.org/10.1016/J.JCONREL.2011.10.2009.

Caliceti, P., Veronese, F.M., 2003. Pharmacokinetic and biodistribution properties of poly(ethylene glycol)-protein conjugates. Adv. Drug Deliv. Rev. 55, 1261–1277. http://dx.doi.org/10.1016/S0169-409X(03)00108-X.

Chen, H., Kim, S., He, W., Wang, H., Low, P.S., Park, K., Cheng, J.X., 2008. Fast release of lipophilic agents from circulating PEG-PDLLA micelles revealed by in vivo forster resonance energy transfer imaging. Langmuir 24, 5213–5217. http://dx.doi.org/10.1021/la703570m.

Chen, J., Park, H., Park, K., 1999. Synthesis of superporous hydrogels: hydrogels with fast swelling and superabsorbent properties. J. Biomed. Mater. Res. 44, 53–62. http://dx.doi.org/10.1002/(SICI)1097-4636(199901)44.

Chnari, E., Nikitczuk, J.S., Uhrich, K.E., Moghe, P.V., 2006a. Nanoscale anionic macromolecules can inhibit cellular uptake of differentially oxidized LDL. Biomacromolecules 7, 597–603. http://dx.doi.org/10.1021/bm0506905.

Chnari, E., Nikitczuk, J.S., Wang, J., Uhrich, K.E., Moghe, P.V., 2006b. Engineered polymeric nanoparticles for receptor-targeted blockage of oxidized low density lipoprotein uptake and atherogenesis in macrophages. Biomacromolecules 7, 1796–1805. http://dx.doi.org/10.1021/bm0600872.

Conforti, A., Bertani, S., Lussignoli, S., Grigolini, L., Terzi, M., Lora, S., Caliceti, P., Marsilio, F., Veronese, F.M., 1996. Anti-inflammatory activity of polyphosphazene-based naproxen slow-release systems. J. Pharm. Pharmacol. 48, 468–473. http://dx.doi.org/10.1111/j.2042-7158.1996.tb05956.x.

Dang, J., Leong, K., 2006. Natural polymers for gene delivery and tissue engineering. Adv. Drug Deliv. Rev. 58, 487–499. http://dx.doi.org/10.1016/J.ADDR.2006.03.001.

Dang, W., Colvin, O.M., Brem, H., Saltzman, W.M., 1994. Covalent coupling of methotrexate to dextran enhances the penetration of cytotoxicity into a tissue-like matrix. Cancer Res. 54, 1729–1735.

Davis, J.R., 2003. Handbook of Materials for Medical Devices. ASM International.

de Duve, C., de Barsy, T., Poole, B., Trouet, A., Tulkens, P., Van Hoof, F., 1974. Commentary. Lysosomotropic agents. Biochem. Pharmacol. 23, 2495–2531.

Dhal, P., Holmes-Farley, S.R., Huval, C., Jozefiak, T., 2006. Polymers as drugs. In: Satchi-Fainaro, R., Duncan, R. (Eds.), Polymer Therapeutics I. Springer Berlin Heidelberg. http://dx.doi.org/10.1007/12_020.

Dhal, P.K., Polomoscanik, S.C., Avila, L.Z., Holmes-Farley, S.R., Miller, R.J., 2009. Functional polymers as therapeutic agents: concept to market place. Adv. Drug Deliv. Rev. 61, 1121–1130. http://dx.doi.org/10.1016/j.addr.2009.05.004.

Duncan, R., 2003. The dawning era of polymer therapeutics. Nat. Rev. Drug Discov. 2, 347–360. http://dx.doi.org/10.1038/nrd1088.

Duncan, R., Ringsdorf, H., Satchi-Fainaro, R., 2006. Polymer therapeutics: polymers as drugs, drug and protein conjugates and gene delivery systems: past, present and future opportunities. In: Satchi-Fainaro, R., Duncan, R. (Eds.), Polymer Therapeutics I. Springer Berlin Heidelberg. http://dx.doi.org/10.1007/12_037.

Etrych, T., Jelinkova, M., Rihova, B., Ulbrich, K., 2001. New HPMA copolymers containing doxorubicin bound via pH-sensitive linkage: synthesis and preliminary in vitro and in vivo biological properties. J. Control. Release 73, 89–102. http://dx.doi.org/10.1016/S0168-3659(01)00281-4.

Falk, R., Randolph, T.W., Meyers, J.D., Kelly, R.M., Manning, M.C., 1997. Controlled release of ionic compounds from poly (L-lactide) microspheres produced by precipitation with a compressed antisolvent. J. Control. Release 44, 77–85. http://dx.doi.org/10.1016/S0168-3659(96)01508-8.

Fichter, K.M., Zhang, L., Kiick, K.L., Reineke, T.M., 2008. Peptide-functionalized poly(ethylene glycol) star polymers: DNA delivery vehicles with multivalent molecular architecture. Bioconjug. Chem. 19, 76–88. http://dx.doi.org/10.1021/bc0701141.

Fire, A., Xu, S., Montgomery, M.K., Kostas, S.A., Driver, S.E., Mello, C.C., 1998. Potent and specific genetic interference by double-stranded RNA in *Caenorhabditis elegans*. Nature 391, 806–811.

Fischbach, C., Mooney, D.J., 2007. Polymers for pro- and anti-angiogenic therapy. Biomaterials 28, 2069–2076. http://dx.doi.org/10.1016/j.biomaterials.2006.12.029.

Gindy, M.E., Panagiotopoulos, A.Z., Prud'homme, R.K., 2008. Composite block copolymer stabilized nanoparticles: simultaneous encapsulation of organic actives and inorganic nanostructures. Langmuir 24, 83–90. http://dx.doi.org/10.1021/la702902b.

Godwin, A., Bolina, K., Clochard, M., Dinand, E., Rankin, S., Simic, S., Brocchini, S., 2001. New strategies for polymer development in pharmaceutical science–a short review. J. Pharm. Pharmacol. 53, 1175–1184. http://dx.doi.org/10.1211/0022357011776612.

Gooding, M., Browne, L.P., Quinteiro, F.M., Selwood, D.L., 2012. siRNA delivery: from lipids to cell-penetrating peptides and their mimics. Chem. Biol. Drug Des. 80, 787–809. http://dx.doi.org/10.101111/CBDD.12052.

Greenwald, R.B., 2001. PEG drugs: an overview. J. Control. Release 74, 159–171. http://dx.doi.org/10.1016/S0168-3659(01)00331-5.
Greenwald, R.B., Choe, Y.H., Mcguire, J., Conover, C.D., 2003. Effective drug delivery by PEGylated drug conjugates. Adv. Drug Deliv. Rev. 55, 217–250. http://dx.doi.org/10.1016/S0169-409X(02)00180-1.
Greenwald, R.B., Conover, C.D., Choe, Y.H., 2000. Poly(ethylene glycol) conjugated drugs and prodrugs: a comprehensive review. Crit. Rev. Ther. Drug Carrier Syst. 17, 101–161.
Gregoriadis, G., Florence, A.T., 1993. Liposomes in drug delivery. Clinical, diagnostic and ophthalmic potential. Drugs 45, 15–28. http://dx.doi.org/10.2165/00003495-199345010-00003.
Greish, K., Fang, J., Inutsuka, T., Nagamitsu, A., Maeda, H., 2003. Macromolecular therapeutics: advantages and prospects with special emphasis on solid tumour targeting. Clin. Pharmacokinet. 42, 1089–1105. http://dx.doi.org/10.2165/00003088-200342130-00002.
Gu, L., Nusblat, L.M., Tishbic, N., Noblec, S.C., Pinsonc, C.M., Mintzer, E., Roth, C.M., Uhrich, K.E., 2013. Cationic amphiphilic macromolecule (CAM)-lipid complexes for efficient siRNA gene silencing. J. Control. Release 184, 28–35.
Haag, R., Kratz, F., 2006. Polymer therapeutics: concepts and applications. Angew. Chem. Int. Ed. Engl. 45, 1198–1215. http://dx.doi.org/10.1002/anie.200502113.
Haensler, J., Szoka Jr., F.C., 1993. Polyamidoamine cascade polymers mediate efficient transfection of cells in culture. Bioconjug. Chem. 4, 372–379. http://dx.doi.org/10.1021/BC00023A012.
Harris, J.M., Chess, R.B., 2003. Effect of pegylation on pharmaceuticals. Nat. Rev. Drug Discov. 2, 214–221. http://dx.doi.org/10.1038/nrd1033.
Hubbell, J.A., 2003. Materials science. Enhancing drug function. Science 300, 595–596. http://dx.doi.org/10.1126/science.1083625.
Iverson, N.M., Sparks, S.M., Demirdirek, B., Uhrich, K.E., Moghe, P.V., 2010. Controllable inhibition of cellular uptake of oxidized low-density lipoprotein: structure-function relationships for nanoscale amphiphilic polymers. Acta Biomater. 6, 3081–3091. http://dx.doi.org/10.1016/j.actbio.2010.02.019.
Joester, D., Losson, M., Pugin, R., Heinzelmann, H., Walter, E., Merkle, H.P., Diederich, F., 2003. Amphiphilic dendrimers: novel self-assembling vectors for efficient gene delivery. Angew. Chem. Int. Ed. Engl. 42, 1486–1490. http://dx.doi.org/10.1002/anie.200250284.
Johnson, O.L., Cleland, J.L., Lee, H.J., Charnis, M., Duenas, E., Jaworowicz, W., Shepard, D., Shahzamani, A., Jones, A.J., Putney, S.D., 1996. A month-long effect from a single injection of microencapsulated human growth hormone. Nat. Med. 2, 795–799. http://dx.doi.org/10.1038/nm0796-795.
Jones, M.C., Ranger, M., Leroux, J.C., 2003. pH-sensitive unimolecular polymeric micelles: synthesis of a novel drug carrier. Bioconjug. Chem. 14, 774–781. http://dx.doi.org/10.1021/bc020041f.
Kataoka, K., Harada, A., Nagasaki, Y., 2001. Block copolymer micelles for drug delivery: design, characterization and biological significance. Adv. Drug Deliv. Rev. 47, 113–131. http://dx.doi.org/10.1016/S0169-409X(00)00124-1.
Katayama, N., Hughes, S.J., Persaud, S.J., Jones, P.M., Howell, S.L., 1995. Insulin secretion from islets of GK rats is not impaired after energy generating steps. Mol. Cell Endocrinol. 111, 125–128. http://dx.doi.org/10.1016/0303-7207(95)03560-T.
Keys, K.B., Andreopoulos, F.M., Peppas, N.A., 1998. Poly(ethylene glycol) star polymer hydrogels. Macromolecules 31, 8149–8156. http://dx.doi.org/10.1021/ma980999z.
Khandare, J., Minko, T., 2006. Polymer–drug conjugates: progress in polymeric prodrugs. Prog. Polym. Sci. 31, 359–397. http://dx.doi.org/10.1016/j.progpolymsci.2005.09.004.

Kiick, K.L., 2007. Materials science. Polymer therapeutics. Science 317, 1182–1183. http://dx.doi.org/10.1126/science.1145951.
Kim, S., Shi, Y., Kim, J.Y., Park, K., Cheng, J.X., 2010. Overcoming the barriers in micellar drug delivery: loading efficiency, in vivo stability, and micelle-cell interaction. Expert Opin. Drug Deliv. 7, 49–62. http://dx.doi.org/10.1517/17425240903380446.
Knop, K., Hoogenboom, R., Fischer, D., Schubert, U.S., 2010. Poly(ethylene glycol) in drug delivery: pros and cons as well as potential alternatives. Angew. Chem. Int. Ed. Engl. 49, 6288–6308. http://dx.doi.org/10.1002/anie.200902672.
Kopecek, J., Kopeckova, P., Minko, T., Lu, Z., 2000. HPMA copolymer-anticancer drug conjugates: design, activity, and mechanism of action. Eur. J. Pharm. Biopharm. 50, 61–81. http://dx.doi.org/10.1016/j.ejps.2009.03.011.
Kukowska-Latallo, J.F., Bielinska, A.U., Johnson, J., Spindler, R., Tomalia, D.A., Baker Jr., J.R., 1996. Efficient transfer of genetic material into mammalian cells using starburst polyamidoamine dendrimers. Proc. Natl. Acad. Sci. U.S.A. 93, 4897–4902.
Kwon, G.S., Kataoka, K., 1995. Block copolymer micelles as long-circulating drug vehicles. Adv. Drug Deliv. Rev. 16, 295–309. http://dx.doi.org/10.1016/0169-409X(95)00031-2.
Langer, R., 1995. 1994 Whitaker lecture: polymers for drug delivery and tissue engineering. Ann. Biomed. Eng. 23, 101–111. http://dx.doi.org/10.1007/BF02368317.
Langer, R., Tirrell, D.A., 2004. Designing materials for biology and medicine. Nature 428, 487–492. http://dx.doi.org/10.1038/nature02388.
Langer, R.S., Peppas, N.A., 1981. Present and future applications of biomaterials in controlled drug delivery systems. Biomaterials 2, 201–214. http://dx.doi.org/10.1016/0142-9612(81)90059-4.
Lim, F., Sun, A.M., 1980. Microencapsulated islets as bioartificial endocrine pancreas. Science 210, 908–910. http://dx.doi.org/10.10126/science.6776628.
Liu, S., Maheshwari, R., Kiick, K.L., 2009. Polymer-based therapeutics. Macromolecules 42, 3–13. http://dx.doi.org/10.1021/ma801782q.
Lutolf, M.P., Hubbell, J.A., 2005. Synthetic biomaterials as instructive extracellular microenvironments for morphogenesis in tissue engineering. Nat. Biotechnol. 23, 47–55. http://dx.doi.org/10.1038/nbt1055.
Maeda, H., Matsumura, Y., 1989. Tumoritropic and lymphotropic principles of macromolecular drugs. Crit. Rev. Ther. Drug Carrier Syst. 6, 193–210.
Maeda, H., Sawa, T., Konno, T., 2001. Mechanism of tumor-targeted delivery of macromolecular drugs, including the EPR effect in solid tumor and clinical overview of the prototype polymeric drug SMANCS. J. Control. Release 74, 47–61. http://dx.doi.org/10.1016/S0168-3659(01)00309-1.
Maeda, H., Wu, J., Sawa, T., Matsumura, Y., Hori, K., 2000. Tumor vascular permeability and the EPR effect in macromolecular therapeutics: a review. J. Control. Release 65, 271–284. http://dx.doi.org/10.1016/S0168-3659(99)00248-5.
Mcgee, J.P., Davis, S.S., O'hagan, D.T., 1994. The immunogenicity of a model protein entrapped in poly(lactide-*co*-glycolide) microparticles prepared by a novel phase separation technique. J. Control. Release 31, 55–60. http://dx.doi.org/10.1016/0168-3659(94)90251-8.
Mukherjee, S., Ghosh, R.N., Maxfield, F.R., 1997. Endocytosis. Physiol. Rev. 77, 759–803.
Murthy, N., Campbell, J., Fausto, N., Hoffman, A.S., Stayton, P.S., 2003. Bioinspired pH-responsive polymers for the intracellular delivery of biomolecular drugs. Bioconjug. Chem. 14, 412–419. http://dx.doi.org/10.1021/bc020056d.

Oh, J.K., Siegwart, D.J., Lee, H.I., Sherwood, G., Peteanu, L., Hollinger, J.O., Kataoka, K., Matyjaszewski, K., 2007. Biodegradable nanogels prepared by atom transfer radical polymerization as potential drug delivery carriers: synthesis, biodegradation, in vitro release, and bioconjugation. J. Am. Chem. Soc. 129, 5939–5945. http://dx.doi.org/10.1021/ja069150l.

Ouimet, M.A., Griffin, J., Carbone-Howell, A.L., Wu, W.H., Stebbins, N.D., Di, R., Uhrich, K.E., 2013. Biodegradable ferulic acid-containing poly(anhydride-ester): degradation products with controlled release and sustained antioxidant activity. Biomacromolecules 14, 854–861. http://dx.doi.org/10.1021/bm3018998.

Park, E.S., Maniar, M., Shah, J.C., 1998. Biodegradable polyanhydride devices of cefazolin sodium, bupivacaine, and taxol for local drug delivery: preparation, and kinetics and mechanism of in vitro release. J. Control. Release 52, 179–189. http://dx.doi.org/10.1016/S0168-3659(96)00223-X.

Pechar, M., Ulbrich, K., Subr, V., Seymour, L.W., Schacht, E.H., 2000. Poly(ethylene glycol) multiblock copolymer as a carrier of anti-cancer drug doxorubicin. Bioconjug. Chem. 11, 131–139. http://dx.doi.org/10.1021/bc9900921.

Pedder, S.C., 2003. Pegylation of interferon alfa: structural and pharmacokinetic properties. Semin. Liver Dis. 23 (Suppl 1), 19–22. http://dx.doi.org/10.1055/s-2003-41635.

Prudencio, A., Uhrich, K.E., 2009. Ampicillin and Amoxicillin-based Poly(Anhydride-Amides). Google Patents.

Putnam, D.A., Shiah, J.G., Kopecek, J., 1996. Intracellularly biorecognizable derivatives of 5-fluorouracil. Implications for site-specific delivery in the human condition. Biochem. Pharmacol. 52, 957–962. http://dx.doi.org/10.1016/0006-2952(96)00410-8.

Rejmanova, P., Kopecek, J., Duncan, R., Lloyd, J.B., 1985. Stability in rat plasma and serum of lysosomally degradable oligopeptide sequences in *N*-(2-hydroxypropyl) methacrylamide copolymers. Biomaterials 6, 45–48. http://dx.doi.org/10.1016/0142-9612(85)90037-7.

Richardson, S.C., Kolbe, H.V., Duncan, R., 1999. Potential of low molecular mass chitosan as a DNA delivery system: biocompatibility, body distribution and ability to complex and protect DNA. Int. J. Pharm. 178, 231–243. http://dx.doi.org/10.1016/S0378-5173(98)00378-0.

Rihova, B., Kubackova, K., 2003. Clinical implications of *N*-(2-hydroxypropyl)methacrylamide copolymers. Curr. Pharm. Biotechnol. 4, 311–322.

Rosario-Meléndez, R., Harris, C.L., Delgado-Rivera, R., Yu, L., Uhrich, K.E., 2012. PolyMorphine: an innovative biodegradable polymer drug for extended pain relief. J. Control. Release 162, 538–544. http://dx.doi.org/10.1016/j.jconrel.2012.07.033.

Rosario-Melendez, R., Yu, W., Uhrich, K.E., 2013. Biodegradable polyesters containing ibuprofen and naproxen as pendant groups. Biomacromolecules 14, 3542–3548. http://dx.doi.org/10.1021/bm400889a.

Satchi-Fainaro, R., 2002. Targeting tumor vasculature: reality or a dream? J. Drug Target. 10, 529–533. http://dx.doi.org/10.1080/1061186021000051062.

Schierholz, J.M., Steinhauser, H., Rump, A.F., Berkels, R., Pulverer, G., 1997. Controlled release of antibiotics from biomedical polyurethanes: morphological and structural features. Biomaterials 18, 839–844. http://dx.doi.org/10.1016/S0142-9612(96)00199-8.

Schmeltzer, R.C., Anastasiou, T.J., Uhrich, K.E., 2003. Optimized synthesis of salicylate-based poly(anhydride-esters). Polym. Bull. 49, 441–448. http://dx.doi.org/10.1007/s00289-003-0123-6.

Seymour, L.W., 1991. Synthetic polymers with intrinsic anticancer activity. J. Bioact. Comp. Polym. 6, 178–216. http://dx.doi.org/10.1177/088391159100600205.

Shamis, M., Lode, H.N., Shabat, D., 2004. Bioactivation of self-immolative dendritic prodrugs by catalytic antibody 38C2. J. Am. Chem. Soc. 126, 1726–1731. http://dx.doi.org/10.1021/ja039052p.

Sparks, S.M., Waite, C.L., Harmon, A.M., Nusblat, L.M., Roth, C.M., Uhrich, K.E., 2011. Efficient intracellular siRNA delivery by ethyleneimine-modified amphiphilic macromolecules. Macromol. Biosci. 11, 1192–1200. http://dx.doi.org/10.1002/mabi.201100064.

Srinivasachari, S., Liu, Y., Prevette, L.E., Reineke, T.M., 2007. Effects of trehalose click polymer length on pDNA complex stability and delivery efficacy. Biomaterials 28, 2885–2898. http://dx.doi.org/10.1016/j.biomaterials.2007.01.037.

Srinivasachari, S., Liu, Y., Zhang, G., Prevette, L., Reineke, T.M., 2006. Trehalose click polymers inhibit nanoparticle aggregation and promote pDNA delivery in serum. J. Am. Chem. Soc. 128, 8176–8184. http://dx.doi.org/10.1021/ja0585580.

Topchieva, I.N., Efremova, N.V., Khvorov, N.V., Magretova, N.N., 1995. Synthesis and physicochemical properties of protein conjugates with water-soluble poly(alkylene oxides). Bioconjug. Chem. 6, 380–388. http://dx.doi.org/10.1021/bc00034a007.

Torchilin, V., 2012. Liposomes in drug delivery. In: Siepmann, J., Siegel, R.A., Rathbone, M.J. (Eds.), Fundamentals and Applications of Controlled Release Drug Delivery. Springer, USA. http://dx.doi.org/10.1007/978-1-4614-0881-9_11.

Uhrich, K.E., Cannizzaro, S.M., Langer, R.S., Shakesheff, K.M., 1999. Polymeric systems for controlled drug release. Chem. Rev. 99, 3181–3198. http://dx.doi.org/10.1021/cr940351u.

Wagenaar, B.W., Muller, B.W., 1994. Piroxicam release from spray-dried biodegradable microspheres. Biomaterials 15, 49–54. http://dx.doi.org/10.1016/0142-9612(94)90196-1.

Walter, K.A., Tamargo, R.J., Olivi, A., Burger, P.C., Brem, H., 1995. Intratumoral chemotherapy. Neurosurgery 37, 1128–1145.

Watson, K.J., Anderson, D.R., Nguyen, S.T., 2001. Toward polymeric anticancer drug cocktails from ring-opening metathesis polymerization. macromolecules 34, 3507–3509. http://dx.doi.org/10.1021/ma001916t.

Wolff, J.A., 2002. The "grand" problem of synthetic delivery. Nat. Biotechnol. 20, 768–769. http://dx.doi.org/10.1038/nbt0802-768.

Ye, W.P., Chien, Y.W., 1996. Dual-controlled drug delivery across biodegradable copolymer. I. Delivery kinetics of levonorgestrel and estradiol through (caprolactone/lactide) block copolymer. Pharm. Dev. Technol. 1, 1–9. http://dx.doi.org/10.3109/10837459609031412.

Part Two

Coatings and surface modifications

Bio-inspired antimicrobial polymers

4

T.D. Michl[1,*], K.E.S. Locock[2,*], S.S. Griesser[1,*], M. Haeussler[2], L. Meagher[2], H.J. Griesser[3]
[1]Ian Wark Research Institute, University of South Australia, Mawson Lakes, SA, Australia; [2]CSIRO Materials Science and Engineering, Clayton, VIC, Australia; [3]Mawson Institute, University of South Australia, Mawson Lakes, SA, Australia

4.1 Introduction

In modern human and veterinary health care, a prominent topic is the threat that bacterial, fungal and polymicrobial infections pose. Microbial infections have long plagued humanity, and countermeasures date back to ancient civilisations that used antibiotics from plants or silver or copper, in the form of drinking vessels and other implements, to combat infections. With the advent of microbiology and the development of molecularly designed antibiotics optimised by chemical synthesis, there seemed to be a reason to believe that the battle could be won. However, these molecules do not affect slow-growing or dormant bacteria (Hurdle et al., 2011). More critically, bacteria in particular can develop different strains rapidly, and gene swapping occurs between bacteria; thus, bacteria resistant to many commonly used antibiotics have emerged. They are often termed 'superbugs', and their increased occurrence has raised alarm among healthcare professionals as well as being the subject of popular science media.

In addition to direct invasion of, for example, the cardiovascular system, microbes can also cause other health problems. A well-known problem is the formation of bacterial, fungal or mixed biofilms on biomedical devices (O'Gara and Humphreys, 2001; Harris and Richards, 2006; Arciola et al., 2012; Subbiahdoss et al., 2009). For example, almost 100% of urinary catheters become infected within 7 days (Richards et al., 1999). Microbes attach onto the surface of devices and implants, and once a sufficient density is obtained, the attached bacteria convert to a biofilm-forming phenotype. This leads to the growth of biofilm colonies, protected from the immune system by a slimy extracellular matrix (ECM) (Figure 4.1) that contains various biopolymers with a high proportion of polysaccharides (O'Gara and Humphreys, 2001; Hall-Stoodley et al., 2004; O'Toole et al., 2000). This ECM also provides a barrier that slows or prevents in-diffusion of conventional antibiotics, thus mandating much larger therapeutic doses to combat biofilms compared with non-sessile bacteria (Hall-Stoodley et al., 2004).

Such biofilms can cause direct problems such as infection of knee and hip implants that require subsequent surgical interventions. A more insidious attack, however, takes

* These authors contributed equally.

Biosynthetic Polymers for Medical Applications. http://dx.doi.org/10.1016/B978-1-78242-105-4.00004-3

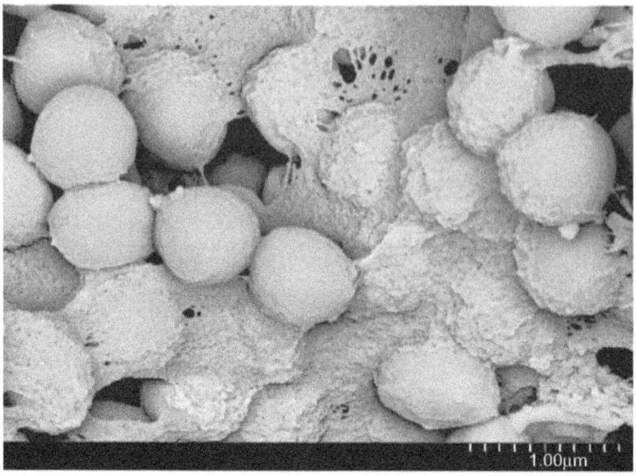

Figure 4.1 SEM image of a staphylococcal biofilm. Note the multiple layers of bacteria covered partially with a (desiccated) polysaccharide matrix (Harris and Richards, 2006).

place when the biofilm does not give rise to a clinically manifest health problem at first but grows for a time, eventually releasing daughter cells that are distributed by the cardiovascular system throughout the body, looking for new places to form further colonies. This is a particular concern with *Candida* fungal species that cause persistent invasive candidiasis, which can, in turn, complicate other issues such as wound healing (Douglas, 2003).

Nature has developed a variety of solutions to combat microbial attack or the settlement of microbial biofilms on multicellular animals and plants. Scientists have for a long time studied those natural mechanisms and agents in order to derive bio-inspired solutions for human health care. A well-known early example is the fungal-derived penicillin. Examples from the plant world are macro-algae that use furanones to deter microbial colonisation and Australian plants in the *Eremophila* genus that use serrulatane diterpenes to combat fungal colonisation (Hentzer et al., 2002; Ndi et al., 2007). However, antimicrobial compounds derived from plants often are not as specific and selective as is desirable for pharmaceuticals for application with much more biochemically and metabolically complex mammalian environments. Thus there is considerable interest in bio-inspired leads derived from natural antimicrobial compounds found in amphibians and mammals, and the adaption of those leads into fully synthetic analogues that may be easier to produce or have advantageous biomedical properties. Such novel compounds could be envisaged for use both as antibiotics per se, administered in the same way as current therapies, or as molecular layers coated onto the surface of biomedical devices in order to render them resistant to biofilm formation.

We will first discuss those natural leads, focusing on polymeric compounds rather than low molecular weight (Mw) compounds, and in particular on antimicrobial peptides (AMPs) that have been found to provide a first line of defence in many animals to microbial attack, before the immune system can respond. Some of those natural peptides are at advanced stages of incorporation into products. However, peptides are inherently susceptible to enzymatic attack, though this is thought to be slower in the case of AMPs than for other peptides for structural reasons. The design of fully synthetic polymers which do not contain amino acids is thought to provide a means of circumventing the issue of enzymatic degradation; however, the challenge then becomes replication of the evolved selectivity of natural AMPs with synthetic polymers.

Nature also has evolved another approach for the prevention of microbial settlement, which consists of the provision of a nontoxic, highly hydrated barrier layer to which microbes cannot attach due to their fluid-like surface composed of mobile polymer chains. These polymer chains give rise to an entropic barrier to attachment. This approach of applying a passive, fouling-resistant coating is also of interest for equipping biomedical devices, as well as membranes and many other non-biomedical products, with resistance to biofilm formation.

4.2 Naturally occurring AMPs

AMPs are an abundant group of naturally occurring molecules and are part of the innate immune system. They form the first line of defence against bacterial invasion for multicellular organisms. AMPs are highly diverse and have been isolated from a wide variety of animals, plants, bacteria, fungi and viruses (Brogden, 2005). Despite their name, they exhibit the typical multifunctionality of most proteins, functioning both as antimicrobial agents and as modulators of the immune system (Barns and Weisshaar, 2013). Many bodily secretions and fluids are known to have antibacterial properties, and in the 1950s the existence of antimicrobial substances in normal tissues and fluids of the human body was first identified and proposed as an integral mechanism of natural and adaptive immunity (Skarnes and Watson, 1957). For example, lysozyme is a common antibacterial protein found throughout the body; it was first isolated from oral mucosa by Fleming in 1922 (Aoki et al., 2012), but it provides protection in many other body sites, for example, as a major component of the human tear fluid protecting the eye against bacterial invasion of its surface. This is necessary as the eye is an avascular tissue which has limited access to the defences of the immune system.

AMPs are highly diverse structurally yet have three characteristics that are shared by almost all known AMPs: their relatively low Mw (10–20 amino acids), a highly cationic character and an amphipathic nature (Costa et al., 2011). They are of intense interest because it appears that they combat even multidrug resistant superbug bacteria effectively. AMPs thus offer many significant potential advantages over conventional low Mw synthetic drugs in that they have broad spectrum activity across a wide range of Gram-positive and Gram-negative bacteria including drug-resistant strains and are also active against clinically relevant fungi (Wimley and Hristova, 2011). The latter is particularly significant given the recognition that many infectious biofilms are polymicrobial in nature (Peleg et al., 2008). It seems reasonable to suspect that clinical failure to achieve complete eradication of biofilm infections may be due, in some cases, to the targeting of bacteria and not fungi with the antibiotic used in treating the infection. This enhances the opportunity for coexisting fungal colonies to bloom. AMPs might provide a more effective weapon in the treatment of, for example, biofilms in open and chronic wounds.

Many AMPs target bacterial membrane functions (Figure 4.2) rather than specific protein binding sites (Brogden, 2005; Wimley and Hristova, 2011). Antimicrobial strategies that target the bacterial membrane by disrupting it or interfering with the proteins that are integral to membrane function are promising alternatives to antibiotics which target intracellular proteins or DNA as their primary mode of action. Membrane-active agents can provide a new means of eradication of recalcitrant, nongrowing bacteria (Hurdle et al., 2011). Secondly, antibiotics covalently grafted onto biomedical devices may be unlikely to reach intracellular targets. Hence membrane activity appears to be the approach to take for resistance to microbial attachment and biofilm formation on solid materials surfaces. This makes AMPs highly advantageous, and, unlike conventional antibiotics that interfere with active metabolic processes, they can kill bacteria in both growing and nongrowing states, as well as in dormancy. Such membrane activity also is believed to avoid induction of resistance, and this conjecture is supported by the observable fact that AMPs continue to be a viable line of defence for the wide range of organisms that employ them against a wide range of microbial attackers.

One disadvantage, however, is that the bioavailability of AMPs is reduced because they cannot be taken orally in the same way as many conventional antibiotics. However, AMPs are excellent candidates for topical applications, such as onto open infected wounds, and as components of protective layers attached onto biomedical devices to deter biofilm formation. Some studies have shown that AMPs grafted

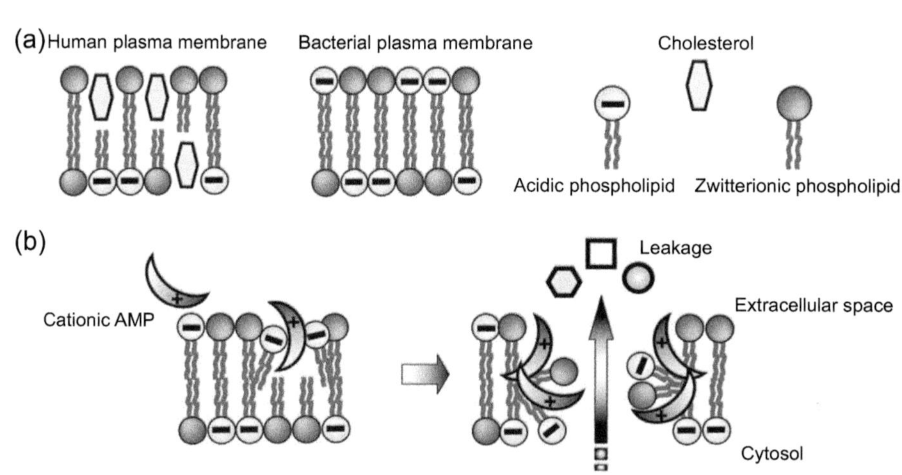

Figure 4.2 Mode of action and bacterial selectivity of AMPs. (a) Composition of human and bacterial plasma membranes. (b) Disruption of bacterial plasma membrane by cationic AMPs. Cationic AMPs show preference for bacterial plasma membranes depending on the membrane composition and electrical charge of the outer cell membrane. Positively charged AMPs are selectively attracted to the negatively charged bacterial cell membrane, and disrupt the membrane integrity (Aoki et al., 2012).

onto solid material surfaces resist infectious biofilm formation (Kazemzadeh-Narbat et al., 2013; Basu et al., 2013; Chen et al., 2012).

The molecular mechanisms of action of AMPs continues to be the subject of much active research, and part of the reason for some inconsistencies in the literature may well be that not all AMPs act the same way. While AMPs generally have both membrane and intracellular modes of killing and lysis, it is the membrane activity which most interests developers of new antibiotics (Brogden, 2005). While this membrane permeabilising mechanism is still not well understood, the advantages are attractive. They act without high biochemical specificity towards a protein target, which reduces the likelihood of induced resistance (Wimley and Hristova, 2011). Linear amphipathic peptides have a well-defined distribution of polar and hydrophobic residues, which regulate interaction of the peptide with the phospholipid membrane; this disturbs the bilayer integrity through defects, disruption or pore formation. Various models have been proposed to explain the action of AMPs; the models can generally be placed broadly into two categories, the *transmembrane pore models* and the *nonpore models*.

There are two main models of membrane permeation by peptides involved in the formation of membrane-spanning pores, the barrel-stave pore model and the toroidal pore model. The barrel-stave model is the simplest model and is also known as the helical-bundle model. The model proposes that peptides self-assemble to form the lining of a pore enclosing a channel, much like a protein ion channel (Rapaport and Shai, 1991; Bechinger, 1999; Pieta et al., 2012). In the toroidal pore model, the peptides affect the curvature of the membrane, causing tension and openings into which the peptides can insert themselves and partially line the opening (Henzler Wildman et al., 2003; Mihajlovic and Lazaridis, 2012). The nonpore models involve destabilisation of the bacterial membrane. In the Carpet Model, peptides accumulate on the membrane surface until they reach a critical mass and permeabilisation occurs via global destabilisation (Gazit et al., 1996). The detergent model is used to describe the destabilisation observed with many AMPs and describes a direct peptide–lipid interaction causing a collapse of the membrane (Bechinger and Lohner, 2006) (Figure 4.3).

There have been other models reported which have been proposed to explain the various observations in AMP membrane disruption; however, the exact molecular effects on the geometry and structural arrangement and stability of the lipid bilayer remain under investigation. Recent investigations into these aspects have furnished many interesting observations. Peptides other than AMPs have also been found to affect biological membranes and they are now discussed as a group referred to as *membrane-active peptides* which, according to their distinct biological functions, are generally classified as antimicrobial (AMP), cell-penetration (CPP) or fusion peptides (Wadhwani et al., 2012; Moiset et al., 2013). AMPs and CPPs are known to have some structural and physicochemical similarities; however, fusogenic peptides tend to possess different features and sequences (Wadhwani et al., 2012). Yet, many AMPs and CPPs exhibit pronounced fusogenic activity. Magainin, a potent AMP isolated from the African clawed frog, has been found to accumulate on the membrane surface and produce toroidal type pores; it has also been found to be mildly fusogenic but it does not translocate across the membrane, so is not cell-penetrating

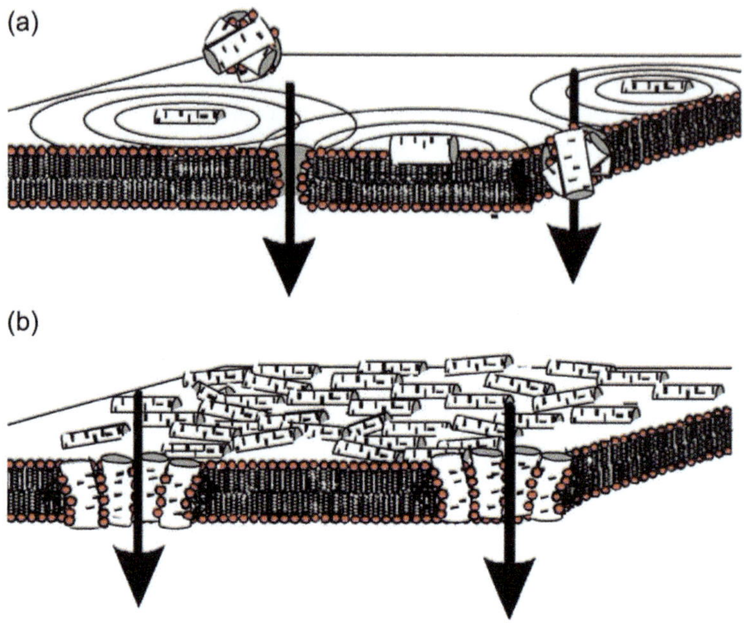

Figure 4.3 Models describing the interactions of linear, cationic amphipathic peptides with membranes. (a) At low concentrations three effects of detergent-like molecules are shown. A peptide micelle contacts the membrane, few lipid molecules are adsorbed, concomitant with pore formation (top). The micelle can also insert in the membrane, resulting in a micellar aggregate channel (right side). Furthermore, in the presence of detergents, in-plane oriented amphipathic peptides destabilise the membrane within a diameter of several nanometres (circles). Lateral diffusion of the peptides along the membrane surface results in transient changes in local peptide density and the temporary collapse of the membrane's ohmic resistance when peptides approach each other. (b) At higher concentrations the membrane disintegrates as described by the carpet, toroidal pore or wormhole models (Bechinger and Lohner, 2006).

(Wadhwani et al., 2012; Almeida and Pokorny, 2009). Other AMPs such as melittin are highly pore-forming yet also translocate across membranes (Almeida and Pokorny, 2009; Krauson et al., 2012). LL37 is a very important and widely researched AMP found in human macrophages and polymorphonuclear leukocytes and is found throughout the human body. It was thought to be pore forming but has been shown to permeabilise membranes through destabilisation and does not form pores. Despite the many contributions being made towards understanding membrane-active peptides, we still do not know how many fundamentally different mechanisms of activity exist, what the membrane binding activity and strength are, and how data from, for example, model vesicle leakage experiments can be correlated with antimicrobial activity.

To further complicate matters, it is now known that some chemokines also have antimicrobial activity (Yang et al., 2004). Chemokines are a small group of chemotactic cytokines that play an important role in the innate and adaptive immune system. Their main function is related to the recruitment of white blood cells to the site of infection, where they bind to chemokine receptors, subsequently triggering signalling pathways in the leukocytes. Some AMPs have been shown to be involved in the regulation of the immune response as well, by binding to these same receptors (Zaat and Hiemstra, 2013). It is interesting to consider what the interplay might be between the naturally occurring AMPs and chemokines, particularly in the area of wound repair where it has long been hypothesised that they both have a role in healing. A new group of synthetic variants, termed innate defence regulators, have been developed; they are synthetic immunomodulatory versions of AMPs based on the immunomodulatory activities of natural peptides and are specifically aimed at wound healing (Steinstraesser et al., 2012).

Despite these gaps in understanding, a number of biotechnology companies have pursued and are pursuing the development of novel antibacterial pharmaceutical approaches utilising AMPs. While AMPs have thought to have enormous potential as antimicrobials, their commercial clinical development has been hampered by incomplete understanding of the modes of action and, perhaps even more importantly, by high production costs. There have also been issues with bioavailability, which is hampered due to toxicity when administered conventionally. However this disadvantage can likely be overcome with further research. The best potential for AMPs appears to be for topical and device surface applications (Fox, 2013; Wimley and Hristova, 2011; Zaat and Hiemstra, 2013). A number of products are being developed for topical application using AMPs including a Magainin-based product for diabetic foot ulcers, and OP-145 based on LL-37 for chronic inner ear infections (Fox, 2013).

Peptides are inherently susceptible to enzymatic proteolysis. While it is generally considered that proteolysis of AMPs is slower than for many other proteins or peptides, proteolytic degradation must be considered in relation to potential applications, particularly in the wound healing environment where a highly enzymatically active environment may exist. Yet, AMPs have been shown to be expressed at wound edges and studies with LL-37, an endogenous human peptide which is known to be present in wounds, have shown it to be relatively resistant to degradation in chronic wound fluid, possibly because of the action of endogenous proteinase inhibitors (Grönberg et al., 2011).

There has been much interest in utilising AMPs as molecularly thin protective layers against infection of biomedical devices. Due to their high solubility in aqueous media and diffusion rates, they must be anchored covalently if longer-duration protection is desired. The fact that AMPs affect the membrane of bacteria, rather than having to enter the bacterial cytoplasm, makes them well suited to the constraints of activity between a solid material surface and bacterial cells approaching the medical device. Antimicrobial surface coatings can be generated from many antibiotics that kill bacteria attempting to colonise them, but a major problem is the lack of selectivity as many antibacterial compounds are also cytotoxic. In some applications this might not be a problem, but for many biomedical device applications, particularly for implants, a surface coating must deter bacterial colonisation while integrating well with human tissue without damage to mammalian cells. This requirement of specific bacterial toxicity with no cytotoxicity is a major challenge in the development of antimicrobial coatings. The highly effective low Mw antibiotics in current use act intracellularly on bacterial proteins or DNA and hence become ineffective when covalently attached to a biomedical device surface, as they can no longer diffuse into the bacterial cell. In contrast, surface-coated broad-spectrum antiseptics kill approaching bacteria but also mammalian cells with the same effectiveness. AMPs offer a rare case of the prospect of specific antimicrobial activity when surface-attached, as many AMPs are not cytotoxic (in appropriate doses).

For studies of AMPs as coatings for biomedical devices and implants, AMPs must be selected that are known from solution studies to be nontoxic and do not initiate an immune response. Implantable biomaterials may also require a surface that can encourage tissue growth and integration. AMPs have been immobilised onto solid substrates using two main strategies: physically via absorption into layer by layer (LBL) thin films and gels, or chemically, where AMPs were covalently tethered using bonding interlayers prepared by self-assembly, plasma polymerisation (Onaizi and Leong, 2011; Glinel et al., 2012) or poly(ethylene glycol) (PEG) linkers. A number of reports have described studies with AMPs as surface coatings but reviews have highlighted the lack of rigour in many studies; often there is no or poor surface analysis data to speak to the uniformity, density and integrity of the desired coating. The importance has been emphasised of essential surface analysis for tethering parameters such as peptide orientation, surface concentration and proof of covalent attachment (Costa et al., 2011; Onaizi and Leong, 2011).

LBL assembly of polymeric films with AMPs embedded in the layers allows for high and controllable amounts of AMPs to be loaded within the film (Figure 4.4).

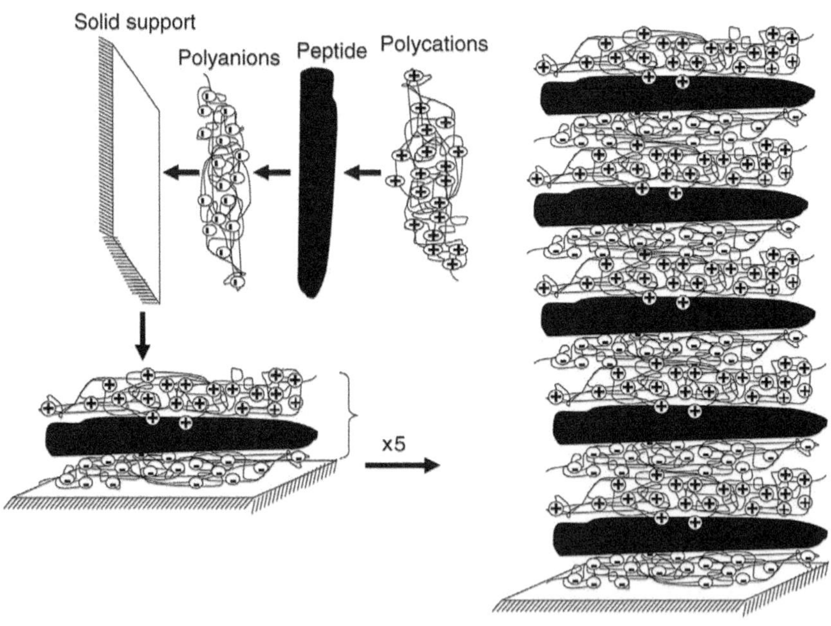

Figure 4.4 Layer-by-layer assembly (not drawn to scale or exact structure) of polyionic materials containing antimicrobial peptides (AMPs). The peptide is sandwiched between two layers of oppositely charged polyions, which can be achieved by sequential dipping of the solid support in polyanion, AMP and polycation solutions (Onaizi and Leong, 2011).

Release is through diffusion, which may be affected by electrostatic interactions between the peptides and the polyelectrolyte matrix. Control of the diffusion process can be difficult, the release duration being typically limited to hours or a couple of days, and the long-term stability of such films has not been tested sufficiently (Onaizi and Leong, 2011).

Covalent anchoring techniques require a solid material surface with a reactive chemical group that can bind to the AMP via a gentle chemical reaction that does not affect its bioactivity and binds it in a geometry that allows the AMP to retain functionality. Such surface coatings are advantageous in providing extended activity due to no loss via release, in that the amounts of surface-attached AMPs can be controlled and confirmed through the use of surface analysis techniques, and the AMPs can interact directly with bacteria. Self-assembled monolayers (SAMs) of reactive compounds on a suitable substrate provide an easy and effective method to produce an antimicrobial coating (Onaizi and Leong, 2011). However, there are practical limitations to the use of SAMs on gold or metal oxide surfaces (e.g. cost, stability and the use of gold or metal oxide bonding layer limits its applicability). Peptides can be modified, for example, with a group such as cysteine and reacted with maleimide-functionalised solid surface, which produces a highly effective antimicrobial surface (Figure 4.5) (Chen et al., 2012). These authors have also shown that the orientation of the AMP is important, as different ways of covalent anchoring gave different activities.

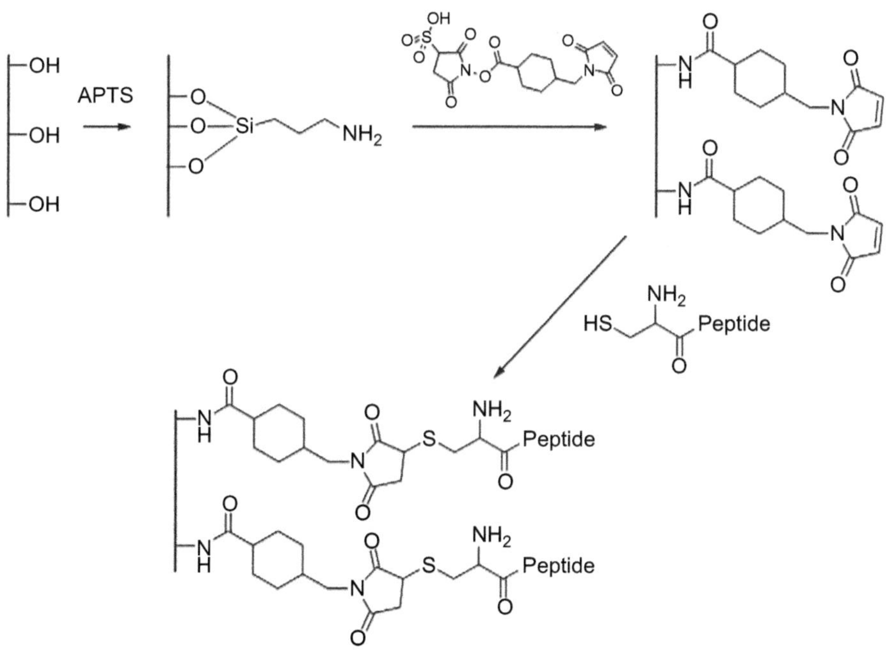

Figure 4.5 Site-directed attachment of cysteine-modified melamine on maleimide-functionalised glass (Chen et al., 2012).

SAM surfaces also allow for the use of spacers and functionalised PEG or other 'brushes' (Onaizi and Leong, 2011). PEG is commonly used because of its low nonspecific adsorptive, anti-adhesive properties; however, there may be some confusion between the role that the antibacterial molecules and the underlying low-fouling surfaces play. For example, a reduction in bacterial attachment can arise from the presence of a low-fouling surface (discussed later), with no antibacterial effect arising from the presence of an antibacterial molecule such as an AMP. The bacteria-resistant activity of some PEG layers, however, can be short term (Kingshott et al., 2003) and in such cases the addition of an active antimicrobial compound may be beneficial.

Plasma polymerisation is a method widely used in industry to covalently modify material surfaces by the application of ultrathin coatings. It provides excellent long-term covalent attachment of peptides, which is adaptable to many devices and highly reproducible. It has been used to covalently attach nisin onto biomaterials surfaces using amine groups (Duday et al., 2013) and has been used by Griesser (2015) to coat wound healing products and implantable biomaterials with a number of surface active AMPs bound via aldehyde, epoxide and amine groups. Immobilisation of AMPs onto a range of solid biomaterial surfaces functionalised with aldehyde groups has been used to covalently bind AMPs via the formation of imine bond between the functionalised surfaces and the peptide molecules. The imine bond is then reduced using sodium cyanoborohydride ($NaBH_3CN$) to convert imine into amide bonds and thus stabilise the attachment of the peptide to the surface. AMPs bearing accessible amines of lysine residues or −SH of cysteine residues can be readily immobilised onto epoxide functionalised surfaces in a catalyst-free coupling process. The peptide coupling to the surface is through nucleophilic ring-opening of the epoxide by thiol or primary amino groups of the peptide. Alternatively, immobilisation of AMPs onto amine-functionalised surfaces can be achieved using carbodiimide (EDC) and *N*-hydroxysuccinimide (NHS) activation of carboxylic acids, analogous to the peptide coupling onto carboxyl-functionalised surfaces. Surface-bound LL-37 and magainin have shown excellent antimicrobial activity, with almost complete reduction of bacterial colonisation on the surface and dead bacteria visible using a Live/Dead Baclight stain (Griesser, 2015). The AMP Parasin was also active and killed bacteria but with time, live bacteria were found to grow on large numbers of dead bacteria that remained attached on the sample surface. This comparison shows that it is difficult to generalise, as the rate of killing versus bacterial adhesion appears important. This result could be an indication of the mode of killing, as studies using Parasin have found that membrane permeabilising anchors imbed themselves into the bacterial wall (Koo et al., 2008). These results raise the question as to whether the mechanism is simply membrane permeabilisation, or fusion as suggested by the numbers of dead bacteria that remain on the surface.

In summary, AMPs provide valuable bio-inspired leads for the development of novel antimicrobial compounds and coatings. Analysis and understanding of their modes of action enable rational optimisation of leads. Yet, challenges remain in terms of detailed understanding of mechanisms of action as a function of the detailed molecular composition and structure of AMPs, their cost of production, and the question of their susceptibility to enzymatic proteolysis. These challenges have led to investigations into alternative approaches comprising synthetic analogues, as discussed next, while those approaches have derived many design principles from studies of AMPs.

4.3 Synthetic polymer mimics of AMPs

While AMPs represent a promising lead in the development of novel antimicrobial drugs, their transition from the bench to the clinic has been hampered by the fact that peptides have limited chemical and pharmacokinetic stability and can be expensive to produce on a large scale (Zasloff, 2002). One breakthrough in this area has been the development of synthetic AMP-mimicking polymers. These polymers, constructed from appropriate monomers, can be seen to have a repeating backbone structure with pendant functional groups likened to that of the peptide backbone and amino acid side chains of the AMPs. While typically unable to adopt the secondary structures of AMPs such as α-helices, evidence has shown that well-defined secondary structures are not essential for potent antimicrobial effects (Mowery et al., 2007; Hong et al., 1999; Wieprecht et al., 1999; Sharon et al., 1999). It was hence postulated that the amphiphilic nature of the AMPs is the dominating reason behind their selective antimicrobial effects and thus could be replicated within a polymeric, random coil structure. Owing to the wide array of monomers, polymerisation techniques and post-polymerisation chemistries available for polymers compared with AMPs, a body of work has developed investigating the relationship between structure and antimicrobial effects and toxicity systematically. This has ultimately led to AMP-mimicking polymers with highly potent broad-spectrum effects and low inherent human cell toxicity. An overview of the different approaches adopted by various groups and relevant findings will be provided in the following sections.

4.3.1 Generation of amphiphilicity

Evidence suggests that it is the amphiphilic mixture of cationic and lipophilic functional groups, of AMPs that is essential for the conferment of selective antimicrobial effects to polymers. As this activity does not appear to be hampered by the need to adopt ordered secondary conformations, the generation of amphiphilicity within polymers can be achieved using a variety of methods. Three such major architectures have been detailed below.

4.3.1.1 Single pendants: the use of monomers bearing a single hydrophobic or cationic pendant group

Such monomers can be assembled into either random or block copolymers to give a final amphiphilic structure whereby charges are spatially separated (Figure 4.6). The global amphiphilicity of the polymer is hence easily controlled through a simple adjustment of the monomer ratios used, and is not restricted to a 1:1 ratio as in other methods.

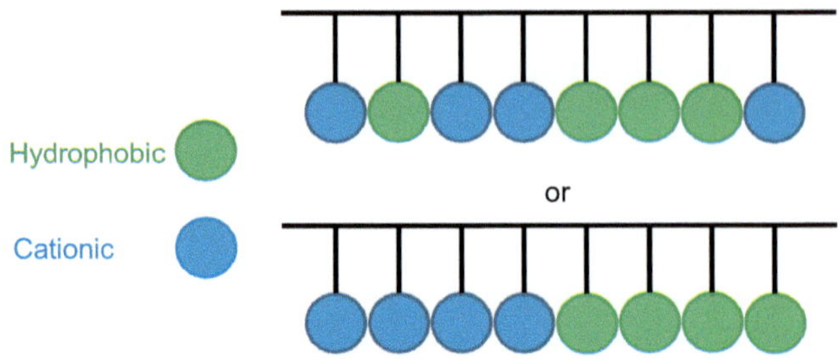

Figure 4.6 Differing-centre amphiphilic polymer structures: random and block copolymers.

4.3.1.2 Dual pendants: the use of monomers that contain both hydrophilic and cationic pendant groups connected to the same centre

Here, the hydrophilic/cationic character of the polymer was adjusted within the original monomer and then reacted to give homopolymers. This approach allowed the investigation of two different architectures, one where pendant groups are attached on the same face of the polymer chain, the other with pendant groups on opposite sides of the backbone as seen in Figure 4.7.

4.3.1.3 Serial pendants: the use of monomers that contain both hydrophilic and cationic groups joined in series within one monomer unit

The reasoning behind this approach is that the hydrophilic head and hydrophobic tail more closely resemble the phospholipid bilayer of membranes, thus facilitating insertion and cell lysis (Figure 4.8).

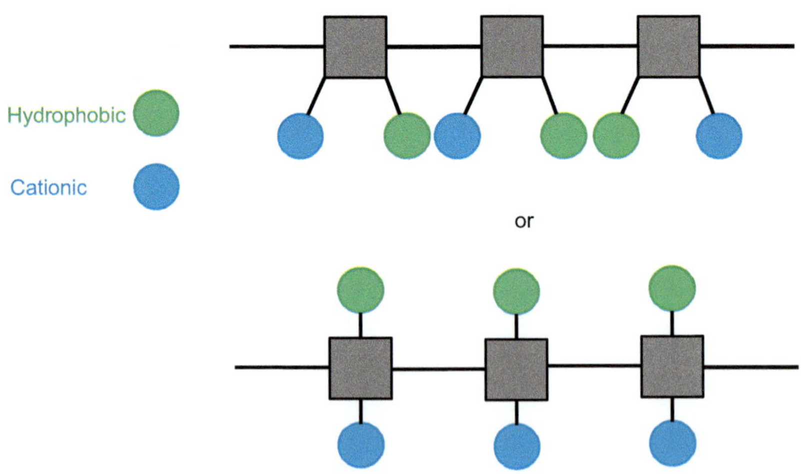

Figure 4.7 Same-centre amphiphilic polymers: same-face and opposite-face.

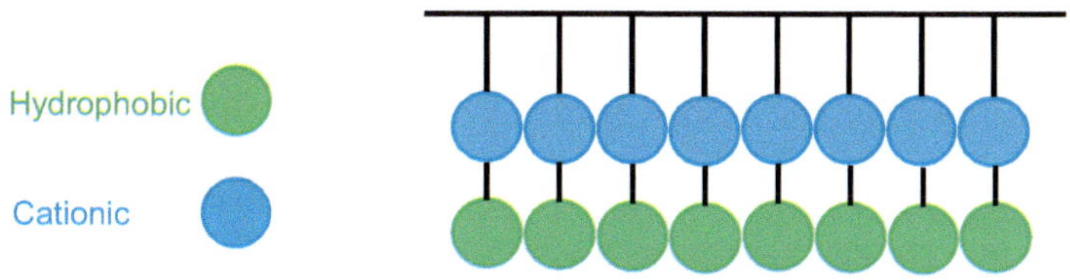

Figure 4.8 Series amphiphilic polymer structures: connected hydrophobic and hydrophilic moieties.

4.3.2 Polymerisation methods

While there are three major architectures that researchers have adopted to introduce amphiphilicity into their AMP mimics, the polymerisation methods that can be utilised to achieve these are varied. This section overviews the major approaches adopted by various research groups, while leaving the detailed examination of structure–activity relationships to later sections.

Initial work on AMP mimicking polymers was aimed at maintaining the peptide linkage seen in the naturally occurring AMPs. One method to achieve this is through the ring-opening polymerisation of α-aminoacid-*N*-carboxyanhydrides to give structures as seen in Figure 4.9 (Engler et al., 2011; Zhou et al., 2009). This represents a facile, one-step synthesis of an α-peptide linked polymer, in contrast with traditional solid-phase peptide synthesis. This method does, however, give less control over chain polydispersity. Zhou and colleagues created a series of random copolymers using this method, using a lysine-mimicking monomer bearing a primary amine in combination with a hydrophobic monomer containing pendant alkyl or aryl groups (Figure 4.9(a)) (Zhou et al., 2009). Engler et al. applied the same polymerisation method for a serial pendant approach. Here, homopolymers were first created using monomers bearing terminal alkyne groups. These then underwent click-reactions with azides, functionalised with primary amines or various *N*-alkyl derivatives to give the final amphiphilic polymers (Figure 4.9(b)) (Engler et al., 2011).

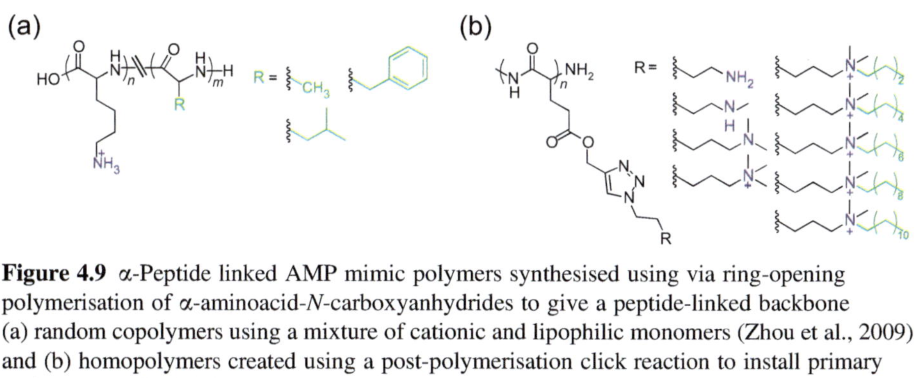

Figure 4.9 α-Peptide linked AMP mimic polymers synthesised using via ring-opening polymerisation of α-aminoacid-*N*-carboxyanhydrides to give a peptide-linked backbone (a) random copolymers using a mixture of cationic and lipophilic monomers (Zhou et al., 2009) and (b) homopolymers created using a post-polymerisation click reaction to install primary amines or *N*-alkyl derivatives (Engler et al., 2011).

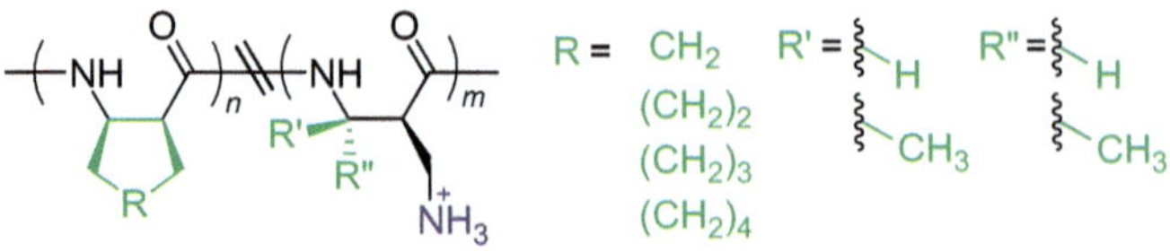

Figure 4.10 β-Peptide linked AMP mimic polymers synthesised using via ring-opening polymerisation of β-lactams (Mowery et al., 2007; Liu et al., 2013).

Owing to the ready enzymatic degradation of α-peptides, Mowery and colleagues turned towards the use of β-peptides (Nylon-3, Figure 4.10) (Mowery et al., 2007, 2009). These can be readily achieved by the ring-opening polymerisation of β-lactams. Random copolymers were synthesised using a mixture of hydrophobic monomers bearing cyclic alkane groups (cyclopentane to cyclooctane) with another bearing a primary amine. Additional series were also investigated that introduced further hydrophobic character to the polymer by incorporating an additional one or two methyl groups adjacent to the amine.

Breaking away from the peptide backbone, Ilker and colleagues created a series of amphiphilic polynorbonenes, through a ruthenium catalyzed metathesis polymerisation mechanism (Ilker et al., 2004). The choice of norbornene as a backbone allowed for the incorporation of both cationic and hydrophobic functional groups within the monomer, giving dual pendant amphiphilic homopolymers as depicted in Figure 4.7. The advantage of using this backbone is the number of locations within which can be chemically modified in order to generate the amphiphilic character. This has allowed the investigation of both same-faced (Figure 4.11(a)) (Lienkamp et al., 2008) and

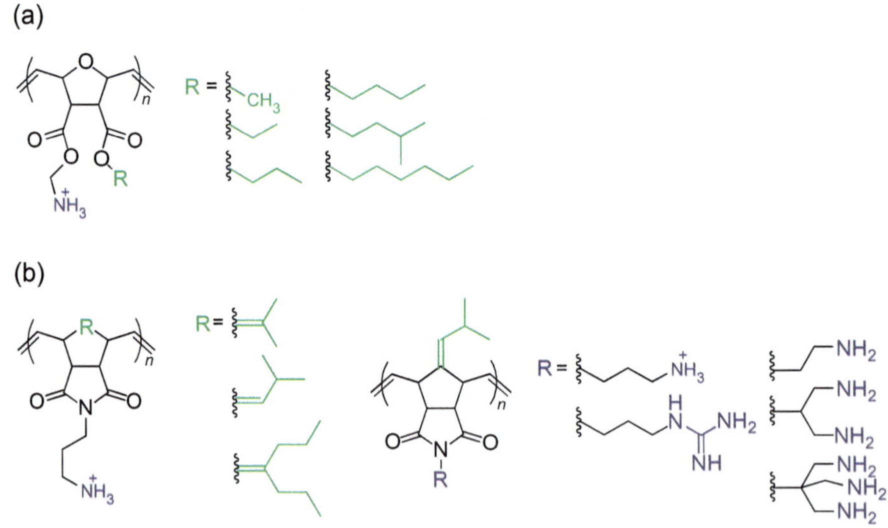

Figure 4.11 Amphiphilic polynorbornenes with same-centre architectures displaying either (a) same-faced (Lienkamp et al., 2008) or (b) facially amphiphilic structures (Ilker et al., 2004; Al-Badri et al., 2008; Gabriel et al., 2008).

opposite-faced (Figure 4.11(b)) (Ilker et al., 2004; Al-Badri et al., 2008; Gabriel et al., 2008) architectures.

Free radical polymerisation is a method applicable to a wide range of functional groups to generate random, block and homopolymers. This method has been utilised by Sen and co-workers, to copolymerise 4-vinylpyridine and methacrylates, to produce a series of random copolymers as detailed in Figure 4.12(a) (Sambhy et al., 2008). A corresponding series was created through *N*-alkylation of the pyridinyl group with alkyl chains of matched length. This approach made it possible to generate and compare amphiphilic polymers in which the hydrophobic and cationic components were either spatially separated (single pendant) or directly connected to each other (dual pendant), the results of which will be discussed in a later section.

Hu, Takahashi and colleagues have performed extensive and systematic investigation of the structure–activity relationships governing a random copolymer series of amphiphilic polymethacrylates (Figure 4.12(b)) (Hu et al., 2013; Takahashi et al., 2013). This synthetic method involves the copolymerisation of one monomer, bearing a protected terminal amine, along with a hydrophobic monomer with various *O*-alkyl and *O*-aryl groups. This allows a straightforward control over the relative cationic or hydrophobic character of the polymer through the relative proportion of each monomer used. Such work has been important in establishing the relative contribution of such structural properties to both antimicrobial activity and human cell toxicity. The polymethacrylate class was further explored in work by Locock and Michl et al. (Locock et al., 2013, 2014a,b; Michl et al., 2014) whereby reversible addition–fragmentation chain transfer (RAFT) polymerisation methods were used to derive a series of amine polymers with low polydispersity (Figure 4.12(c) and (d)). In a post-polymerisation method, these polymers were converted directly into a correspondingly matched guanidine series. This allowed for the direct comparison of the effect of the cation source, amine versus guanidine, on activity and toxicity profiles (Locock et al., 2013).

4.3.3 Cationic to hydrophobic balance

There is a growing body of evidence in this field that the dominant factor giving rise to a highly potent antimicrobial polymer with minimal human cell toxicity lies within striking the correct balance between cationic charge and hydrophobic character. Polymers with high cationic charge, for instance, typically display the undesirable agglutination of human red blood cells (Oda et al., 2011). Higher degrees of hydrophobic character on the other hand usually leads to increased haemolytic behaviour (Mowery et al., 2007; Oda et al., 2011; Kuroda et al., 2009; Locock et al., 2013). These principles are further demonstrated with examples such as the quaternary ammonium cationic molecules that show little lytic selectivity between bacterial or mammalian cells, killing each cell type indiscriminately (Engler et al., 2011; Palermo et al., 2010; Muñoz-Bonilla and Fernández-García, 2012).

An explanation for such observations has been put forward in light of the proposed mechanism for AMPs and hence that of their polymeric mimics. It is thought that the cationic component is responsible for binding to negatively charged phosphate head

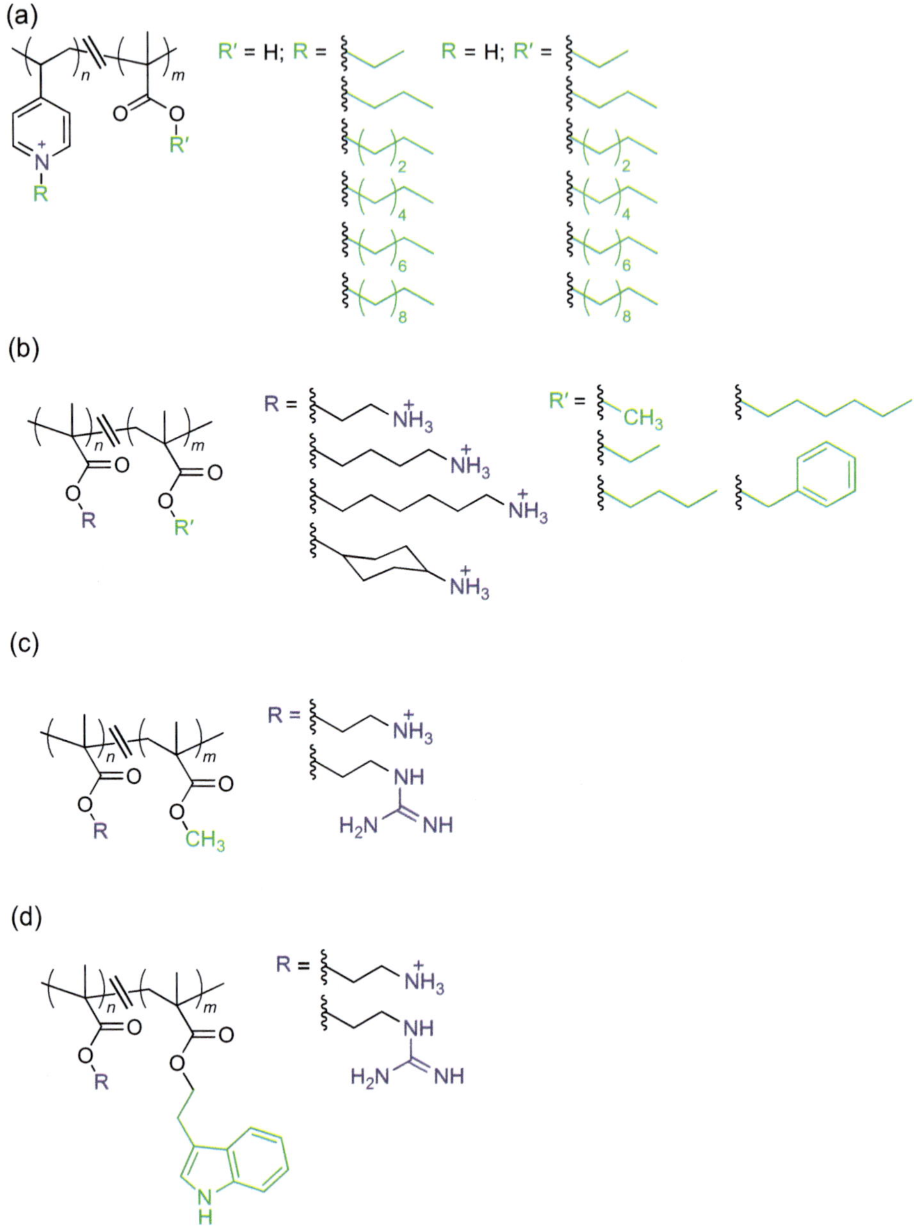

Figure 4.12 Amphiphilic polymers from the (a) copolymerisation of 4-vinylpyridine and alkyl methacrylates (Sambhy et al., 2008), (b) amine-based cationic and alkyl or aryl methacrylates, (c) RAFT-derived amine and guanidine polymethacrylates and (d) RAFT-derived indole polymethacrylates (Takahashi et al., 2013; Hu et al., 2013; Kuroda et al., 2009; Palermo et al., 2010; Locock et al., 2013).

groups located at the bacterial membrane, following which, insertion of lipophilic groups bring about cell lysis. As both aspects of polymer structure are heavily involved in this mechanism, it follows that if the percentage of either component in the polymer chains is too high or too low that a loss of activity or selectivity will occur. As an example, Mowery and co-workers found that their random Nylon-3 copolymers with a mole fraction of approximately 60% cationic monomer exhibited the optimum balance between haemolytic behaviour and antibacterial activity. An increase by as little as 10% of the cationic monomer to an overall content of 70% lead to a loss of activity against *Escherichia coli* by an order of magnitude. On the other hand, decreasing the cationic monomer percentage by 10% to a total of 50% lead to an increase of haemolysis by an order of magnitude (Mowery et al., 2007). As another example, Locock and co-workers showed that for methacrylate-based copolymers, a 30% molar ratio of the hydrophobic methyl methacrylate to cationic groups was optimal in respect to activity and low toxicity (Locock et al., 2014a). In a follow-up study, a series of polymers were produced that were inspired by AMPs which are rich in the amino acid tryptophan (Locock et al., 2014b). These polymers incorporated a novel indole-based methacrylate monomer, synthesised so as to mimic the structure of tryptophan (Figure 4.12(d)). It was found that polymer activity and toxicity for these polymers was optimal when only a very small amount of indole methacrylate was incorporated, at 5–6%. This is a much lower level than that found for the methylmethacrylate copolymers (Figure 4.12(c)), presumably because the indole group offers a much more significant hydrophobic character in comparison.

4.3.4 Source and location of charge

Not all amines are equal. Interestingly, the location and type of amine used in the synthetic polymer has a profound effect on activity and selectivity. Palermo et al. have synthesised random copolymers which differed in the type of amine group; that is, primary, secondary or quaternary amines (Palermo et al., 2010). Potentiometric titrations revealed that a higher proportion of amine groups were protonated at physiological pH in the case of primary amines than secondary amines. Even for primary amines, the level of protonation was only approximately 90% at a pH 7. One would expect almost complete protonation of primary amines at this pH given their pK_a of approximately 10 (Perrin, 1972). This observation may in part be explained by the proximity of hydrophobic groups, which decreases the relative basicity of the amine groups. The level of protonation affects the overall hydrophobicity of the AMP mimicking polymers and the degree of alkylation of the amine affects the specific interaction with the phospholipid head group via hydrogen bonds. Thus, polymers containing primary amines have been shown to be more selective than their alkylated analogues across a variety of polymer backbones (Palermo et al., 2010; Engler et al., 2011; Muñoz-Bonilla and Fernández-García, 2012). Gabriel et al. went further and compared the activity and selectivity of one of their polynorbornenes containing a primary amine to one which contained a guanidine group. The amine polymer was shown to be inactive, while its direct guanidine analogue was highly potent and specific (Gabriel et al., 2008). These results were also echoed in the polymethacrylate class. Locock, Michl and

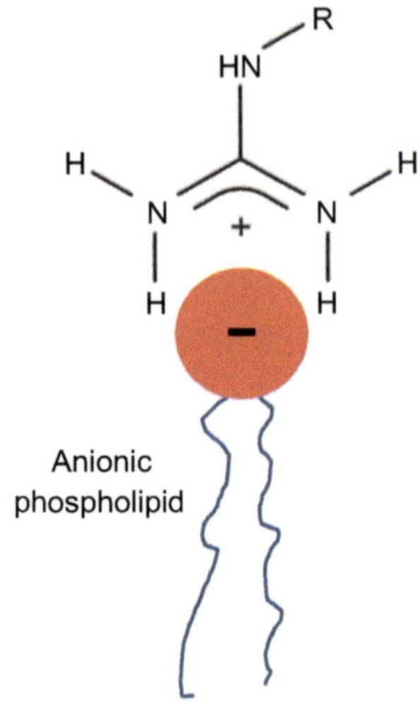

Figure 4.13 The guanidine group and its chelating properties with a phospholipid headgroup.

co-workers prepared series of polymethacrylates bearing either primary amine or guanidine cations. Without exception, the guanidine analogues exhibited higher potency and lower haemolytic behaviour than their direct amine counterparts (Locock et al., 2013).

The high pK_a of 12.5 of a guanidine group leads to a complete protonation at physiological pH, which in turn causes a higher polymer charge density (Perrin, 1972). Furthermore, the guanidine can act as a bidentate ligand to the anionic phospholipid headgroup (Figure 4.13), thus increasing the affinity for this interaction (Dietrich et al., 1979).

Al-Badri et al. also investigated how charge density affected the activity of polynorbonene-based AMP mimicking polymers. Figure 4.11(b) depicts the series, in which the number of primary amine groups per monomer unit was increased incrementally (Al-Badri et al., 2008). In certain cases an improvement of bactericidal activity was observed, especially against the Gram-positive bacteria *Staphylococcus aureus*. The biggest change noted was decreased haemolytic activity, which correlated with an increasing number of primary amines per monomer. A haemagglutination test though was unfortunately not conducted. In follow-up work, the role of the counter-ion was investigated, revealing that introduction of increased hydrophobicity through complete anion exchange did not change the activity significantly (Lienkamp et al., 2009). This is surprising given the previously noted strong correlation between polymer hydrophobicity and activity and toxicity profiles.

Sen and co-workers designed a series of polymers to investigate what effect the spatial separation of charge and linker chain length has on polymer activity and selectivity (Sambhy et al., 2008). For this purpose, the alkyl chain was either chemically attached directly to the nitrogen in the pyridinium ring (serially attached) or to the methacrylate (spatially separated); as depicted in Figure 4.12(a). The resulting copolymers were almost identical in their global level of cationic to hydrophobic ratio but their relative activity and selectivity was observed to differ. The copolymers with spatially separated charge and alkyl chain showed slightly more potency against *E. coli* and *Bacillus subtilis*; however, they also exhibited strong haemolytic behaviour. Their same-centre counterparts on the other hand displayed a greater than 3000-fold reduction in haemolysis. This observation may be explained by the fact that when the cationic head and hydrophobic tail are connected in series, they are better able to mimic the anionic phosphate lipids found in bacterial membranes. This lock-and-key principle would also lead to a mismatch in the case of the uncharged phospholipids which are present in mammalian cells, hence resulting in the increased selectivity observed.

In addition to the type of cation and its relative location to hydrophobic groups, work from Palermo and colleagues has shown that the spatial separation between charge and polymer backbone can play an important role (Palermo et al., 2012). Depicted in Figure 4.12(b) is a series of monomers that vary in linker length between the acrylate group and terminal amine, by two, four or six carbons bonds. A linker of four carbons was found to be optimal, providing maximal antimicrobial effects with minimal toxicity. A possible explanation for this is that the increased conformational flexibility introduced by the longer spacer assists in the adoption of a facially amphiphilic conformation by the polymer chains. This in turn may enable deeper insertion into the membrane and allow a more favourable interaction.

4.3.5 Random, block and homopolymer architectures

Analysis of studies in the literature suggest that a highly potent and selective AMP mimicking polymer may be generated via random, block and homopolymer architectures if suitable monomers are selected. Oda and colleagues compared a random polyvinylether copolymer, modified with hydrophilic amine and hydrophobic isobutyl groups, with its block-copolymer version (Oda et al., 2011). With the cationic to hydrophilic ratio optimised, the random copolymers displayed superior activity against *E. coli* while the block copolymers were found to be less haemolytic (Figure 4.14).

The current hypothesis behind this behaviour is that the block copolymers were able to adopt a folded conformation in aqueous environments such that; hydrophobic moieties, held within the core were shielded by protonated amine groups. This led to haemagglutination occurring preferentially over haemolysis. The random copolymer counterparts, on the other hand, were thought to adopt a random coil structure and hence participate in haemolytic mechanisms of toxicity (Oda et al., 2011). Such mechanisms have not been established for the more conformationally rigid polymethacrylates.

These results were echoed in a study by Gabriel and co-workers that compared facially amphiphilic homopolymer and amphiphilic random copolymer polynorbornenes (Gabriel et al., 2009). Facially amphiphilic polymers were found to be both more potent and selective, thought to stem from an enhanced interaction with bacterial membranes. It is, however, difficult to draw any conclusions as to which of the polymer architectures was most successful, as the antibacterial and haemolysis activities are often confounded by the flexibility and bulk of the polymer backbone used.

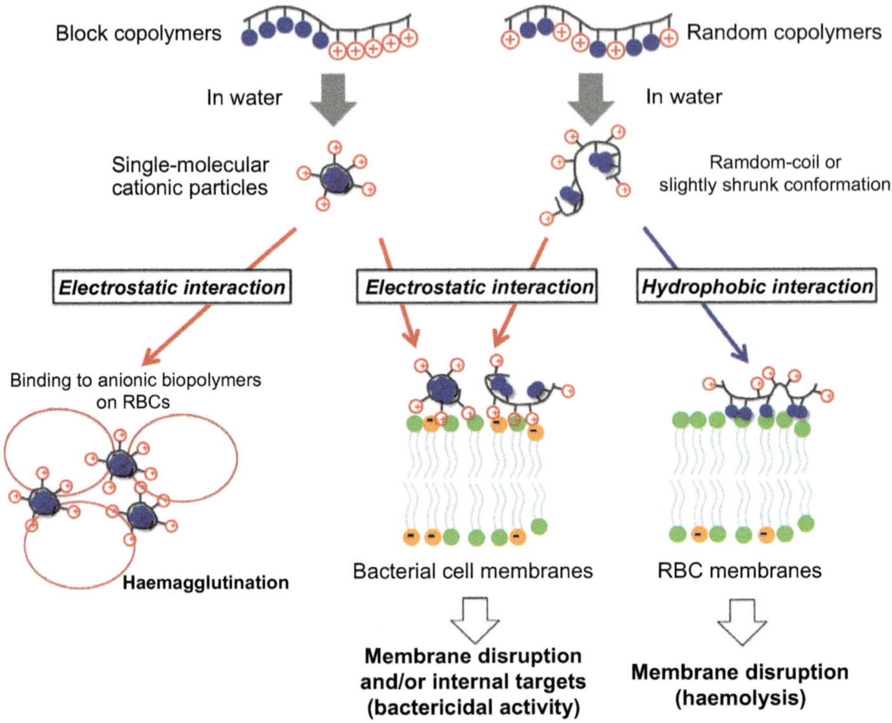

Figure 4.14 Schematic representation of proposed antibacterial and haemolytic activities. Reprinted with permission from Oda et al. (2011). Copyright (2011) American Chemical Society.

4.3.6 Polymer length and dispersity

Owing to the typically low Mw of naturally occurring AMPs, it would follow that the relative length of polymer chain may also play a role in the activity and selectivity of AMP mimicking polymers. The major issue in this area is that work to date has typically involved polymers synthesised using conventional polymerisation methods. These provide limited control over the corresponding distribution of polymer Mw obtained or polydispersity. While trends may be observed with such candidates, it becomes difficult to draw concrete conclusions. Hence there are some discrepancies when such aspects of the structure–activity relationship are examined.

Kuroda and colleagues found general trends towards higher activity and haemolysis with increasing Mw for their amine-based random polymethacrylates (Kuroda et al., 2009). Such trends were more clearly elucidated in work by Locock and Michl et al. which involved the use of RAFT polymerisation methods to derive highly monodisperse cationic polymethacrylates. These results showed that both the amine and guanidine polymers displayed an increased level of haemolytic toxicity with increasing polymer chain length. There appeared to be no such relationship for the antibacterial activity of amine polymers, while the guanidine polymers were found to be most potent at lower Mw. This led to a suggestion that amine and guanidine polymers may possibly be eliciting their antibacterial actions via different mechanisms (Locock et al., 2013).

In line with these results, Gabriel and co-workers found that for a random copolymer polynorbornene series, the highest activity and lowest haemolysis was obtained for shorter random copolymers with segregated hydrophilic and hydrophobic units (Gabriel et al., 2009). This differed to results obtained using their facially amphiphilic polymers where there appeared to be no direct correlation between polymer length and antibacterial or haemolytic activity (Ilker et al., 2004). Making matters more complex, Engler et al. found a decrease in haemolysis with increasing polymer chain length for their α-peptide-based polymers bearing quaternary ammonium groups; but with the opposite behaviour for primary amine AMP polymer mimics (Engler et al., 2011). Mowery et al. elucidated that for Nylon-3 copolymers, an increase in polymer Mw directly correlated with increased haemolysis without improving the anti-bacterial activity (Mowery et al., 2009). This was further confirmed following the testing of polymer samples separated into lower and higher Mw fractions via dialysis, with the lower Mw polymers demonstrating less haemolytic effects than the higher Mw.

Overall, it appears that the length of polymer chain does play a role in the activity and selectivity profile of AMP polymer mimics. As to the size and direction of this relationship, further studies will need to be carried out before such conclusions can be drawn. One key may be to utilise polymerisation methods such as atom transfer radical polymerisation (ATRP) or RAFT that provide greater control over the rate of chain growth. Such methods have the potential to lead to polymers with very discrete Mw distributions (low polydispersity), the examination of which may help to deconvolute the relationship between Mw and activity profiles for AMP-mimicking polymers.

4.3.7 End-group effect

In contrast to their natural counterparts, which are always carboxy and amine terminated, a broad variety of terminating groups appear to be able to be accommodated in AMP-mimicking polymers while retaining activity. While data on this topic are fairly limited, it does appear that the location and identity of end groups can affect both the activity and toxicity of amphiphilic polymers. Initial work by Mowery and colleagues has shown that a minimum length of alkyl chain with six to eight carbons at the polymer N-terminus was necessary to achieve antimicrobial potency but that increasing it beyond C16 led to an increase in haemolytic and self-aggregating behaviour (Mowery et al., 2009). This may indicate that the alkyl group could be involved in assisting with polymer-membrane orientation during initial interaction. In a follow-up study, Zhang et al. examined the relative importance of the location of end groups to activity/toxicity profiles (Zhang et al., 2011). The incorporation of a hydrophobic group at the N-terminus resulted in a potent and selective antimicrobial polymer; however, when this group was instead installed at the C-terminus, this led to a complete

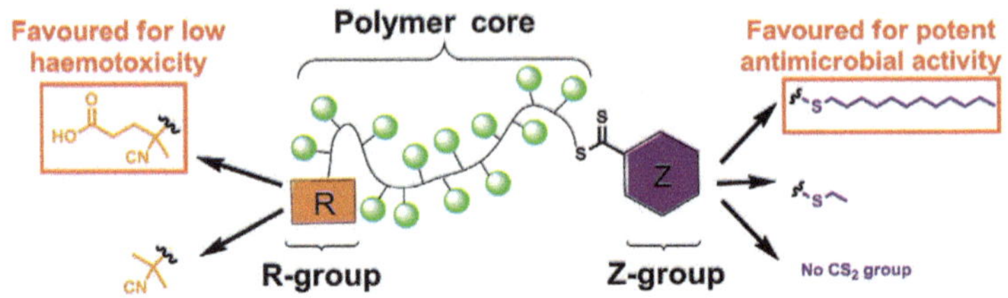

Figure 4.15 Effects of different R- and Z-groups on haemotoxicity and antimicrobial activity Michl et al. (2014).

loss of selectivity. It is thought that these observations may be explained by the relative influence of end groups on the cationic and hydrophilic monomer distribution during polymerisation.

Michl and co-workers systematically investigated the impact of end groups on biological activity by varying the R and Z end groups of RAFT-derived methyl methacrylates bearing either amine or guanidine groups. Results showed that removal of the cyanovaleric acid group from the R terminus resulted in an increase in haemolytic behaviour of 9% for guanidine and 25% for amine polymers. It was also shown that a hydrophobic alkyl chain at the Z-terminus appeared to improve antimicrobial activity (Michl et al., 2014) (Figure 4.15).

It appears that the incorporation of optimal end groups may not be an essential structural characteristic to derive potent and selective AMP-mimicking polymers; however, it does represent another valuable avenue for the optimisation of polymer characteristics. Further work needs to be carried out within a wider array of polymeric architectures before clear rules can be derived which describe the role that end groups may play in the mechanism of action.

4.3.8 Immobilisation onto surfaces

The vast majority of work conducted on AMP-mimicking polymers has thus far been based on activity in solution. There is great potential for the immobilisation of polymers to create antimicrobial surfaces. Such polymer coating technologies could be inexpensively and easily produced for integration into medical implants, thus leading to an effective method to combat device-related infections. Such approaches lead to a more targeted antimicrobial application than systemic antibiotics; thus increasing effectiveness, reducing potential toxicity and the propensity for bacterial resistance. The major problem with this approach is that the translation from a three-dimensional environment in solution, to that of an essentially two-dimensional surface, may give rise to a very different picture of the relationship between polymer structure and activity. For example, Lee and co-workers immobilised their Nylon-3 polymers onto surfaces bearing carboxy acid groups. The primary amines of the antibacterial polymers were thus covalently bonded via peptide bonds in a 'side-on' manner to the surface. Those surfaces showed protein adsorption and NIH 3T3 cell proliferation superior to the used controls, even under serum-free conditions. These observations

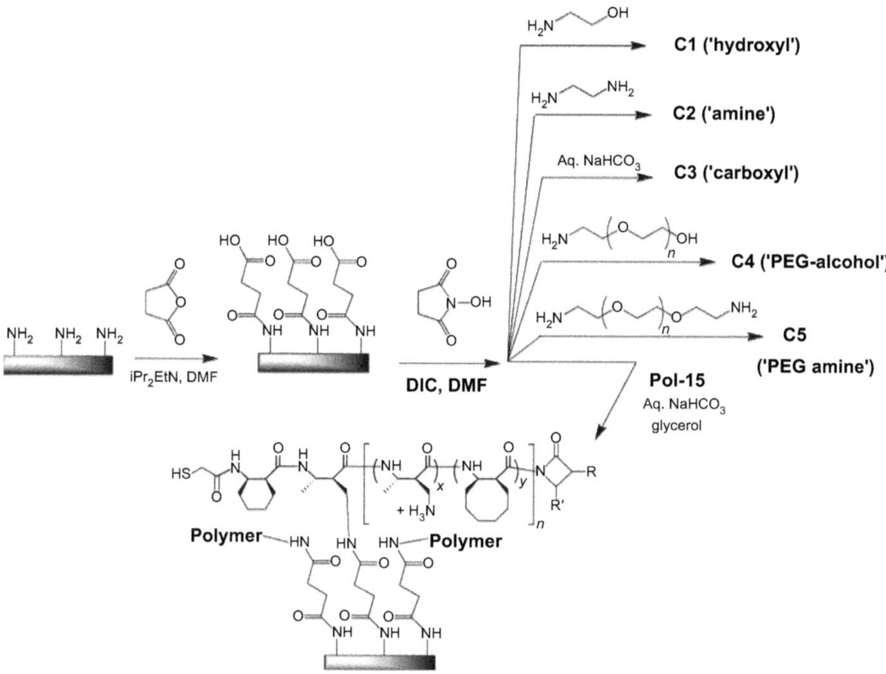

Figure 4.16 Preparation of functionalised glass surfaces.
Reprinted with permission from Lee et al. (2009). Copyright (2009) American Chemical Society

could be explained by the peptide-like backbone of the Nylon-3 polymers used, favouring interactions with natural proteins and peptides (Lee et al., 2009) (Figure 4.16).

In a follow-up study, it was found that longer polymer chains of less hydrophobic nature provided best conditions for cell adhesion (Liu et al., 2012). There was no examination of the antibacterial activity of surfaces however. Braun et al. used a dip-coating method to coat surgical sutures with polymethacrylate antimicrobial polymers. The resulting sutures showed superior kill efficacy at lower loadings compared to Triclosan coated commercially used ones. Unfortunately no study of the biocompatibility or human cell proliferation on the surfaces was carried out (Li et al., 2012).

A surface-based antibacterial study was also conducted by Engler and co-workers involving spin cast solutions onto surfaces of their peptide polymers bearing quaternary ammonium groups with alkyl chains of various lengths. In the case of *E. coli*, the most potent polymer in solution with a medium length alkyl chain also showed best efficacy on surfaces. Interestingly, for *S. aureus*, polymers with long alkyl chains were most efficient in solution whereas on surfaces a medium length was found to be optimal (Engler et al., 2011).

While data are limited in the area of surface immobilisation of AMP mimicking polymers, there is a growing body of evidence to suggest that such work could lead to the development of robust and safe for use antimicrobial surfaces for integration into medical devices. To achieve this, the same careful and systematic investigation of the relationships between polymer structure and antimicrobial potency and selectivity that were performed in solution will need to be replicated at the surface.

4.4 Chitosan – a natural antimicrobial polysaccharide

Similarly to AMPs, naturally occurring polysaccharides have been found that also display antimicrobial activities. Chitosan (CS) is a linear hydrophilic and biocompatible aminopolysaccharide biopolymer, soluble only in aqueous solutions with a pH < 6.5. It is structurally related to cellulose, where the hydroxyl group at the C-2 position has been replaced by an amino group. CS is derived as an *N*-deacetylated product of chitin, found in the shell of crustaceans, making it the second most abundant natural polysaccharide in the ecosphere after cellulose. Chitin is a waste product of the seafood industry thus making CS a readily available and relatively cheap renewable material (Figure 4.17).

4.4.1 Antimicrobial activity of chitosan

Chitosan has been reported to exhibit broad-spectrum antimicrobial activity against Gram-positive and Gram-negative bacteria, spoilage yeasts and hyphae-forming fungi. The latter are particularly interesting for the food industry since CS has shown good potency against fungi by suppressing sporulation and spore germination (Hernández-Lauzardo et al., 2008).

This is in contrast to its antibacterial activity, where different results have been reported in the literature. In some studies CS appears to be more active against Gram-positive than Gram-negative bacteria (Zhong et al., 2008), while in others the opposing effect has been found (Chung et al., 2004; No et al., 2002). The authors of various review articles on the subject have come to opposing conclusions (Goy et al., 2009; Raafat and Sahl, 2009). Furthermore, studies are available where no significant difference was detected between the two bacteria types (Wang et al., 2004).

Early research also claimed bacteriocidal activity against pathogens, meaning that CS kills live bacteria (Goy et al., 2009). Work suggests CS as being more bacteriostatic and thus hindering the growth of bacteria, although the exact mechanism is not fully understood. The fact that bacteria can rapidly regrow after removal from the chitosan solution, however, suggests irreversible binding of CS to the microbial cell walls, rendering it inactive against residual pathogens (Rhoades and Roller, 2000).

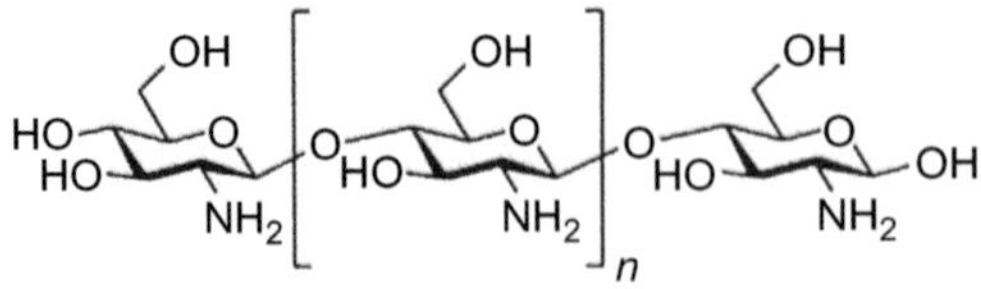

Figure 4.17 The chemical structure of chitosan.

Perhaps the lack of standardised testing conditions together with varying initial starting materials has contributed to these controversial findings. Nevertheless, from all the studies it appears that CS in general is more active against fungi than bacteria (Roller and Covill, 1999; Kong et al., 2010).

4.4.2 Factors affecting activity

Compared to its completely inactive congener cellulose, it is easy to conclude that the antimicrobial activity of chitosan must originate from its amino functionality, in particular upon protonation in acidic media. In general a higher charge density (associated with a higher degree of deacetylation) relates to a stronger antimicrobial activity (Shigemasa and Minami, 1995; Fei Liu et al., 2001). However, other factors such as Mw, derivatisation, solvent and concentration as well as environmental conditions, for example, test strain and its physiological state, culture medium, pH, temperature, ionic strength and the presence of small molecules and metal ions likely play a role (Raafat and Sahl, 2009). Excellent literature reviews have been published on this subject and the interested reader is referred to those for a more detailed discussion (Raafat and Sahl, 2009; Goy et al., 2009; Pillai et al., 2009; Honarkar and Barikani, 2009; Nejati Hafdani and Sadeghinia, 2011). Here, we will only summarise the highlights and briefly discuss the potential of chitosan for biomedical applications.

As mentioned above, with an increase in protonated amine groups along the backbone, the antimicrobial potency of CS increases. This most likely originates from the interaction between the positive charges of CS with the negatively charged bacterial cell walls. Indeed, Raafat et al. identified a correlation between the availability of teichoic acid, an essential polyanionic polymer of the cell wall of Gram-positive bacteria, on the susceptibility of *S. aureus* to chitosan (Raafat et al., 2008). Comparing various mutants, the bacteria strain with missing or reduced teichoic acid moieties, and consequently less negatively charged cell walls, were most resistant to CS (up to fivefold higher minimum inhibitory concentration (MIC) compared to the wild strain). On the contrary, a mutant which lacked a D-alanine modification in teichoic acid and exhibited thus a higher negative charge, was almost 100 times more susceptible to CS with an MIC value as low as 0.9 μg/mL. Similar findings were observed by Helander et al. using mutants of *Salmonella typhimurium* (Helander et al., 2001).

After the initial contact between the polycationic CS and the anionic-rich bacterial cell walls through electrostatic interaction, the next steps in the chain of events are still unclear and quite controversial. A number of researchers consider CS as membrane-perturbing, inducing frayed cell walls or even pore formation (Muzzarelli et al., 1990; Vishu Kumar et al., 2005). Other mechanisms suggest that the interaction between CS and the cell wall interferes with dynamic processes within the cytoplasmic membrane and hence alter its optimal functionality leading to metabolic imbalance and impaired ionic homeostasis (Raafat et al., 2008). Such a process might be accompanied by a growth inhibition pathway through CS deposition onto the surface of the bacteria and thereby blocking the mass transfer and nutrient flow, and suppressing the

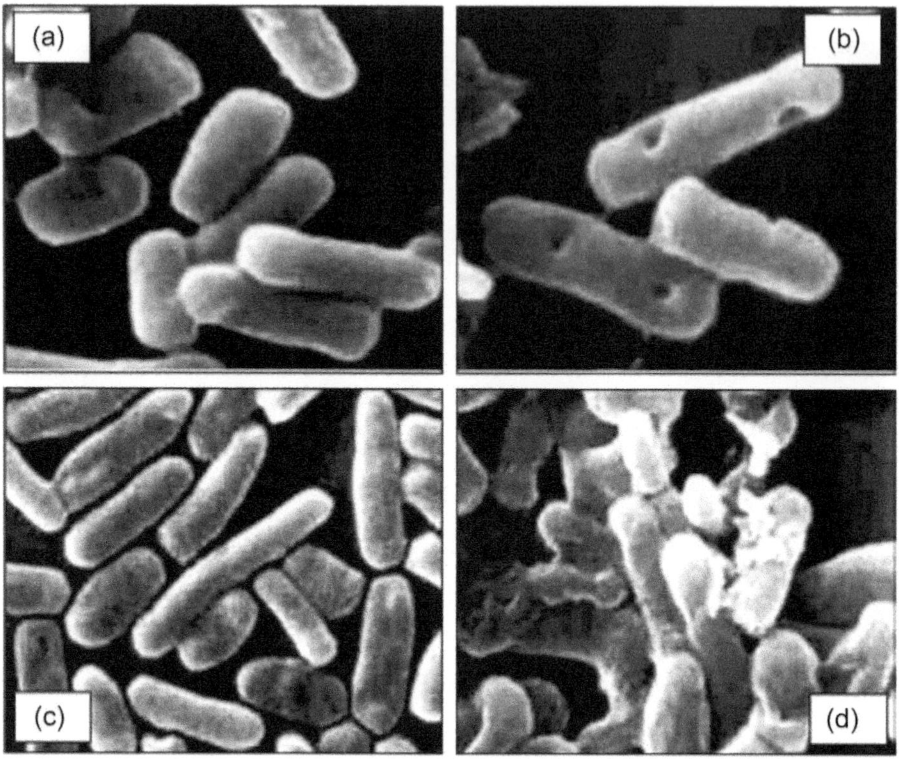

Figure 4.18 SEM of *Bacillus cereus* and *Escherichia coli* before (a and c, respectively) and after (b and d, respectively) treatment with chito-oligomeric–monomeric mixture (Vishu Kumar et al., 2005).

metabolic activity (Sudarshan et al., 1992; Tokura et al., 1997; Vishu Kumar et al., 2005) (Figure 4.18).

Surveying the available literature, it appears that the antimicrobial activity of CS is further affected by its Mw only to the point that there seems to be a minimum degree of polymerisation necessary to render it active. The Mw cut-off is around 10 kDa as oligosaccharides and glucosamine as well as small Mw degradation products of CS appear to be non or only weakly active (Rhoades and Roller, 2000; No et al., 2002; Raafat et al., 2008; Jeon et al., 2001). These findings are in good agreement with the grow inhibition model, where a certain Mw would be necessary to cover to surface of the bacteria.

The remaining important factors increasing the activity of CS are lower pH, higher temperature and the presence of ethylene diamine tetraacetate (Tsai and Su, 1999; Jumaa et al., 2002; No et al., 2002). Metal ions other than silver or zinc dramatically reduce the antimicrobial activity, most likely due to complex formation between the amine groups and the metal ion (Tsai and Su, 1999; Bhatia and Ravi, 2003; Wang et al., 2004).

4.4.3 Potential use of chitosan for biomedical applications

Chitosan, as a biocompatible polymer, is an ideal material for biomedical applications. It is approved by the Food and Drug Administration, USA and exhibits, as described above, antimicrobial properties in solution. Transferring its potency into the solid state, however, appears to be very difficult and it seems that CS diminishes or even completely loses its bacteriostatic or bacteriocidal activity (Foster and Butt, 2011; Yuan et al., 2013). This is understandable since the potency of CS relies on the electrostatic interaction between positively charged amine groups and the negative microbial cell walls. Such interactions can only take place if the CS polymer chains are sufficiently hydrated and have a certain degree of flexibility to interact with the pathogen. Nevertheless, chitosan has been utilised commercially mainly in blends with other natural as well as synthetic polymers such as cellulose, viscose cellulose (trade name: Crabion®), starch, poly(lactic acid), poly (acrylic acid), polyurethane, poly(vinylpyrrolidone), poly(ethylene oxide) and poly(ethylene terephthalate) (Pillai et al., 2009; Shih and Huang, 2003; Yeh et al., 2006; Li et al., 2010; Zivanovic et al., 2007; Jung et al., 2007; Kuorwel et al., 2011). Commercial products are many fold and include fibres for wound dressing badges (CS has also been found to be haemostatic) (Malette et al., 1983; Ramya et al., 2012) and sutures as well as scaffolds for tissue engineering and for regenerative medicine (Honarkar and Barikani, 2009). Commercial products include HemCon® bandages and ChitoFlex wound dressings (HemCon Medical Technologies, UK) and CELOX™ (Medtrade Products, UK) (Raafat and Sahl, 2009). These properties, however, are often due to its excellent biocompatibility, biodegradability, nontoxicity and low immunogenicity rather than its antimicrobial properties.

Personal and oral care may be other interesting fields of biomedical application. Chitosonic® acid, carboxymethyl hexanoyl chitosan or carboxymethyl caprooyl chitosan, has been recently accepted by the Personal Care Products Council as a preservative in personal care formulations. A 2% solution showed very high antimicrobial activity against Gram-negative bacteria as well as good activity against gram-positive bacteria and fungi (Lee et al., 2013). In a similar way, chitooligosaccharides as well as higher Mw chitosan have been tested against oral pathogens (Choi et al., 2001; Ikinci et al., 2002). Approximately 2 log colony forming units (CFU)/mL of *Aggregatibacter actinomycetemcomitans* were inactivated by 0.1% of oligochitosan after 30 min, while 120 min exposure inactivated about 4.5 log CFU/mL of this organism. Additionally, the higher Mw chitosan has shown to have an antimicrobial activity against *Porphyromonas gingialis*. The combination of chitosan with chlorhexidine gluconate (Chx) showed a higher activity when compared with that of Chx alone, which would provide Chx application at lower concentrations thus avoiding its unwanted side effects.

Chitosan is a renewable biopolymer and has been shown to exhibit broad antimicrobial activities against bacteria, yeasts and fungi. Apart from the initial electrostatic interaction between the cationic amine groups with the anionic head groups of the pathogen cell wall, the detailed mechanism of the activity is still not clear and different pathways have been postulated. Nevertheless, a number of applications in the biomedical field have been proposed and commercial products are already successfully placed on the market.

4.5 Neutral polymer brush layers for reducing bacterial attachment

Nature commonly uses polymeric materials at interfaces to modify interactions with surrounding aqueous media. For example, the corneal surface of the eye is coated with a mucin 'polymer brush-like' layer which helps to modify the way tears wet the corneal surface (Mantelli and Argueso, 2008; Watanabe, 2002) and reduce any bacterial attachment (Guzman-Aranguez and Argueso, 2010). These mucin layers are strongly hydrated and contain *O*-linked sugars which enhance the anti-adhesive nature of these layers (Sumiyoshi et al., 2008). Another example of the use of net neutral chemical entities which are strongly hydrated and which act to reduce nonspecific interactions are the phosphorylcholine head groups of the lipids in cell wall membranes (Vermette and Meagher, 2003). Researchers have taken some of these concepts from nature and applied them to produce synthetic coatings and surface modifications which have some of the same properties.

Many materials used in biomedical applications have appropriate bulk properties for their particular application but rarely have optimum surface properties, for example a surface onto which bacterial colonisation is minimised. In addition, the surface properties which result in reduced bacterial attachment may be required to persist either for a relatively short period (e.g. short-term catheter use) or for long time periods (e.g. pacing leads, heart values, cochlea implants) depending on the application or whether the medical device is to be used externally or internally (Figure 4.19) (Campoccia et al., 2013). In many of these cases, surface modification of the bulk material will most likely be required.

Over the last decade or so there has been increasing interest in the use of polymer brush layers to modify the interactions between biomolecules and cells with surfaces. Most of the developmental work has been in the area of designing surface treatments which either encourage or discourage eukaryotic cell attachment and growth (Coad et al., 2012a,b; Ayres, 2010; Barbey et al., 2009), for example, in the area of polymeric scaffolds for tissue engineering, surfaces for ex vivo growth of cells or coatings to reduce protein adsorption (Senaratne et al., 2005) associated with the early stages of the foreign body response.

In this context the term polymer brush has a quite specific meaning, as described by de Gennes (1987) and refined later by Milner (1991). In order to use this type of surface coatings to effectively modify the interactions between biomolecules/cell and surfaces, there are some key design rules. These are

- The polymer molecules are either strongly physically adsorbed or more likely, chemically attached to the surface via an end group, particularly for biomedical applications.
- The monomers used to form the polymer brush layers need to be hydrophilic and net neutral. Uncharged and zwitterionic monomers seem to work the best in these applications.

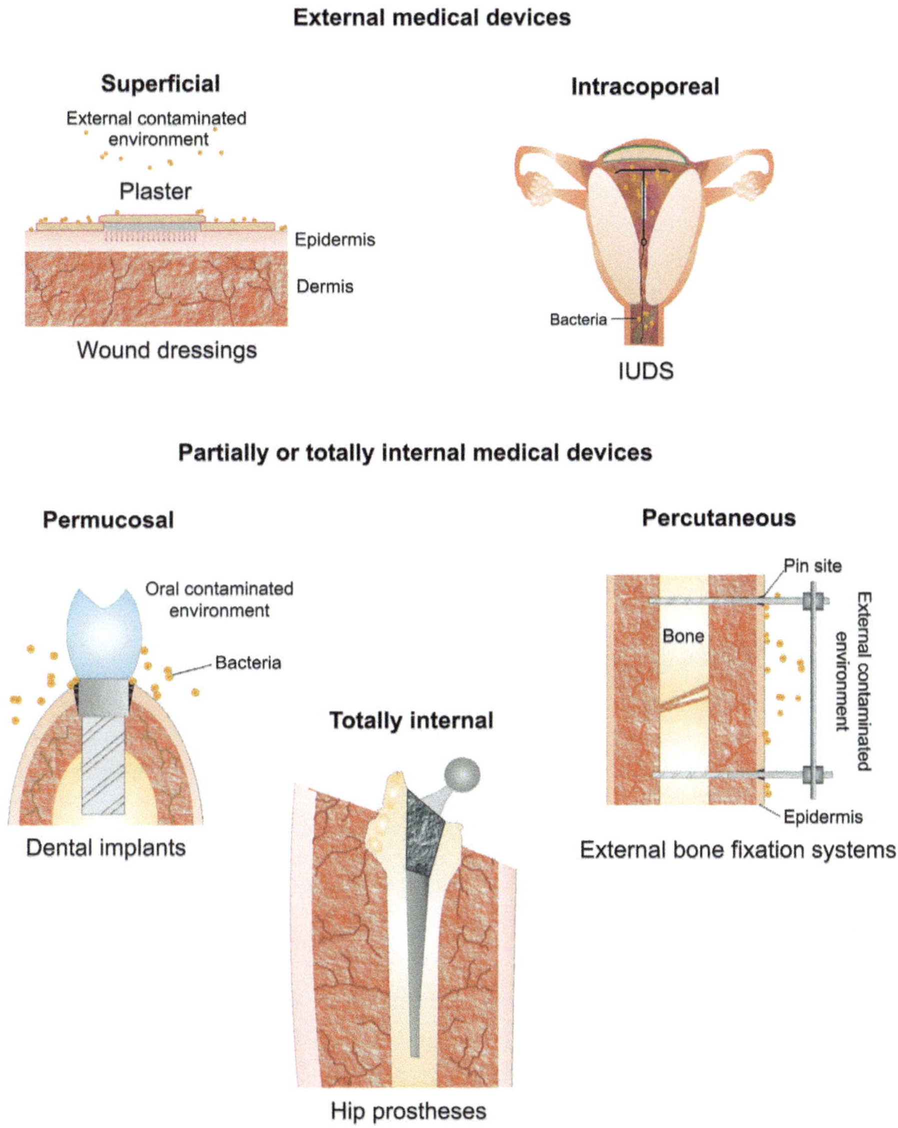

Figure 4.19 Examples of medical devices with different anatomic locations and degree of tissue invasiveness (Campoccia et al., 2013).

- The surface density of the polymer molecules attached to the surface needs to be high. By high we mean that the distance between the attachment points needs to be less than twice the radius of gyration of the polymer molecule, that is the polymer chains are strongly overlapping.

The approach to achieving the grafting densities which are necessary to form polymer brush coatings can either be 'grafting-to', where the polymer molecules are

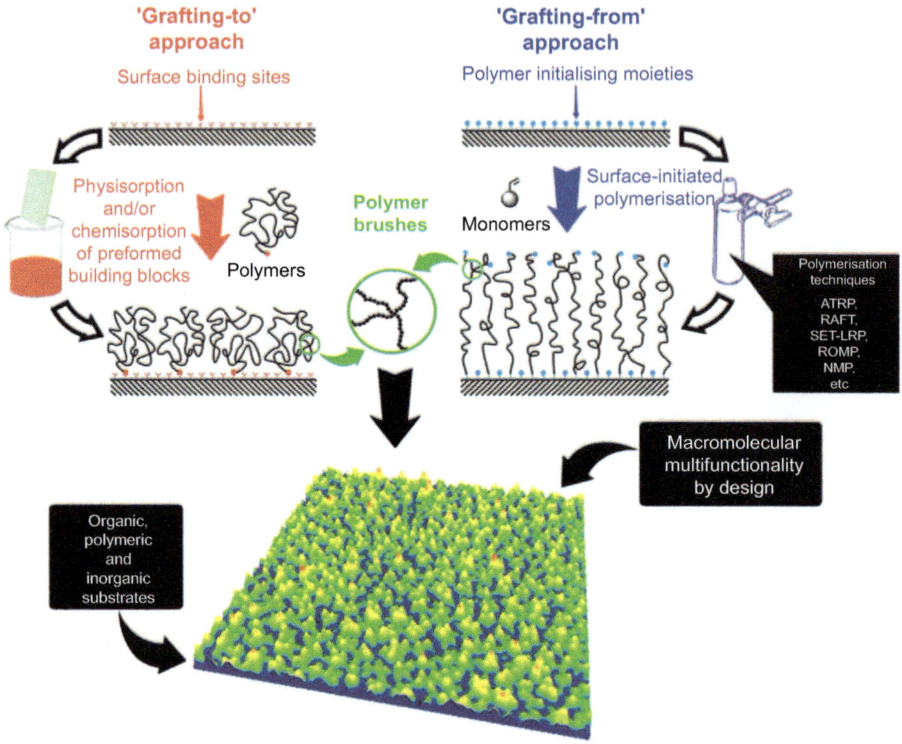

Figure 4.20 Conceptual illustration of the chemical strategies (grafting-to and grafting-from approaches) used to tether functional polymer brushes on a wide variety of substrates. The figure also includes an atomic force microscopy image (500 × 500 nm^2) of poly(2-(methacryloyloxy)-ethyl-trimethyl-ammonium chloride) brushes grown on a silicon substrate via surface-initiated atom transfer radical polymerisation (SI-ATRP) (Azzaroni, 2012).

preformed and adsorbed or coupled chemically to the surface or the 'grafting-from' approach where polymer chains are grown from surface coupled initiators or control agents such as chain transfer agents. For an in-depth review of these two approaches, there are a number of excellent review articles which can be consulted (Azzaroni, 2012) (Figure 4.20).

The rationale behind these design rules is to produce surfaces or coatings that (i) do not have functional groups which might interact nonspecifically (e.g. by hydrogen bonding, hydrophobic or electrostatic interactions) or specifically with proteins and other biomolecules (ligand–receptor interactions), (ii) when grafted (either via a grafting-from or grafting-to approach) to the surface, the polymer molecules interact strongly with water and are highly hydrated and (iii) approaching biomolecules which compress the polymer layer are repelled from the surface. These repulsive interactions are primarily due to the strong entropic forces and local polymer segment density effects that result from chains that have a strongly stretched conformation normal to the surface, as a result of sufficiently high packing densities. Whilst there is still some controversy surrounding the exact mechanisms of action, these three features appear to provide the most effective low-fouling properties. The key hypothesis is that if the nonspecific adsorption of biomolecules that encourage bacterial attachment can be prevented, then the bacterial attachment will be prevented. In some cases, for example with self-assembled alkane thiol coatings containing chemistries from which most polymer brush coatings are constructed (e.g. PEG, zwitterions or other neutral groups), this hypothesis has been called into question (Ostuni et al., 2001). One must bear in mind in this case that even though the chemistries tested were similar, the structure of SAMs are very different to polymer brushes and the mechanisms of action, although related may be quite different.

Using these design principles, a number of groups have investigated how surface modifications such as these, resulting in densely packed, hydrophilic polymer brush layers might result in reduced bacterial attachment. In most cases, the polymer used was PEG. Some of the earlier work used surface coatings which were not covalently immobilised (Kingshott et al., 2003; Vacheethasanee and Marchant, 2000) or where the polymers (PEG in all cases) were chemically attached via a grafting-to approach (Cunliffe et al., 1999; Kingshott et al., 2003; Park et al., 1998; Zdyrko et al., 2009). In most cases, the presence of the surface coatings were only able to reduce bacterial attachment by one to two orders of magnitude and for relatively short time periods (e.g. hours). From these works one can infer that covalent attachment and a high grafting density are essential (Kingshott et al., 2003). Indeed Kingshott et al. (2003) were able to demonstrate that a four order of magnitude reduction in the adhesion of *Pseudomonas* sp. was possible using grafting to PEG coatings of high grafting density for up to 5 h. For PEG graft to coatings, where the Mw of the PEG molecules was 5000 g/mol, grafting densities in the order of 0.2−0.3 molecules nm^2 were achievable (Hamilton-Brown et al., 2009). Similar reductions in bacterial attachment were also obtained for zwitterionic polymers such as poly(sulfobetaine) using a grafting-to approach which was effective for over three days (Jiang and Cao, 2010). Approaches using adsorbed PEG-based diblock copolymer coatings on ultrafiltration membranes gave very significant reductions in the attachment of *E. coli* and *Staphylococcus epidermidis* over 24 h (Lin et al., 2013) (Figure 4.21).

A variant on the grafting-to approach is to preform a 'bottle-brush' or comb polymer and either chemically attach or adsorb the polymer onto a substrate surface. Often the backbone is poly(L-lysine) with polymer chains of Mw for 1000−5000 g/mol grafted onto the backbone. The multiple electrostatic interactions between the substrate and the positively charged backbone serve to stabilise the adsorbed comb polymers resulting in significantly denser polymer brushes than can ready be achieved by adsorbing or coupling linear polymers. Using this approach, poly(2-oxazoline) polymer brushes were shown to reduce the attachment of *E. coli* by at least three orders of magnitude (Tauhardt et al., 2013), although longer term stability would most likely be an issue in this case. Gon et al. (2012) used this sort of approach to show that PEG-based polymer brushes which had low bacterial attachment could be made attractive to bacteria by including small positively charged patches. Under the ionic strength conditions utilised, the only way the bacteria could increase their interaction with the positively charged patches was to compress the polymer brushes. The authors suggest

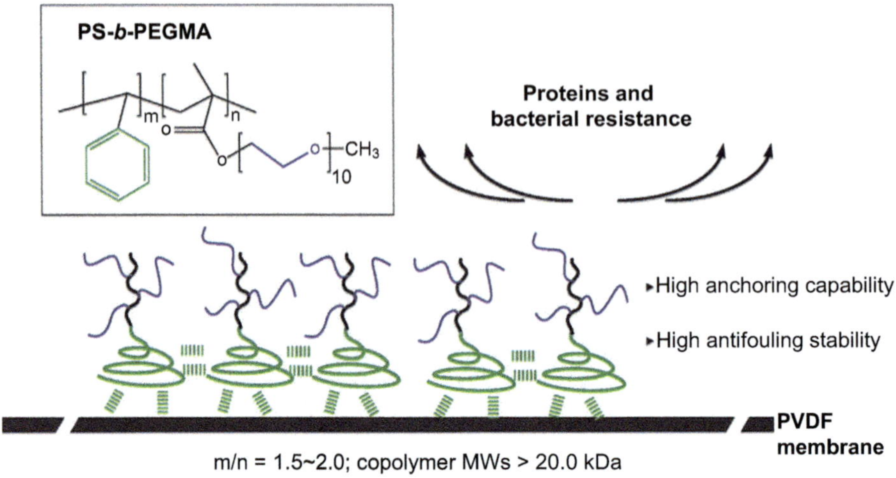

Figure 4.21 Hydrophobically driven anchoring of PS-b-PEGMA copolymers on PVDF membrane surfaces with various PS/PEGMA ratios.

that bacterial colonisation of surfaces could occur via this mechanism if small flaws in the surface coating were present.

Other simpler casting methods used to apply coatings gave much lower reductions in bacterial adhesion (one order of magnitude) for clinically isolated bacterial strains for time periods of up to approximately 170 h (Fernandez et al., 2007). However, these coatings had the advantage that they were much easier to apply than some of the more complex methodologies which rely on the presence of complementary surface chemical functional groups or reasonably sophisticated methods to modify the surface chemistry of the substrate materials so that chemical reactions could be carried out. Here, the relevant question is whether the reduction of one order of magnitude with respect to bacterial attachment would be useful clinically.

While some progress has been made with graft to polymer coatings, in many cases it is simply not possible to achieve the grafting densities that may be readily achieved using the grafting-from approach. Using this approach it is possible to achieve much higher grafting densities (in the order of 0.4 chains/nm^2) and much high Mw (Feng et al., 2006) that can conceivably be grafted using the grafting-to approach. Most groups using a grafting-from approach have used a controlled method of radical polymerisation, for example, ATRP to grow chains from surfaces. Generally speaking the monomers used fall into several chemical types: that is oligomeric PEG (meth)acrylates, zwitterionic monomers such as carboxybetaine (meth)acrylates, sulfobetaine meth(acrylates) and methacrylphosphorylcholine and hydroxylated monomers such as hydroxypropyl methacrylamide (HPMA), hydroxyethyl acrylamide (HEA) and hydroxyethyl methacrylate (HEMA).

In the case of polymer brushes prepared from oligomeric PEG monomers, short-term studies indicate that the coatings were highly effective (at least one order of magnitude) (Cheng et al., 2007). In the same study, poly(sulfobetaine) coatings performed equally well. This work was extended to longer term studies using poly(carboxybetaine) coatings (Cheng et al., 2009). After an initial 24 h attachment phase, the zwitterionic coatings reduced biofilm formation of *Pseudomonas aeruginosa* and *Pseudomonas pudita* by 93% at 37 °C for 64 h and 95% at 30 °C for 192 h, respectively, compared to biofilm formation on glass substrates. Kuang and Messersmith (Kuang and Messersmith, 2012) observed two to three orders of magnitude reductions in the attachment of *P. aeruginosa* and *S. epidermidis* on poly(sulfobetaine) coated substrates over a 24 h period. Li et al. (2008) observed similar reductions in the attachment of *P. aeruginosa* onto poly(sulfobetaine) coated substrates over a three-day time period, although the reduction observed by Yang et al. (2012) were more modest for *Pseudomonas* sp. and *S. aureus* in a 24 h study. Cao et al. (2012) observed a three order of magnitude reduction in *E. coli* attachment for poly(carboxybetaine) coated substrates in very short-term studies.

A comparative study of poly(HEA), poly(HEMA) and poly(HPMA) coatings was carried out by Zhao and Zheng. In this case, all three coating chemistries afforded a one to two order of magnitude reduction in the attachment of *S. epidermidis* and *E. coli* attachment over three days. Similar overall bacterial attachment results have been observed in shorter term (2 h) studies with *Cytophaga lytica* for poly(HEMA), poly(HPMA) and poly(sulfobetaine) coated substrates (Zhao and Zheng, 2011; Zhao et al., 2011).

There are some key differences in performance of these various coatings (one to three orders of magnitude reduction in bacterial attachment) which is most likely related to the grafting density and Mw but which can only be teased apart by careful consideration of the various coupling strategies used and close examination of the surface characterisation data.

Key issues that need to be addressed are (i) performance over relatively long timeframes that are relevant to longer term biomedical implants (not just a few hours days), (ii) the ability to apply the coatings to a wide variety of substrates (metals, polymers, ceramic, flexible, rigid) which are of relevance to biomedical implants, (iii) performance in the presence of human serum and the elimination of coating flaws which are of relevance to biomedical implants and (iii) performance in the presence of human serum.

References

Al-Badri, Z.M., Som, A., Lyon, S., Nelson, C.F., Nüsslein, K., Tew, G.N., 2008. Investigating the effect of increasing charge density on the hemolytic activity of synthetic antimicrobial polymers. Biomacromolecules 9, 2805–2810.

Almeida, P.F., Pokorny, A., 2009. Mechanisms of antimicrobial, cytolytic, and cell-penetrating peptides: from kinetics to thermodynamics. Biochemistry 48, 8083–8093.

Aoki, W., Kuroda, K., Ueda, M., 2012. Next generation of antimicrobial peptides as molecular targeted medicines. J. Biosci. Bioeng. 114, 365–370.

Arciola, C.R., Campoccia, D., Speziale, P., Montanaro, L., Costerton, J.W., 2012. Biofilm formation in *Staphylococcus* implant infections. A review of molecular mechanisms and implications for biofilm-resistant materials. Biomaterials 33, 5967–5982.

Ayres, N., 2010. Polymer brushes: applications in biomaterials and nanotechnology. Polym. Chem. 1, 769–777.

Azzaroni, O., 2012. Polymer brushes here, there, and everywhere: recent advances in their practical applications and emerging opportunities in multiple research fields. J. Polym. Sci., Part A-1: Polym. Chem. 50, 3225–3258.

Barbey, R., Lavanant, L., Paripovic, D., Schuwer, N., Sugnaux, C., Tugulu, S., Klok, H.A., 2009. Polymer brushes via surface-initiated controlled radical polymerization: synthesis, characterization, properties, and applications. Chem. Rev. 109, 5437–5527.

Barns, K.J., Weisshaar, J.C., 2013. Real-time attack of LL-37 on single *Bacillus subtilis* cells. Biochim. Biophys. Acta 1828, 1511–1520.

Basu, A., Mishra, B., Leong, S.S.J., 2013. Immobilization of polybia-MPI by allyl glycidyl ether based brush chemistry to generate a novel antimicrobial surface. J. Mater. Chem. B 1, 4746–4755.

Bechinger, B., 1999. The structure, dynamics and orientation of antimicrobial peptides in membranes by multidimensional solid-state NMR spectroscopy. Biochim. Biophys. Acta 1462, 157–183.

Bechinger, B., Lohner, K., 2006. Detergent-like actions of linear amphipathic cationic antimicrobial peptides. Biochim. Biophys. Acta. 1758, 1529–1539.

Bhatia, S.C., Ravi, N., 2003. A Mössbauer study of the interaction of chitosan and D-glucosamine with iron and its relevance to other metalloenzymes. Biomacromolecules 4, 723–727.

Brogden, K.A., 2005. Antimicrobial peptides: pore formers or metabolic inhibitors in bacteria? Nat. Rev. Microbiol. 3, 238–250.

Campoccia, D., Montanaro, L., Arciola, C.R., 2013. A review of the clinical implications of anti-infective biomaterials and infection-resistant surfaces. Biomaterials 34, 8018–8029.

Cao, Z.Q., Mi, L., Mendiola, J., Ella-Menye, J.R., Zhang, L., Xue, H., Jiang, S.Y., 2012. Reversibly switching the function of a surface between attacking and defending against bacteria. Angew. Chem., Int. Ed. 51, 2602–2605.

Chen, R., Willcox, M.D.P., Cole, N., Ho, K.K.K., Rasul, R., Denman, J.A., Kumar, N., 2012. Characterization of chemoselective surface attachment of the cationic peptide melimine and its effects on antimicrobial activity. Acta Biomater. 8, 4371–4379.

Cheng, G., Li, G.Z., Xue, H., Chen, S.F., Bryers, J.D., Jiang, S.Y., 2009. Zwitterionic carboxybetaine polymer surfaces and their resistance to long-term biofilm formation. Biomaterials 30, 5234–5240.

Cheng, G., Zhang, Z., Chen, S.F., Bryers, J.D., Jiang, S.Y., 2007. Inhibition of bacterial adhesion and biofilm formation on zwitterionic surfaces. Biomaterials 28, 4192–4199.

Choi, B.-K., Kim, K.-Y., Yoo, Y.-J., Oh, S.-J., Choi, J.-H., Kim, C.-Y., 2001. In vitro antimicrobial activity of a chitooligosaccharide mixture against *Actinobacillus actinomycetemcomitans* and *Streptococcus mutans*. Int. J. Antimicrob. Agents 18, 553–557.

Chung, Y.-C., Su, Y.-P., Chen, C.-C., Jia, G., Wang, H.-L., Wu, J.C.G., Lin, J.-G., 2004. Relationship between antibacterial activity of chitosan and surface characteristics of cell wall. Acta Pharmacol. Sin. 25, 932–936.

Coad, B.R., Lu, Y., Glattauer, V., Meagher, L., 2012a. Substrate-independent method for growing and modulating the density of polymer brushes from surfaces by ATRP. ACS Appl. Mater. Interfaces 4, 2811–2823.

Coad, B.R., Lu, Y., Meagher, L., 2012b. A substrate-independent method for surface grafting polymer layers by atom transfer radical polymerization: reduction of protein adsorption. Acta Biomater. 8, 608–618.

Costa, F., Carvalho, I.F., Montelaro, R.C., Gomes, P., Martins, M.C.L., 2011. Covalent immobilization of antimicrobial peptides (AMPs) onto biomaterial surfaces. Acta Biomater. 7, 1431–1440.

Cunliffe, D., Smart, C.A., Alexander, C., Vulfson, E.N., 1999. Bacterial adhesion at synthetic surfaces. Appl. Environ. Microbiol. 65, 4995–5002.

De Gennes, P.G., 1987. Polymers at an interface: a simplified view. Adv. Colloid Interface Sci. 27, 189–209.

Dietrich, B., Fyles, D.L., Fyles, T.M., Lehn, J.-M., 1979. Anion coordination chemistry: polyguanidinium salts as anion complexones. Helv. Chim. Acta 62, 2763–2787.

Douglas, L.J., 2003. Candida biofilms and their role in infection. Trends Microbiol. 11, 30–36.

Duday, D., Vreuls, C., Moreno, M., Frache, G., Boscher, N.D., Zocchi, G., Archambeau, C., Van De Weerdt, C., Martial, J., Choquet, P., 2013. Atmospheric pressure plasma modified surfaces for immobilization of antimicrobial nisin peptides. Surf. Coat. Technol. 218, 152–161.

Engler, A.C., Shukla, A., Puranam, S., Buss, H.G., Jreige, N., Hammond, P.T., 2011. Effects of side group functionality and molecular weight on the activity of synthetic antimicrobial polypeptides. Biomacromolecules 12, 1666–1674.

Fei Liu, X., Lin Guan, Y., Zhi Yang, D., Li, Z., De Yao, K., 2001. Antibacterial action of chitosan and carboxymethylated chitosan. J. Appl. Polym. Sci. 79, 1324–1335.

Feng, W., Zhu, S.P., Ishihara, K., Brash, J.L., 2006. Protein resistant surfaces: comparison of acrylate graft polymers bearing oligo-ethylene oxide and phosphorylcholine side chains. Biointerphases 1, 50–60.

Fernandez, I.C.S., Van Der Mei, H.C., Lochhead, M.J., Grainger, D.W., Busscher, H.J., 2007. The inhibition of the adhesion of clinically isolated bacterial strains on multi-component cross-linked poly(ethylene glycol)-based polymer coatings. Biomaterials 28, 4105–4112.

Foster, L.J.R., Butt, J., 2011. Chitosan films are NOT antimicrobial. Biotechnol. Lett. 33, 417–421.

Fox, J.L., 2013. Antimicrobial peptides stage a comeback. Nat. Biotechnol. 31, 379–382.

Gabriel, G.J., Madkour, A.E., Dabkowski, J.M., Nelson, C.F., NüSslein, K., Tew, G.N., 2008. Synthetic mimic of antimicrobial peptide with nonmembrane-disrupting antibacterial properties. Biomacromolecules 9, 2980–2983.

Gabriel, G.J., Maegerlein, J.A., Nelson, C.F., Dabkowski, J.M., Eren, T., Nüsslein, K., Tew, G.N., 2009. Comparison of facially amphiphilic versus segregated monomers in the design of antibacterial copolymers. Chem. – Eur. J. 15, 433–439.

Gazit, E., Miller, I.R., Biggin, P.C., Sansom, M.S.P., Shai, Y., 1996. Structure and orientation of the mammalian antibacterial peptide cecropin P1 within phospholipid membranes. J. Mol. Biol. 258, 860–870.

Glinel, K., Thebault, P., Humblot, V., Pradier, C.M., Jouenne, T., 2012. Antibacterial surfaces developed from bio-inspired approaches. Acta Biomater. 8, 1670–1684.

Gon, S., Kumar, K.N., Nusslein, K., Santore, M.M., 2012. How bacteria adhere to brushy PEG surfaces: clinging to flaws and compressing the brush. Macromolecules 45, 8373–8381.

Goy, R.C., De Britto, D., Assis, O.B.G., 2009. A review of the antimicrobial activity of chitosan. Polím. Ciênc. Tecnol. 19, 1–7.

Griesser, S., 2015. (PhD Thesis). University of South Australia.

Grönberg, A., Zettergren, L., Agren, M.S., 2011. Stability of the cathelicidin peptide LL-37 in a non-healing wound environment. Acta Derm. Venereol. 91, 511.

Guzman-Aranguez, A., Argueso, P., 2010. Structure and biological roles of mucin-type O-glycans at the ocular surface. Ocul. Surf. 8, 8–17.
Hall-Stoodley, L., Costerton, J.W., Stoodley, P., 2004. Bacterial biofilms: from the natural environment to infectious diseases. Nat. Rev. Microbiol. 2, 95–108.
Hamilton-Brown, P., Gengebach, T., Griesser, H.J., Meagher, L., 2009. End terminal, poly (ethylene oxide) graft layers: surface forces and protein adsorption. Langmuir 25, 9149–9156.
Harris, L.G., Richards, R.G., 2006. Staphylococci and implant surfaces: a review. Injury 37, S3–S14.
Helander, I.M., Nurmiaho-Lassila, E.L., Ahvenainen, R., Rhoades, J., Roller, S., 2001. Chitosan disrupts the barrier properties of the outer membrane of Gram-negative bacteria. Int. J. Food Microbiol. 71, 235–244.
Hentzer, M., Riedel, K., Rasmussen, T.B., Heydorn, A., Andersen, J.B., Parsek, M.R., Rice, S.A., Eberl, L., Molin, S., Høiby, N., Kjelleberg, S., Givskov, M., 2002. Inhibition of quorum sensing in *Pseudomonas aeruginosa* biofilm bacteria by a halogenated furanone compound. Microbiology 148, 87–102.
Henzler Wildman, K.A., Lee, D.-K., Ramamoorthy, A., 2003. Mechanism of lipid bilayer disruption by the human antimicrobial peptide, LL-37. Biochemistry 42, 6545–6558.
Hernández-Lauzardo, A.N., Bautista-Baños, S., Velázquez-Del Valle, M.G., Méndez-Montealvo, M.G., Sánchez-Rivera, M.M., Bello-Pérez, L.A., 2008. Antifungal effects of chitosan with different molecular weights on in vitro development of *Rhizopus stolonifer* (Ehrenb.:Fr.) Vuill. Carbohydr. Polym. 73, 541–547.
Honarkar, H., Barikani, M., 2009. Applications of biopolymers I: chitosan. Monatsh. Chem. 140, 1403–1420.
Hong, J., Oren, Z., Shai, Y., 1999. Structure and organization of hemolytic and nonhemolytic diastereomers of antimicrobial peptides in membranes. Biochemistry 38, 16963–16973.
Hu, K., Schmidt, N.W., Zhu, R., Jiang, Y., Lai, G.H., Wei, G., Palermo, E.F., Kuroda, K., Wong, G.C.L., Yang, L., 2013. A critical evaluation of random copolymer mimesis of homogeneous antimicrobial peptides. Macromolecules 46, 1908–1915.
Hurdle, J.G., O'neill, A.J., Chopra, I., Lee, R.E., 2011. Targeting bacterial membrane function: an underexploited mechanism for treating persistent infections. Nat. Rev. Microbiol. 9, 62–75.
Ikinci, G., Şenel, S., AKINCIBAY, H., Kaş, S., Erciş, S., Wilson, C.G., Hincal, A.A., 2002. Effect of chitosan on a periodontal pathogen *Porphyromonas gingivalis*. Int. J. Pharm 235, 121–127.
Ilker, M.F., Nüsslein, K., Tew, G.N., Coughlin, E.B., 2004. Tuning the hemolytic and antibacterial activities of amphiphilic polynorbornene derivatives. J. Am. Chem. Soc. 126, 15870–15875.
Jeon, Y.-J., Park, P.-J., Kim, S.-K., 2001. Antimicrobial effect of chitooligosaccharides produced by bioreactor. Carbohydr. Polym. 44, 71–76.
Jiang, S.Y., Cao, Z.Q., 2010. Ultralow-fouling, functionalizable, and hydrolyzable zwitterionic materials and their derivatives for biological applications. Adv. Mater. 22, 920–932.
Jumaa, M., Furkert, F.H., Müller, B.W., 2002. A new lipid emulsion formulation with high antimicrobial efficacy using chitosan. Eur. J. Pharm. Biopharm. 53, 115–123.
Jung, K.-H., Huh, M.-W., Meng, W., Yuan, J., Hyun, S.H., Bae, J.-S., Hudson, S.M., Kang, I.-K., 2007. Preparation and antibacterial activity of PET/chitosan nanofibrous mats using an electrospinning technique. J. Appl. Polym. Sci. 105, 2816–2823.
Kazemzadeh-Narbat, M., Lai, B.F.L., Ding, C.F., Kizhakkedathu, J.N., Hancock, R.E.W., Wang, R.Z., 2013. Multilayered coating on titanium for controlled release of antimicrobial peptides for the prevention of implant-associated infections. Biomaterials 34, 5969–5977.

Kingshott, P., Wei, J., Bagge-Ravn, D., Gadegaard, N., Gram, L., 2003. Covalent attachment of poly(ethylene glycol) to surfaces, critical for reducing bacterial adhesion. Langmuir 19, 6912–6921.

Kong, M., Chen, X.G., Xing, K., Park, H.J., 2010. Antimicrobial properties of chitosan and mode of action: a state of the art review. Int. J. Food Microbiol. 144, 51–63.

Koo, Y.S., Kim, J.M., Park, I.Y., Yu, B.J., Jang, S.A., Kim, K.-S., Park, C.B., Cho, J.H., Kim, S.C., 2008. Structure-activity relations of parasin I, a histone H2A-derived antimicrobial peptide. Peptides 29, 1102–1108.

Krauson, A.J., He, J., Wimley, W.C., 2012. Determining the mechanism of membrane permeabilizing peptides: identification of potent, equilibrium pore-formers. Biochim. Biophys. Acta 1818, 1625–1632.

Kuang, J.H., Messersmith, P.B., 2012. Universal surface-initiated polymerization of antifouling zwitterionic brushes using a mussel-mimetic peptide initiator. Langmuir 28, 7258–7266.

Kuorwel, K.K., Cran, M.J., Sonneveld, K., Miltz, J., Bigger, S.W., 2011. Antimicrobial activity of biodegradable polysaccharide and protein-based films containing active agents. J. Food Sci. 76, R90–R102.

Kuroda, K., Caputo, G.A., Degrado, W.F., 2009. The role of hydrophobicity in the antimicrobial and hemolytic activities of polymethacrylate derivatives. Chemistry 15, 1123–1133.

Lee, M.-R., Stahl, S.S., Gellman, S.H., Masters, K.S., 2009. Nylon-3 copolymers that generate cell-adhesive surfaces identified by library screening. J. Am. Chem. Soc. 131, 16779–16789.

Lee, S.-M., Liu, K.-H., Liu, Y.-Y., Chang, Y.-P., Lin, C.-C., Chen, Y.-S., 2013. Chitosonic (R) acid as a novel cosmetic ingredient: evaluation of its antimicrobial, antioxidant and hydration activities. Materials 6, 1391–1402.

Li, G.Z., Cheng, G., Xue, H., Chen, S.F., Zhang, F.B., Jiang, S.Y., 2008. Ultra low fouling zwitterionic polymers with a biomimetic adhesive group. Biomaterials 29, 4592–4597.

Li, J., Zivanovic, S., Davidson, P.M., Kit, K., 2010. Characterization and comparison of chitosan/PVP and chitosan/PEO blend films. Carbohydr. Polym. 79, 786–791.

Li, Y., Kumar, K.N., Dabkowski, J.M., Corrigan, M., Scott, R.W., Nüsslein, K., Tew, G.N., 2012. New bactericidal surgical suture coating. Langmuir 28, 12134–12139.

Lienkamp, K., Madkour, A.E., Kumar, K.-N., Nüsslein, K., Tew, G.N., 2009. Antimicrobial polymers prepared by ring-opening metathesis polymerization: manipulating antimicrobial properties by organic counterion and charge density variation. Chemistry 15, 11715–11722.

Lienkamp, K., Madkour, A.E., Musante, A., Nelson, C.F., NüSslein, K., Tew, G.N., 2008. Antimicrobial polymers prepared by ROMP with unprecedented selectivity: a molecular construction kit approach. J. Am. Chem. Soc. 130, 9836–9843.

Lin, N.J., Yang, H.S., Chang, Y., Tung, K.L., Chen, W.H., Cheng, H.W., Hsiao, S.W., Aimar, P., Yamamoto, K., Lai, J.Y., 2013. Surface self-assembled PEGylation of fluoro-based PVDF membranes via hydrophobic-driven copolymer anchoring for ultra-stable biofouling resistance. Langmuir 29, 10183–10193.

Liu, R., Chen, X., Hayouka, Z., Chakraborty, S., Falk, S.P., Weisblum, B., Masters, K.S., Gellman, S.H., 2013. Nylon-3 polymers with selective antifungal activity. J. Am. Chem. Soc. 135, 5270–5273.

Liu, R., Masters, K.S., Gellman, S.H., 2012. Polymer chain length effects on fibroblast attachment on nylon-3-modified surfaces. Biomacromolecules 13, 1100–1105.

Locock, K.E.S., Michl, T.D., Griesser, H.J., Haeussler, M., Meagher, L., 2014a. Structure-activity relationships of guanylated antimicrobial polymethacrylates. Pure Appl. Chem. 86 (8), 1281.

Locock, K.E.S., Michl, T.D., Stevens, N., Hayball, J.D., Vasilev, K., Postma, A., Griesser, H.J., Meagher, L., Haeussler, M., 2014b. Antimicrobial polymethacrylates synthesized as mimics of tryptophan-rich cationic peptides. ACS Macro Lett. 3, 319–323.

Locock, K.E.S., Michl, T.D., Valentin, J.D.P., Vasilev, K., Hayball, J.D., Qu, Y., Traven, A., Griesser, H.J., Meagher, L., Haeussler, M., 2013. Guanylated polymethacrylates: a class of potent antimicrobial polymers with low haemolytic activity. Biomacromolecules 14, 4021–4031.

Malette, W.G., Quigley, H.J., Gaines, R.D., Johnson, N.D., Rainer, W.G., 1983. Chitosan: a new hemostatic. Ann. Thorac. Surg. 36, 55–58.

Mantelli, F., Argueso, P., 2008. Functions of ocular surface mucins in health and disease. Curr. Opin. Allergy Clin. Immunol. 8, 477–483.

Michl, T.D., Locock, K.E.S., Stevens, N.E., Hayball, J.D., Vasilev, K., Postma, A., Qu, Y., Traven, A., Haeussler, M., Meagher, L., Griesser, H.J., 2014. RAFT-derived antimicrobial polymethacrylates: elucidating the impact of end-groups on activity and cytotoxicity. Polym. Chem. 5, 5813–5822.

Mihajlovic, M., Lazaridis, T., 2012. Charge distribution and imperfect amphipathicity affect pore formation by antimicrobial peptides. Biochim. Biophys. Acta 1818, 1274–1283.

Milner, S.T., 1991. Polymer brushes. Science 251, 905–914.

Moiset, G., Cirac, A.D., Stuart, M.C.A., Marrink, S.-J., Sengupta, D., Poolman, B., 2013. Dual action of BPC194: a membrane active peptide killing bacterial cells. PLoS One 8, e61541.

Mowery, B.P., Lee, S.E., Kissounko, D.A., Epand, R.F., Epand, R.M., Weisblum, B., Stahl, S.S., Gellman, S.H., 2007. Mimicry of antimicrobial host-defense peptides by random copolymers. J. Am. Chem. Soc. 129, 15474–15476.

Mowery, B.P., Lindner, A.H., Weisblum, B., Stahl, S.S., Gellman, S.H., 2009. Structure–activity relationships among random nylon-3 copolymers that mimic antibacterial host-defense peptides. J. Am. Chem. Soc. 131, 9735–9745.

Muñoz-Bonilla, A., Fernández-García, M., 2012. Polymeric materials with antimicrobial activity. Prog. Polym. Sci. 37, 281–339.

Muzzarelli, R., Tarsi, R., Filippini, O., Giovanetti, E., Biagini, G., Varaldo, P.E., 1990. Antimicrobial properties of N-carboxybutyl chitosan. Antimicrob. Agents Chemother. 34, 2019–2023.

Ndi, C.P., Semple, S.J., Griesser, H.J., Pyke, S.M., Barton, M.D., 2007. Antimicrobial compounds from the Australian desert plant *Eremophila neglecta*. J. Nat. Prod. 70, 1439–1443.

Nejati Hafdani, F., Sadeghinia, N., 2011. A review on application of chitosan as a natural antimicrobial. World Acad. Sci. Eng. Technol. 50, 252–256.

No, H.K., Young Park, N., Ho Lee, S., Meyers, S.P., 2002. Antibacterial activity of chitosans and chitosan oligomers with different molecular weights. Int. J. Food Microbiol. 74, 65–72.

O'Gara, J.P., Humphreys, H., 2001. *Staphylococcus epidermidis* biofilms: importance and implications. J. Med. Microbiol. 50, 582–587.

O'toole, G., Kaplan, H.B., Kolter, R., 2000. Biofilm formation as microbial development. Ann. Rev. Microbiol. 54, 49–79.

Oda, Y., Kanaoka, S., Sato, T., Aoshima, S., Kuroda, K., 2011. Block versus random amphiphilic copolymers as antibacterial agents. Biomacromolecules 12, 3581–3591.

Onaizi, S.A., Leong, S.S.J., 2011. Tethering antimicrobial peptides: current status and potential challenges. Biotechnol. Adv. 29, 67–74.

Ostuni, E., Chapman, R.G., Liang, M.N., Meluleni, G., Pier, G., Ingber, D.E., Whitesides, G.M., 2001. Self-assembled monolayers that resist the adsorption of proteins and the adhesion of bacterial and mammalian cells. Langmuir 17, 6336–6343.

Palermo, E.F., Lee, D.-K., Ramamoorthy, A., Kuroda, K., 2010. Role of cationic group structure in membrane binding and disruption by amphiphilic copolymers. J. Phys. Chem. B 115, 366–375.
Palermo, E.F., Vemparala, S., Kuroda, K., 2012. Cationic spacer arm design strategy for control of antimicrobial activity and conformation of amphiphilic methacrylate random copolymers. Biomacromolecules 13, 1632–1641.
Park, K.D., Kim, Y.S., Han, D.K., Kim, Y.H., Lee, E.H.B., Suh, H., Choi, K.S., 1998. Bacterial adhesion on PEG modified polyurethane surfaces. Biomaterials 19, 851–859.
Peleg, A.Y., Tampakakis, E., Fuchs, B.B., Eliopoulos, G.M., Moellering, R.C., Mylonakis, E., 2008. Prokaryote–eukaryote interactions identified by using *Caenorhabditis elegans*. Proc. Natl. Acad. Sci. U.S.A. 105, 14585–14590.
Perrin, D.D., 1972. Dissociation Constants of Organic Bases in Aqueous Solution. Butterworths, London.
Pieta, P., Mirza, J., Lipkowski, J., 2012. Direct visualization of the alamethicin pore formed in a planar phospholipid matrix. Proc. Natl. Acad. Sci. U.S.A. 109, 21223–21227.
Pillai, C.K.S., Paul, W., Sharma, C.P., 2009. Chitin and chitosan polymers: chemistry, solubility and fiber formation. Prog. Polym. Sci. 34, 641–678.
Raafat, D., Sahl, H.-G., 2009. Chitosan and its antimicrobial potential–a critical literature survey. Microb. Biotechnol. 2, 186–201.
Raafat, D., Von Bargen, K., Haas, A., Sahl, H.-G., 2008. Insights into the mode of action of chitosan as an antibacterial compound. Appl. Environ. Microbiol. 74, 3764–3773.
Ramya, R., Venkatesan, J., Kim, S.K., Sudha, P.N., 2012. Biomedical applications of chitosan: an overview. J. Biomater. Tiss. Eng. 2, 100–111.
Rapaport, D., Shai, Y., 1991. Interaction of fluorescently labeled pardaxin and its analogs with lipid bilayers. J. Biol. Chem. 266, 23769–23775.
Rhoades, J., Roller, S., 2000. Antimicrobial actions of degraded and native chitosan against spoilage organisms in laboratory media and foods. Appl. Environ. Microbiol. 66, 80–86.
Richards, M.J., Edwards, J.R., Culver, D.H., Gaynes, R.P., 1999. Nosocomial infections in medical intensive care units in the United States. National nosocomial infect surveillance system. Crit. Care Med. 27, 887–892.
Roller, S., Covill, N., 1999. The antifungal properties of chitosan in laboratory media and apple juice. Int. J. Food Microbiol. 47, 67–77.
Sambhy, V., Peterson, B.R., Sen, A., 2008. Antibacterial and hemolytic activities of pyridinium polymers as a function of the spatial relationship between the positive charge and the pendant alkyl tail. Angew. Chem., Int. Ed. 47, 1250–1254.
Senaratne, W., Andruzzi, L., Ober, C.K., 2005. Self-assembled monolayers and polymer brushes in biotechnology: current applications and future perspectives. Biomacromolecules 6, 2427–2448.
Sharon, M., Oren, Z., Shai, Y., Anglister, J., 1999. 2D-NMR and ATR-FTIR study of the structure of a cell-selective diastereomer of melittin and its orientation in phospholipids. Biochemistry 38, 15305–15316.
Shigemasa, Y., Minami, S., 1995. Applications of chitin and chitosan as biomaterials. Biotechnol. Genet. Eng. Rev. 13, 383–420.
Shih, C.-Y., Huang, K.-S., 2003. Synthesis of a polyurethane–chitosan blended polymer and a compound process for shrink-proof and antimicrobial woolen fabrics. J. Appl. Polym. Sci. 88, 2356–2363.
Skarnes, R.C., Watson, D.W., 1957. Antimicrobial factors of normal tissues and fluids. Bacteriol. Rev. 21, 273–294.

Steinstraesser, L., Hirsch, T., Schulte, M., Kueckelhaus, M., Jacobsen, F., Mersch, E.A., Stricker, I., Afacan, N., Jenssen, H., Hancock, R.E.W., Kindrachuk, J., 2012. Innate defense regulator peptide 1018 in wound healing and wound infection. PLoS One 7, e39373.

Subbiahdoss, G., Kuijer, R., Grijpma, D.W., Van Der Mei, H.C., Busscher, H.J., 2009. Microbial biofilm growth vs. tissue integration: 'The race for the surface' experimentally studied. Acta Biomater. 5, 1399–1404.

Sudarshan, N.R., Hoover, D.G., Knorr, D., 1992. Antibacterial action of chitosan. Food Biotechnol. 6, 257–272.

Sumiyoshi, M., Ricciuto, J., Tisdale, A., Gipson, I.K., Mantelli, F., Argueso, P., 2008. Antiadhesive character of mucin O-glycans at the apical surface of corneal epithelial cells. Invest. Ophthalmol. Vis. Sci. 49, 197–203.

Takahashi, H., Palermo, E.F., Yasuhara, K., Caputo, G.A., Kuroda, K., 2013. Molecular design, structures, and activity of antimicrobial peptide-mimetic polymers. Macromol. Biosci. 13 (10), 1285–1299 n/a-n/a.

Tauhardt, L., Kempe, K., Gottschaldt, M., Schubert, U.S., 2013. Poly(2-oxazoline) functionalised surfaces: from modification to application. Chem. Soc. Rev. 42, 7998–8011.

Tokura, S., Ueno, K., Miyazaki, S., Nishi, N., 1997. Molecular weight dependent antimicrobial activity by chitosan. Macromol. Symp. 120, 1–9.

Tsai, G.-J., Su, W.-H., 1999. Antibacterial activity of shrimp chitosan against *Escherichia coli*. J. Food Prot. 62, 239–243. http://pub2web.metastore.ingenta.com/ns/.

Vacheethasanee, K., Marchant, R.E., 2000. Surfactant polymers designed to suppress bacterial (*Staphylococcus epidermidis*) adhesion on biomaterials. J. Biomed. Mater. Res. 50, 302–312.

Vermette, P., Meagher, L., 2003. Interactions of phospholipid- and poly(ethylene glycol)-modified surfaces with biological systems: relation to physico-chemical properties and mechanisms. Colloids Surf. B 28, 153–198.

Vishu Kumar, A.B., Varadaraj, M.C., Gowda, L.R., Tharanathan, R.N., 2005. Characterization of chito-oligosaccharides prepared by chitosanolysis with the aid of papain and pronase, and their bactericidal action against *Bacillus cereus* and *Escherichia coli*. Biochem. J. 391, 167–175.

Wadhwani, P., Reichert, J., Buerck, J., Ulrich, A.S., 2012. Antimicrobial and cell-penetrating peptides induce lipid vesicle fusion by folding and aggregation. Eur. Biophys. J. 41, 177–187.

Wang, X., Du, Y., Liu, H., 2004. Preparation, characterization and antimicrobial activity of chitosan–Zn complex. Carbohydr. Polym. 56, 21–26.

Watanabe, H., 2002. Significance of mucin on the ocular surface. Cornea 21, S17–S22.

Wieprecht, T., Beyermann, M., Seelig, J., 1999. Binding of antibacterial magainin peptides to electrically neutral membranes: thermodynamics and structure. Biochemistry 38, 10377–10387.

Wimley, W.C., Hristova, K., 2011. Antimicrobial peptides: successes, challenges and unanswered questions. J. Memb. Biol. 239, 27–34.

Yang, D., Biragyn, A., Hoover, D.M., Lubkowski, J., Oppenheim, J.J., 2004. Multiple roles of antimicrobial defensins, cathelicidins, and eosinophil-derived neurotoxin in host defense. Ann. Rev. Immunol. 22, 181–215.

Yang, W.J., Neoh, K.G., Kang, E.T., Lee, S.S.C., Teo, S.L.M., Rittschof, D., 2012. Functional polymer brushes via surface-initiated atom transfer radical graft polymerization for combating marine biofouling. Biofouling 28, 895–912.

Yeh, J.-T., Chen, C.-L., Huang, K.S., Nien, Y.H., Chen, J.L., Huang, P.Z., 2006. Synthesis, characterization, and application of PVP/chitosan blended polymers. J. Appl. Polym. Sci. 101, 885–891.

Yuan, S., Yin, J., Jiang, W., Liang, B., Pehkonen, S.O., Choong, C., 2013. Enhancing antibacterial activity of surface-grafted chitosan with immobilized lysozyme on bioinspired stainless steel substrates. Colloids Surf. B 106, 11–21.

Zaat, S.A.J., Hiemstra, P.S., 2013. Antimicrobial Peptides and Innate Immunity (electronic Resource). Springer Basel, Basel.

Zasloff, M., 2002. Antimicrobial peptides of multicellular organisms. Nature 415, 389–395.

Zdyrko, B., Klep, V., Li, X.W., Kang, Q., Minko, S., Wen, X.J., Luzinov, I., 2009. Polymer brushes as active nanolayers for tunable bacteria adhesion. Mater. Sci. Eng., C: Biomimetic Supramol. Syst. 29, 680–684.

Zhang, J., Markiewicz, M.J., Mowery, B.P., Weisblum, B., Stahl, S.S., Gellman, S.H., 2011. C-terminal functionalization of nylon-3 polymers: effects of C-terminal groups on antibacterial and hemolytic activities. Biomacromolecules 13, 323–331.

Zhao, C., Li, L.Y., Wang, Q.M., Yu, Q.M., Zheng, J., 2011. Effect of film thickness on the antifouling performance of poly(hydroxy-functional methacrylates) grafted surfaces. Langmuir 27, 4906–4913.

Zhao, C., Zheng, J., 2011. Synthesis and characterization of poly(N-hydroxyethylacrylamide) for long-term antifouling ability. Biomacromolecules 12, 4071–4079.

Zhong, Z., Xing, R., Liu, S., Wang, L., Cai, S., Li, P., 2008. Synthesis of acyl thiourea derivatives of chitosan and their antimicrobial activities in vitro. Carbohydr. Res. 343, 566–570.

Zhou, C., Qi, X., Li, P., Chen, W.N., Mouad, L., Chang, M.W., Leong, S.S.J., Chan-Park, M.B., 2009. High potency and broad-spectrum antimicrobial peptides synthesized via ring-opening polymerization of α-aminoacid-N-carboxyanhydrides. Biomacromolecules 11, 60–67.

Zivanovic, S., Li, J., Davidson, P.M., Kit, K., 2007. Physical, mechanical, and antibacterial properties of chitosan/PEO blend films. Biomacromolecules 8, 1505–1510.

Plasma-based surface modification for the control of biointerfacial interactions

5

H. Thissen
CSIRO Manufacturing Flagship, VIC, Australia

5.1 Introduction

While early work in the area of biomedical devices focused mainly on bulk material properties, such as mechanical properties, transparency and the refractive index of materials, it was soon discovered that the biological response to materials is governed to a large extent by their surface properties, including in particular the surface chemistry and topography [1,2]. In many cases, materials that have suitable bulk properties do not have the desired surface properties, in which case a coating or surface modification is required. Today, much of the research and developmental effort in the area of biomedical devices, including cell culture tools, biosensors and implantable medical devices, has been therefore focused on the optimisation of surface properties.

Here, the requirements are varied, and range from improved biocompatibility to the prevention of cell or pathogen attachment and the display of specific biological signals, such as cell adhesion mediators or antimicrobial compounds. While there are many instances where inorganic or metal-based coatings are applied, polymer-based coatings offer by far the greatest flexibility with regard to performance parameters that can be achieved. There are a range of polymer-based surface modification methods to select from, including dip-coating methods, graft polymerisation methods, solution-based methods, chemical vapour deposition methods as well as plasma-based methods [3].

The reasons to choose one coating method over another again are varied, but common factors that manufacturers will consider include the interfacial adhesion of the deposited layer on the substrate material, the stability and conformity of the deposited coating, the speed and cost of the overall coating process, environmental factors such as the amount of waste products generated and the transferability of the coating method between different substrate materials. An important consideration is also whether complex geometries can be coated. Plasma-based methods have advantages over competing methods with regard to all of these areas and are therefore used by many different manufacturers.

Plasma-based methods can be broadly classified as plasma etching, plasma treatment and plasma polymerisation [5]. The conditions used for processing, such as the type of vapour used, the pressure and energy used, the geometry of the reaction chamber and the way of applying the energy, such as radiofrequency glow discharge

Biosynthetic Polymers for Medical Applications. http://dx.doi.org/10.1016/B978-1-78242-105-4.00005-5

or microwave generators, determine in which class plasma treatment falls. In the biomedical device context, low-pressure and low-temperature plasma treatment and plasma polymerisation are used most frequently and specific examples for these treatments are discussed below. In plasma treatment procedures, gases such as argon, nitrogen, oxygen, ammonia or tetrafluoromethane are used to modify surfaces in regard to the surface energy and functional groups presented at the surface. Plasma polymerisation, on the other hand, is based on the fragmentation of volatile organic compounds and their subsequent crosslinking on the substrate surface. In all cases, the plasma process generates a variety of species such as ions, radicals, electrons and atoms as well as vacuum ultraviolet radiation interacting with the surface. The different plasma processes described in Figure 5.1, which happen simultaneously and compete with each other, have been described by Yasuda as competitive ablation polymerisation [4].

It is important to note that the resulting surface chemistries are somewhat heterogeneous and difficult to describe using traditional chemistry tools. Furthermore, these surfaces undergo post-treatment reactions also described as ageing reactions [6] which have to be taken into account.

Today, plasma-based surface modification is part of established manufacturing processes across many industry sectors, including the aerospace, automotive, energy, information technology and biomedical sector. However, new plasma-based technologies as well as applications are constantly being added. In the biomedical sector, the development of atmospheric plasma treatment options and plasma medicine (the use of

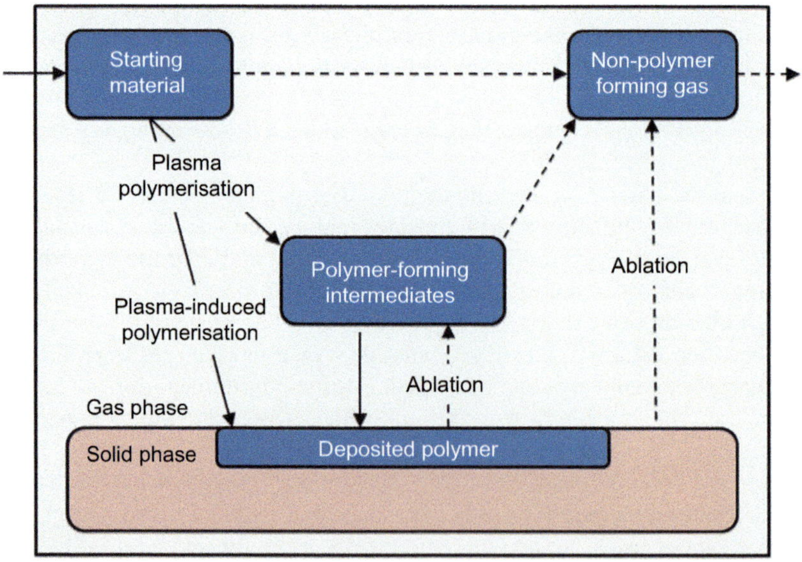

Figure 5.1 Schematic describing the competing processes that play a role in plasma. Adapted from Refs [4,5].

plasma for therapeutic applications), as well as the use of plasma in the sterilisation of biomedical devices, serves as an example.

As the focus of this chapter is on the control of cell–material interactions, it is also important to classify cellular responses to surfaces (Figure 5.2). Equivalent to responses in the natural tissue environment, the cellular response to synthetic materials is governed, in particular, by cell surface receptors, including integrins, a family of transmembrane glycoproteins. Cellular responses such as attachment, spreading, migration and differentiation are guided by the presence of extracellular matrix (ECM) proteins that can be recognised by integrins such as fibronectin, collagen and laminin. Due to the fact that proteins are adsorbed on material surfaces within seconds after implantation *in vivo* or after addition to cell culture media *in vitro*, cellular responses to surfaces are in most cases responses to adsorbed proteins that are present on these surfaces (Figure 5.2(a)). The orientation, nature and ratio of proteins adsorbed on surfaces depend on the chemical nature of the surface, including the presence of functional groups, the surface energy and charge. Therefore, different materials will lead to a different cellular response. However, by using suitable chemistry approaches such as high-density graft polymer coatings, protein adsorption and therefore cell attachment can be reduced or prevented (Figure 5.2(b)). Finally, coatings that prevent nonspecific protein adsorption and therefore cell attachment can be turned into substrates that exclusively provide specific signals to cells by covalent immobilisation of synthetic signals such as peptide sequences that can be detected by integrin receptors or small molecule peptidomimetics (Figure 5.2(c)). Importantly, plasma-based coatings can play a role in all of these scenarios.

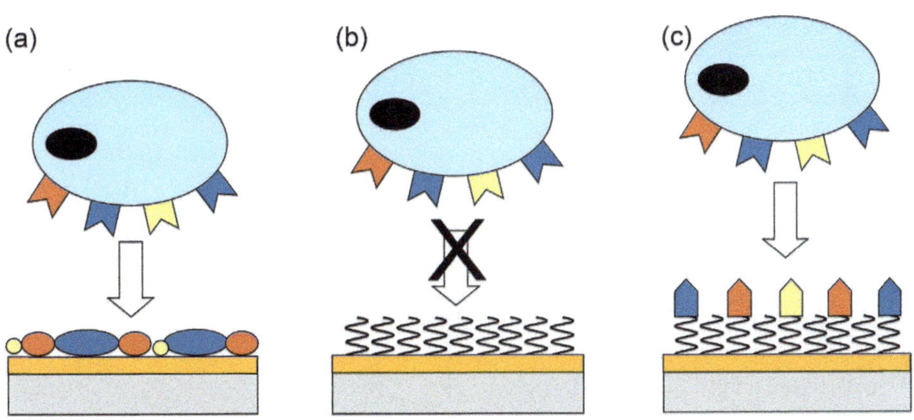

Figure 5.2 Schematic representation of the classification of different coatings and the equivalent cellular response. Different cell surface receptors are represented by different colours. Different adsorbed proteins or synthetic immobilised signals that can be detected by these receptors are also represented by different colours. (a) Cell attachment in response to adsorbed proteins. (b) Cell attachment prevented due to the graft polymer. (c) Cell attachment in response to immobilised signals.

Another important factor that should be considered in the context of plasma-based treatments or coatings is the choice of suitable analytical methods that can be used to verify the success of the surface modification process. Analytical methods must be sufficiently surface sensitive to ensure that surface modifications and deposited coatings, which often have a thickness in the nanometer range, can be verified. Therefore, plasma-treated surfaces as well as plasma-based coatings are often analysed using methods such as water contact angle (CA) measurements, X-ray photoelectron spectroscopy (XPS), atomic force microscopy (AFM), scanning electron microscopy (SEM) and other surface sensitive methods listed below (Table 5.1). In most cases, a reasonable picture of the surface properties before and after treatment can be obtained by using complementary analytical techniques. For example, a surface analysed by CA, XPS and AFM or SEM analysis will provide information in regard to wettability, chemical composition and topography in comparison to suitable control samples such as the untreated substrate material.

5.2 Plasma treatment of material surfaces

Plasma treatment, including atmospheric plasma treatment and the related corona discharge treatment are widely used today in manufacturing processes. Here the

Table 5.1 Surface analytical methods that are typically used for the characterisation of surfaces modified by plasma-based treatments

Method	Abbreviation	Information depth	Information
Contact angle measurement	CA	1 nm	Wettability, surface energy
X-ray photoelectron spectroscopy	XPS	5–10 nm	Chemical composition, imaging
Secondary ion mass spectrometry	SIMS	1 nm	Chemical composition, imaging
Fourier-transform infrared spectroscopy (attenuated total reflection mode)	FTIR-ATR	1 μm	Chemical composition
Atomic force microscopy	AFM	–	Topography, imaging, etc.
Scanning electron microscopy	SEM	–	Topography, imaging

process parameters are selected according to the application and range from plasma etching and plasma cleaning procedures, where material is removed from the surface of the substrate to modulated wettability, surface energy and surface charge of polymers after exposure to for example an oxygen, argon, nitrogen, oxygen, ammonia or tetrafluoromethane plasma. For example, in microfluidics this is used to achieve improved filling of microfluidic channels, in printing to achieve improved printing results on polymer substrates, and in cell culture tools to improve serum protein binding and, more importantly, cell attachment. Since the 1970s, cell biology researchers have been using polystyrene-based cell culture substrates for their experiments, including multiwell plates, dishes, flasks and roller bottles. While polystyrene has many advantages in the context of cell culture applications, such as optical transparency and its compatibility with standard sterilisation protocols, it does not support the attachment of cells at the desired level. The search for a surface modification method of polystyrene that can be used in large-scale manufacturing, is simple, cost-effective and reproducible resulted in plasma treatment and the related corona discharge treatment, which is performed in air, being identified as suitable candidates.

Oxygen plasma treatment, atmospheric plasma treatment or corona discharge treatments all lead to the introduction of oxidised functional groups at the surface of the polystyrene vessels. These functional groups increase the hydrophilicity of the polymer surface and modulate the surface charge. Figure 5.3 shows hydroxyl, aldehyde, ketone and carboxylic acid groups which represent some of the functional groups that have been detected on polystyrene surfaces after these treatments. While the presence of these functional groups is essential for the performance of the modified surfaces, and while an increase in the oxygen content often correlates with improved performance, it is important to control the processing parameters in such a way that the polystyrene is not oxidised too far. Due to the fact that the oxidation also leads to chain scission, eventually highly oxidised smaller molecular weight species are formed at the surface that can be washed off, again exposing the polystyrene substrate material.

In cell culture, the modified polystyrene surface leads to an increased adsorption of ECM proteins from the animal-derived serum used in cell culture. These proteins can in turn be recognised by cell surface receptors as discussed above. Today, tissue culture polystyrene (TCPS) surface coatings remain the gold standard for a wide range

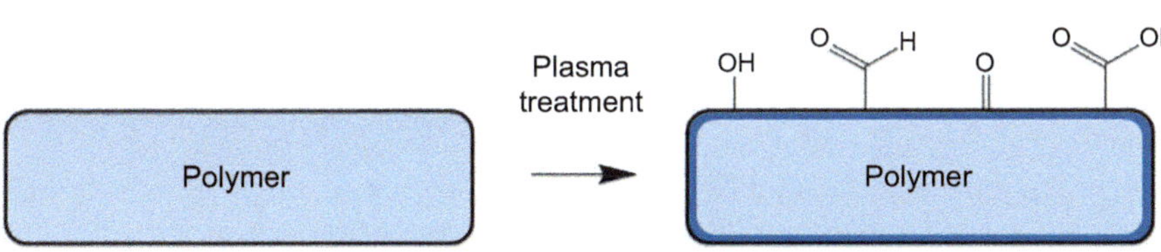

Figure 5.3 Oxygen plasma treatment, atmospheric plasma treatment or corona discharge treatments of cell culture substrates made from polymers such as polystyrene lead to the introduction of oxygen-containing functional groups at the surface. The modulated surface properties, including enhanced wettability, oxygen content and surface charge, lead to enhanced serum protein binding and subsequent cell attachment.

of cell culture applications requiring high cell attachment. However, TCPS surfaces provide only an indirect mechanism for cell attachment. In the absence of proteins provided by serum, the presence of specific attachment factors is required. Therefore, polystyrene-based substrates for cell culture applications are today also available precoated with ECM proteins such as fibronectin, laminin and different types of collagen. In addition, products that display synthetic mimetics of these ECM proteins have now entered the market [7,8]. In most cases, these mimetics consist of relatively short peptide sequences that can be recognised by integrin receptors, such as the RGD, IKVAV or GFOGER sequences found in fibronectin, laminin and collagen, respectively. In the future, this is expected to be extended to the use of small molecule mimetics of these peptides, which can be designed to interact much more specifically with particular integrin subtypes [9].

5.3 Plasma polymer-based coatings

Plasma polymer coatings have been deposited using a wide range of reactor designs, which vary significantly in size. However, in all cases a volatile organic compound (the monomer) is introduced into a chamber via an inlet, and a vacuum is applied using a pump connected to the chamber. Energy is then applied using a radiofrequency glow discharge or microwave generator to induce fragmentation of the monomer, leading to subsequent crosslinking on the substrate surface. In many cases the plasma polymer deposition process is carried out within seconds. Compared with other surface coating methods used in the context of biomedical devices, plasma polymer coatings are not substrate-dependent. This has the advantage that coatings can easily be transferred from one substrate material to another. Suitable substrate materials include a broad range of polymers, metals and inorganic materials. Furthermore, the pinhole-free nature of the plasma polymer films that are obtained leads to evenly coated materials and provides barrier properties.

Compared with many other surface coating methods, plasma polymer coatings are also not based on a 'line of sight' process. In contrast to such methods (such as sputtering or irradiation-based processes), the mass transport phenomena in the low-pressure environment allow the coating of complex geometric shapes, including internal surfaces. Moreover, due to the chemical nature of the highly crosslinked plasma polymer films and the covalent bonds with the substrate that are generated (compare Figure 5.1) the coatings provide excellent substrate adhesion. It is also important to point out that the crosslinked nature of plasma polymers provides coatings that do not introduce leachables, which is a significant advantage in the biomedical context.

One of the most significant differences to other surface coating methods though is the fact that a large range of different surface chemistries, including surface functional groups, can easily be accessed by choosing an appropriate volatile organic compound as the monomer. For example, an amine group contained in monomers such as *n*-heptylamine or allylamine will be reflected on the surface of the resulting plasma polymer [10].

As discussed, the highly reactive environment and chemistry of the plasma polymer deposition process lead to coatings that are highly adhesive and conform well to the contour of the underlying substrate. Figure 5.4 shows the AFM analysis of an *n*-heptylamine plasma polymer coating deposited on a mica surface. Here, an area was masked using a poly(D,L-lactide) polymer mask during coating deposition and analysed after removal of the mask [11]. The AFM section analysis in particular demonstrates the pinhole-free nature of the coating and the fact that the coating follows the contour of the substrate. The section analysis and height histogram also reveal the coating thickness of approximately 49 nm. It is important to emphasise that the coating thickness can be controlled using a range of process parameters, including the deposition time. The typical desired thickness range used in biomedical applications though is in the nanometre range (between approximately 5 and 100 nm).

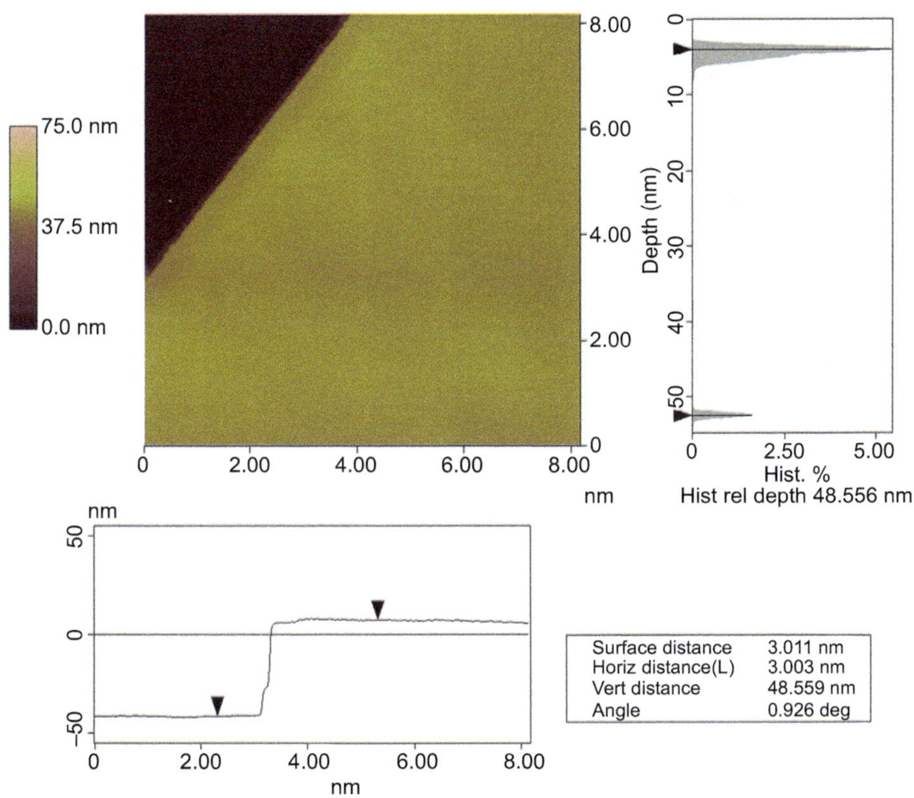

Figure 5.4 AFM image of a heptylamine plasma polymer deposited by radiofrequency glow discharge on a mica surface. A section of the imaged area was masked during coating deposition and the mask subsequently removed. The pinhole-free nature of the coating following the contour of the substrate is evident. In addition, the section analysis and height histogram reveal a coating thickness of approximately 48.6 nm.
Reproduced with permission from Ref. [11].

Plasma polymer coatings are used today in a broad range of biomedical applications where an improved biological response is required. A specific example used in vivo is the use of plasma polymer coatings on silicone hydrogel contact lenses, where the wettability, the biocompatibility and the wearer's comfort are substantially increased by the coating [12]. At this point of time, only a few coating deposition techniques have been developed that match the conformity, adhesive properties and ability to coat complex shapes while providing outstanding biocompatibility. However, the chemical vapour deposition of [2.2]paracyclophanes to yield poly-*p*-xylylenes is an example for a competing technique that has been used commercially (parylene brand) in biomedical devices such as stents, cardiac pacemakers and defibrillators [13]. Plasma polymer coatings combine many aspects that are attractive for the manufacture of biomedical products, as discussed above. However, the fact that a vacuum is required means that the surface modification step needs to be carried out in a batch process, which can be a disadvantage.

5.4 Plasma polymer-based interlayers

In the biomedical context, a large part of the research and development effort involving plasma-based surface modification is focused at this point in time on plasma polymer-based interlayers. The reason for this is that attractive features of plasma polymers, including in particular their excellent adhesion to the substrate material, their pinhole-free nature and stability as well as the provision of functional groups on the surface provide an ideal starting point for subsequent chemical modification reactions.

In many cases where the bulk material is chemically inert (such as commonly used polymers, for example polystyrene, polyethylene and polypropylene) and does not provide suitable functional groups for chemical modification, the covalent immobilisation of desired bioactive compounds or graft polymers is only possible after deposition of a suitable interlayer. Plasma polymer interlayers can be deposited as a coating with defined thickness and can provide the desired functional groups on the surface in a controlled density. In the literature, functional groups such as amine, carboxylic acid and aldehyde groups have been used for interlayer coatings [5]. However, the range of functional groups that can be accessed is only limited by the ability to identify a volatile organic compound carrying the desired functional group (or a precursor) and the stability of this functional group during the plasma polymerisation process. An example of a functional group that has been added to an ever-growing list of functional groups relevant to biomedical applications includes atom transfer radical polymerisation (ATRP) initiators [14].

Here, it is important to emphasise that a balance must often be established between maximising the density of functional groups that are retained and the crosslinking density of the plasma polymer coating. In continuous wave plasma polymers, this balance can be established for example by controlling the power that is applied. At higher power regimes, increased crosslinking within the coating is achieved while the retained density of functional groups compared with the original monomer is low. At lower power regimes, the retained density of functional groups will be higher, but the chemical stability of the resulting coating may not be sufficient. To address these issues, pulsed plasma deposition has been used increasingly. In comparison to continuous wave plasma polymerisation, pulsed plasma polymerisation takes place during short 'on' periods (with a duration of typically milliseconds) while surface reactions continue to occur during the intermediate 'off' periods, leading to enhanced functional group densities [15].

A specific example for the use of a plasma polymer-based interlayer that has been used in the biomedical context is the use of an allylamine plasma polymer (ALAPP) interlayer coating. This coating has frequently been deposited using a radiofrequency glow discharge generator in a continuous deposition process, a power of 20 W and a deposition time of 25 s. The high number of amine functional groups retained in this process were then used in a subsequent high-density polymer grafting reaction of aldehyde terminated poly(ethylene glycol) (PEG). This approach has been demonstrated to provide extremely low protein adsorption [16] and to prevent cell attachment [17] and tissue migration [18]. Furthermore, this plasma polymer interlayer-based coating approach has been successfully translated to silicone hydrogel-based extended wear contact lenses and assessed in controlled clinical studies [19].

The use of the radiofrequency glow discharge deposited plasma polymer allowed the successful transfer of the ALAPP interlayer coating from inorganic substrates such as silicon wafers to a range of polymer substrates without changing the deposition parameters. Importantly, the ALAPP provided amine functional groups at a sufficient surface density to achieve high-density PEG grafting under 'cloud point' conditions. Under these conditions, marginal solvation of the PEG polymer chains leads to reduced chain repulsion during surface immobilisation and accordingly an increase in the surface density of the graft polymer. The influence of the ALAPP interlayer on cell attachment before and after PEG grafting is illustrated in Figure 5.5. Compared with commercially available (plasma treated) tissue culture polystyrene (TCPS), the attachment of bovine corneal epithelial cells was enhanced on the ALAPP coating, while cell attachment was prevented after grafting of an additional high-density PEG layer [17].

Table 5.2 provides an example for the characterisation of the surfaces in Figure 5.5. As mentioned above, XPS analysis is often used in studies related to plasma polymers due to its information depth of approximately 10 nm and the quantitative nature of the resulting data. Here, the complete attenuation of the fluorine signal from the underlying substrate after deposition of the ALAPP interlayer coating demonstrates that a pinhole-free coating with a thickness of more than 10 nm has been deposited. The successful PEG grafting on the other hand is demonstrated by a decrease in the nitrogen signal and an increase in the oxygen signal [17]. In XPS experiments, further information regarding the chemical environment of the elements detected on the surface can also be obtained from high-resolution spectra.

5.5 Plasma polymer-based patterning

In the biomedical context, plasma-based processes such as plasma etching and plasma polymer deposition are also frequently combined with each other and with other

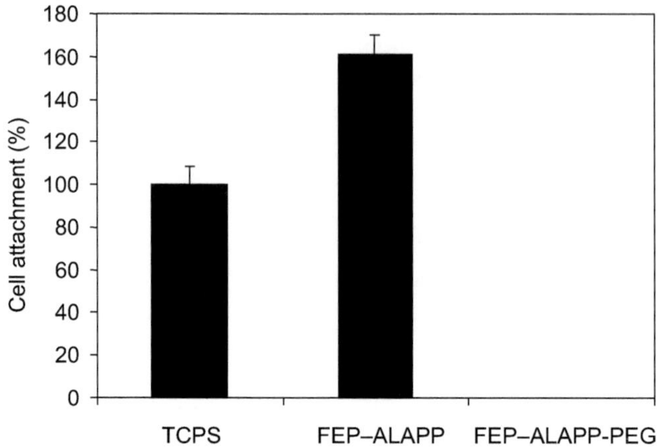

Figure 5.5 Bovine corneal epithelial cell attachment relative to tissue culture polystyrene (TCPS) after 24 h. Fluorinated ethylene propylene (FEP) substrates were coated with ALAPP and subsequently grafted with PEG aldehyde. The enhancement of cell attachment after deposition of the ALAPP and the prevention of cell attachment after PEG grafting is evident. Reproduced from Ref. [17] with permission.

Table 5.2 XPS results obtained on fluorinated ethylene propylene (FEP) substrate materials (% atomic concentration)

Sample	%C	%O	%N	%F
FEP	33.9	–	–	66.1
FEP–ALAPP	77.2	10.2	12.6	–
FEP–ALAPP–PEG	71.3	22.1	6.6	–

surface modification methods, particularly in patterning applications, which are of outstanding interest in applications requiring advanced spatial control over bio-interfacial interactions [20]. An example is provided in Figure 5.6. Here, micrometer-scale arrays containing up to four spatially resolved material regions were fabricated using colloid crystal particle self-assembly in conjunction with multiple surface treatment methods, including plasma etching and 1,7-octadiene plasma polymer (ppOct) deposition [21]. The robustness of the chemical patterning strategy and the accessability of chemically distinct regions was subsequently demonstrated by employing a combination of thiols and silanes that were selectively self-assembled in the Au and SiO_2 regions, respectively.

However, many other patterning methods have been used based on plasma-based methods, including plasma polymer deposition in the presence of a mask or plasma polymerisation combined with photolithography or laser ablation [22]. Furthermore, advanced spatial control over plasma polymer coatings has also been used for the

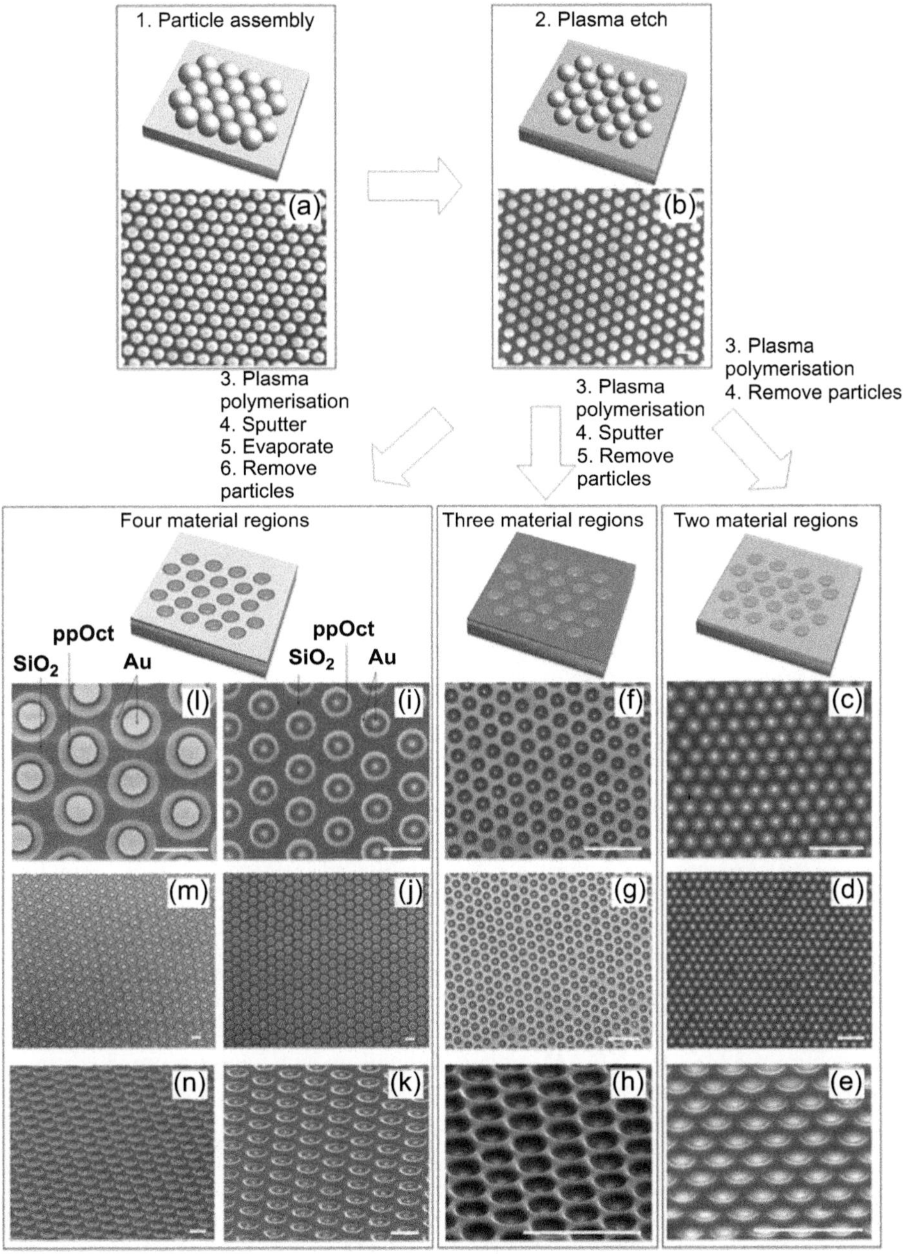

Figure 5.6 Schematic representation of patterning methods leading to spatially controlled surface chemistries and SEM images (a–n) associated with these methods with (a) particles assembled on a substrate, (b) plasma-etched particles to reduce particle size, (c–e) generation of two chemistry regions representing gold (Au, substrate) and ppOct, (f–h) generation of three chemistry regions representing Au (substrate), ppOct and Au (sputtering), and (i–n) generation of four chemistry regions representing Au (substrate), ppOct, Au (sputtered) and SiO_2 (evaporated). Scale bar represents 2 μm.
Reproduced from Ref. [21] with permission.

production of plasma polymer gradients, based for example on the deposition of mixtures of two different monomers. The resulting surfaces are particularly useful in high-throughput screening applications [23].

5.6 Functional plasma polymers

While early work on plasma polymers for biomedical applications was focused on properties such as wettability and protein adsorption, which is related to cell attachment and more generally biocompatibility as discussed above, more recent work has focused on a different approach. Essentially the idea here is that plasma polymers should be able to achieve the beneficial properties of polymer coatings that have been demonstrated by traditional polymer chemistry methods, such as graft polymerisation methods, in a one-step process.

An example for this functional plasma polymer approach is the application of coatings to reduce protein adsorption and cell attachment, as well as biofilm formation (compare Figure 5.2(b)). High-density PEG-based graft polymer coatings have been demonstrated to be effective in this application, as discussed above (compare Figure 5.5). Therefore, plasma polymers derived from monomers reflecting the monomer unit of poly(ethylene glycol), such as diethylene glycol dimethyl ether (diglyme), have been used. Typically deposited using low-power regimes to retain as much of the monomer unit as possible, these plasma polymer coatings have not only been demonstrated to reduce nonspecific protein adsorption and cell attachment but have also been used for the production of patterned coatings which can achieve spatially controlled cell attachment [24,25].

Another example for the functional plasma polymer approach is the deposition of *N*-isopropylacrylamide (NIPAM)-based plasma polymers. The thermoreversible nature of NIPAM-based polymers has been exploited in many biomedical applications, including drug-delivery and tissue culture applications. At physiological temperatures (above 32 °C), NIPAM-based polymers are hydrophobic, which in the case of NIPAM-grafted cell culture substrates leads to the adsorption of ECM proteins from the cell culture medium resulting in cell attachment and growth on the surface. However, when the temperature is reduced below the critical transition temperature of 32 °C, the NIPAM-grafted cell culture substrates become hydrophilic and cells are easily removed from the substrate together with the protein layer at the interface [26]. Okano et al. established an entire area of research and development in the area of regenerative medicine termed 'cell sheet engineering' based on the fact that confluent cell layers can be detached by cooling of cell culture substrates featuring radiation-grafted NIPAM-based polymer coatings [27]. Therefore, plasma polymers have been deposited based on NIPAM, the monomer unit used in NIPAM-based polymers. Again, the functional plasma polymer approach was demonstrated to be effective and coatings were obtained with good retention of the monomer side-chain functionality using low-power deposition conditions. Furthermore, cell adhesion and cell detachment tests also indicated that the surface switches between adhesive and nonadhesive behaviours as a function of temperature [28].

5.7 Antimicrobial plasma polymer coatings

Plasma polymer coatings have also been used to obtain antimicrobial properties [15]. The prevention of biofilm formation following the implantation of permanent and temporary medical devices in vivo is of outstanding importance, as biofilm-related infections associated with such devices remain a common complication in the clinic [29]. However, applications of antimicrobial coatings that prevent biofilm formation range across all industry sectors, from coatings on surfaces in the hospital environment to coatings on water filtration membranes. These coatings can be classified into those that release an antimicrobial agent and those that lead to contact killing. However, coatings providing reduced biofouling can also reduce the occurrence of biofilms due to the fact that the early stages of microbe attachment and colonisation are prevented.

Plasma polymers have been successfully used to produce effective antimicrobial coatings for example by incorporating silver nanoparticles into plasma polymer layers [30], leading to the subsequent slow release of silver ions as the antimicrobial species [31]. Other promising examples for plasma polymer-based antimicrobial coatings include the deposition of isopentyl nitrite-based plasma polymer coatings which lead to the release of nitric oxide at bacteriostatic concentrations [32]. Finally, plasma polymer coatings based on the monomer 1,8-cineole (a component in tea tree oil) have also been successfully and these coatings have shown to provide antimicrobial activity [33].

5.8 Likely future trends

Plasma-based surface modification methods have been extraordinarily successful in providing improved biocompatibility and cellular responses. The effectiveness, reproducibility, convenience and environmental benefits of using a plasma process in comparison to alternatives, such as solution-based processes, will ensure that this class of surface modification procedures will remain attractive to manufacturers in the future. However, the requirement of a vacuum process and the associated fact that a batch process is required have prevented even wider applications. It is therefore likely that the focus will shift further to plasma treatment options that do not require a vacuum and/or batch processing.

In the context of biomedical applications, it is expected that new areas of applications will be explored and adopted. Here, developments in plasma medicine, where a plasma process is used for therapeutic applications, is an example for such a nontraditional application.

In the case of cell culture substrate materials it is expected that, despite many new developments, plasma and corona discharge-based methods will dominate the market for many years to come based on the fact that the progression of many cell-based technologies (such as cell therapies) is highly dependent on cost-effective, highly consistent and chemically defined surfaces that allow companies to comply with the requirements of regulatory agencies.

Furthermore, it is likely that the proportion of surface modification procedures relying on plasma polymer interlayers (rather than simply coatings) will further increase. This is due to the increasingly sophisticated performance requirements in all biomedical products, which often cannot be achieved by a one-step process.

Finally, it is predicted that the functional groups accessed by plasma-based processes will be expanded much further in the future. Here, it is likely that the functional groups accessed will go beyond traditional functional groups (such as carboxylic acid and amine functional groups) and instead also include functional groups representing bioactive signals (such as small molecule mimetics). Again the drivers for this are the increasingly sophisticated performance requirements in all biomedical products.

5.9 Sources of further information

The field of plasma-based surface modification for biomedical applications is closely related to the field of biomaterials. Scientists in this field are represented by societies in Canada, the United States, the European Union, China, Japan, Korea, India and Australasia. The latest research results are shared at annual meetings of these societies. In addition, these societies are unified under the banner of the International Union of Societies for Biomaterials Science and Engineering [34] and a World Biomaterials Congress is held every four years to bring members from all of these societies together. Other conferences that are of particular interest include the American Vacuum Society meetings, which traditionally feature a symposium specifically related to the topic of this book chapter.

International journals that publish peer-reviewed articles on the topic of this book chapter include Biomaterials, Plasma Processes and Polymers, Journal of Biomedical Material Research, Polymer, Biomacromolecules, Macromolecules, Colloids and Surfaces B: Biointerfaces, Journal of Applied Polymer Science, Surface and Coatings Technology, to name just a few. References to some outstanding original articles and reviews from these and other journals pointing to further information have been provided above.

References

[1] K.D.G. Castner, B.D. Ratner, Biomedical surface science: foundations to frontiers, Surf. Sci. 500 (2002) 28–60.

[2] P. Koegler, A. Clayton, H. Thissen, G.N. Santos, P. Kingshott, The influence of nanostructured materials on biointerfacial interactions, Adv. Drug Deliv. Rev. 64 (2012) 1820–1839.

[3] B.D. Ratner, A.S. Hoffman, F.J. Schoen, J.E. Lemons (Eds.), Biomaterials Science, third ed., Elsevier, 2013.

[4] H. Yasuda, Plasma Polymerization, Academic Press, 1985.

[5] K.S. Siow, L. Britcher, S. Kumar, H.J. Griesser, Plasma methods for the generation of chemically reactive surfaces for biomolecule immobilization and cell colonization - a review, Plasma Process. Polym. 3 (2006) 392–418.

[6] T.R. Gengenbach, R.C. Chatelier, H.J. Griesser, Characterization of the ageing of plasma-deposited polymer films: global analysis of X-ray photoelectron spectroscopy data, Surf. Interface Anal. 24 (1996) 271–281.
[7] M. Eisenstein, Thinking outside the dish, Nat. Methods 3 (2006) 1035–1043.
[8] Z. Melkoumian, J.L. Weber, D.M. Weber, A.G. Fadeev, Y. Zhou, P. Dolley-Sonneville, J. Yang, L. Qiu, C.A. Priest, C. Shogbon, A.W. Martin, J. Nelson, P. West, J.P. Beltzer, S. Pal, R. Brandenberger, Synthetic peptide-acrylate surfaces for long-term self-renewal and cardiomyocyte differentiation of human embryonic stem cells, Nat. Biotechnol. 28 (2010) 606–610.
[9] D. Heckmann, H. Kessler, Design and chemical synthesis of integrin ligands, Meth. Enzymol. 426 (2007) 463–503.
[10] H.J. Griesser, P.G. Hartley, S.L. McArthur, K.M. McLean, L. Meagher, H. Thissen, Interfacial properties and protein resistance of nano-scale polysaccharide coatings, Smart Mater. Struct. 11 (2002) 652–661.
[11] P.G. Hartley, H. Thissen, T. Vaithianathan, H.J. Griesser, A surface masking technique for the determination of plasma polymer film thickness by AFM, Plasmas Polym. 5 (2000) 47–60.
[12] D. Sweeney (Ed.), Silicone Hydrogels. The Rebirth of Continuous Wear Contact Lenses, Butterworth Heinemann, 2000.
[13] M. Yoshida, R. Langer, A. Lendlein, J. Lahann, From advanced biomedical coatings to multi-functionalized biomaterials, J. Macromol. Sci. Polym. Rev. 46 (2006) 347–375.
[14] B.R. Coad, K.E. Styan, L. Meagher, One step ATRP initiator immobilization on surfaces leading to gradient-grafted polymer brushes, ACS Appl. Mater. Interfaces 6 (10) (May 28, 2014) 7782–7789.
[15] K. Bazaka, M. Jacob, W. Chrzanowski, K. Ostrikov, Anti-bacterial surfaces: natural agents, mechanisms of action, and plasma surface modification, RSC Adv. 5 (2015) 48739–48759.
[16] P. Kingshott, H. Thissen, H.J. Griesser, Effects of cloud point grafting, chain length, and density of PEG layers on competitive adsorption of ocular proteins, Biomaterials 23 (2002) 2043–2056.
[17] H. Thissen, J.P. Hayes, P. Kingshott, G. Johnson, E.C. Harvey, H.J. Griesser, Nanometer thickness laser ablation for spatial control of cell attachment, Smart Mater. Struct. 11 (2002) 792–799.
[18] H. Thissen, G. Johnson, P.G. Hartley, P. Kingshott, H.J. Griesser, Two-dimensional patterning of thin coatings for the control of tissue outgrowth, Biomaterials 27 (2006) 35–43.
[19] H. Thissen, T. Gengenbach, R. du Toit, D. Sweeney, P. Kingshott, H.J. Griesser, L. Meagher, Clinical observations of biofouling on PEO coated silicone hydrogel contact lenses, Biomaterials 31 (2010) 5510–5519.
[20] M.P. Lutolf, P.M. Gilbert, H.M. Blau, Designing materials to direct stem-cell fate, Nature 462 (2009) 433–441.
[21] R. Ogaki, M.A. Cole, D.S. Sutherland, P. Kingshott, Microcup arrays featuring multiple chemical regions patterned with nanoscale precision, Adv. Mater. 23 (2011) 1876–1881.
[22] D. Falconnet, G. Csucs, H.M. Grandin, M. Textor, Surface engineering approaches to micropattern surfaces for cell-based assays, Biomaterials 27 (2006) 3044–3063.
[23] L.R. Clements, H. Thissen, N.H. Voelcker, High throughput techniques for the investigation of cell–material interactions, in: D. Hutmacher, W. Chrzanowski (Eds.), Biointerfaces: Where Material Meets Biology, The Royal Society of Chemistry, 2014, pp. 257–311.

[24] Q. Cheng, S. Li, K. Komvopoulos, Plasma-assisted surface chemical patterning for single-cell culture, Biomaterials 30 (2009) 4203–4210.

[25] D.J. Menzies, T. Gengenbach, J.S. Forsythe, N. Birbilis, G. Johnson, C. Charles, G. McFarland, R.J. Williams, C. Fong, P. Leech, K. McLean, B.W. Muir, One step multifunctional micropatterning of surfaces using asymmetric glow discharge plasma polymerization, Chem. Commun. 48 (2012) 1907–1909.

[26] M.A. Cole, N.H. Voelcker, H. Thissen, H.J. Griesser, Stimuli-responsive interfaces and systems for the control of protein-surface and cell-surface interactions, Biomaterials 30 (2009) 1827–1850.

[27] T. Owaki, T. Shimizu, M. Yamato, T. Okano, Cell sheet engineering for regenerative medicine: current challenges and strategies, Biotechnol. J. 9 (2014) 904–914.

[28] X. Cheng, Y. Wang, Y. Hanein, K.F. Böhringer, B.D. Ratner, Novel cell patterning using microheater-controlled thermoresponsive plasma films, J. Biomed. Mat. Res. A 70 (2004) 159–168.

[29] M. Salwiczek, Y. Qu, J. Gardiner, R.A. Strugnell, T. Lithgow, K.M. McLean, H. Thissen, Emerging rules for effective antimicrobial coatings, Trends Biotechnol. 32 (2014) 82–90.

[30] L. Ploux, M. Mateescu, K. Anselme, K. Vasilev, Antibacterial properties of silver-loaded plasma polymer coatings, J. Nanomater. 2012 (2012) 9. Article ID 674145.

[31] S. Chernousova, M. Epple, Silver as antibacterial agent: ion, nanoparticle, and metal, Angew. Chem., Int. Ed. 52 (2013) 1636–1653.

[32] T.D. Michl, B.R. Coad, M. Doran, M. Osiecki, M.H. Kafshgari, N.H. Voelcker, A. Hüsler, K. Vasilev, H.J. Griesser, Nitric oxide releasing plasma polymer coating with bacteriostatic properties and no cytotoxic side effects, Chem Commun. (Camb) 51 (2015) 7058–7060.

[33] A. Pegalajar-Jurado, C.D. Easton, K.E. Styan, S.L. McArthur, Antibacterial activity studies of plasma polymerised cineole films, J. Mater. Chem. B 2 (2014) 4993–5002.

[34] www.worldbiomaterials.org.

Stent coatings for blood compatibility

6

K. Udipi
Biopolymer Designs Inc., Santa Rosa, CA, USA

6.1 Introduction

Stents are small, mesh-like tubular devices made of metal or polymer (Figure 6.1) implanted to restore blood flow in blocked arteries. Excessive build-up of plaque over time, and also its hardening and rupture, block the flow of oxygen-rich blood to the heart muscle, leading to myocardial infarction (heart attack).

Surgical intervention in the form of coronary artery bypass grafting (CABG), commonly referred to as bypass surgery, was by far the most favoured mode of restoring blood flow to the heart muscle. In this procedure, a blood vessel is removed from one area of the body and placed around the area or areas of narrowing to 'bypass' the blockages and restore blood flow. However, the procedure is quite invasive, causing pain, bleeding and trauma, and with the potential for infection. It can also involve an extended hospital stay and hence be expensive.

6.2 Stent development

A less invasive interventional procedure called percutaneous transluminal coronary angioplasty (PTCA), developed by Gruentzig (1978), to open up blocked arteries quickly gained favour over bypass surgeries, and the latter were only carried out in

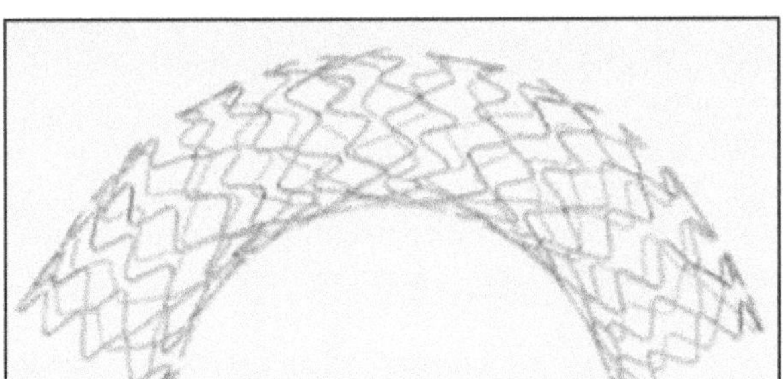

Figure 6.1 Image of a balloon-expandable bare-metal stent.
Courtesy: Medtronic Cardiovascular.

Biosynthetic Polymers for Medical Applications. http://dx.doi.org/10.1016/B978-1-78242-105-4.00006-7

more complex cases. In the PTCA procedure, a catheter with a balloon tip is introduced into an artery generally at the groin or wrist and threaded to the lesion site. The balloon, upon inflation, compresses and flattens the plaque to the arterial wall and restores blood flow. The treated arteries, however, have a tendency to collapse and block the blood flow. In several randomised clinical trials involving PTCA versus CABG, although there was no significant difference in the mortality rates, repeat revascularisation was required much more frequently ($\sim$50% of cases) for PTCA as compared to CABG ($\sim$25%) (Kalynych and King, 1995; King et al., 1994). In order to get around this problem, stents were loaded on balloons and upon deployment would hold the arteries open.

First-generation stents were fabricated from stainless steel. The stent struts were rather thick ($\sim$140 μm) and were adequately radio-opaque to facilitate placement with the aid of radiography. Stent designs have evolved over the years, and there is an ongoing effort to reduce strut thickness, employing stronger cobalt chromium alloys or other alloys containing highly radio-opaque metals like platinum or tungsten. With these thinner struts and suitable design modifications, it is now possible to produce stents that have a high degree of flexibility that was not feasible with thicker stainless steel struts. These changes have also made it possible to treat lesions in highly tortuous arterial settings.

Whereas the stents described above remain in a patient's body all through a patient's lifetime, it is now believed that the stent support is needed only until the arterial segment regains its normal vascular function. Therefore, a bioabsorbable stent would be desirable if it offers the support when needed and then degrades and gets metabolised (Ormiston and Serruys, 2009; Onuma and Serruys, 2011; Gonzalo and Macaya, 2012; Patel and Banning, 2013). This has a number of potential advantages including restoration of normal vasomotor function and physiological responses to stress/exercise and mitigating the long-term consequences related to inflammation, accelerated atherosclerosis and thrombosis. Furthermore, it would allow for revascularisation when required without having to place a stent within a stent.

Bioabsorbable stents are either fabricated from a degradable metal-like magnesium or from a range of bioabsorbable polymers. Magnesium stents studied thus far tend to degrade rapidly and fail to provide the support when needed, leading to some adverse reactions (Haude et al., 2013; Campos et al., 2013; Bowen et al., 2014). Bioabsorbable polymer-based stents, on the other hand, look promising, although the degradation time could approach 2–3 years depending on the polymer and the stent design (Oberhauser et al., 2009; Onuma et al., 2009; Serruys et al., 2009; Gomez-Lara et al., 2010). These polymeric stents are compatible with magnetic resonance imaging, thus avoid employing harmful X-ray radiation during implantation and follow-up procedures.

There are two types of stents: balloon expandable and self-expandable. The former, as described earlier, is loaded on a crimped balloon at the tip of a catheter and is deployed at the lesion site by inflating the balloon. Most coronary stents tend to be balloon expandable and vary in size from 2 to 4 mm in diameter and from 9 to 32 mm in length. The self-expandable stents, made from nitinol wires, are crimped and packed under tension in a plastic sheath. The stent is deployed upon slow removal of the constraint (sheath) at the lesion site. They tend to be larger about 6 mm in diameter and 20–200 mm in length and mostly employed in peripheral applications.

6.3 Thrombosis issue

Thrombosis is a serious issue in patients after stent implantation due to morbidity and mortality (Figure 6.2) (Farb et al., 2003). Patients are required to follow a regimen of relatively expensive antiplatelet therapy for about 90 days to cope with the thrombotic risks. A number of factors lead to thrombus formation, and it seems pertinent to understand the sequence of events taking place when blood comes in contact with a surface and the factors influencing thrombus formation.

6.3.1 Factors influencing thrombus formation

Blood is a complex system consisting of cellular elements suspended in plasma. In addition to the red and white blood cells, blood contains a sizeable population of platelets, which are tiny fragments of cells with no nucleus but rich in enzymes and chemicals necessary for the function of clotting or forming thrombus. Platelets are extremely sensitive, and upon contact with a foreign object or surface get activated. Activation causes platelets to change shape to irregular spheres (Hanson and Tucker, 2013) and secrete sticky granules containing adenosine diphosphate, leading to irreversible platelet aggregation and formation of a fused platelet thrombus. The bloodstream also carries soluble globular proteins and traces of inorganic ions, nutrients, enzymes and hormones. Proteins get deposited instantaneously on a surface upon contact with blood (Vroman, 1988). This process is dynamic in that the adsorbed protein deposition depends on the coating surface characteristics, for example, surface roughness or lack thereof (Hulander et al., 2013); and the chemical composition, specifically electrostatic and hydrophobic interactions and the local increase in entropy due to the displacement

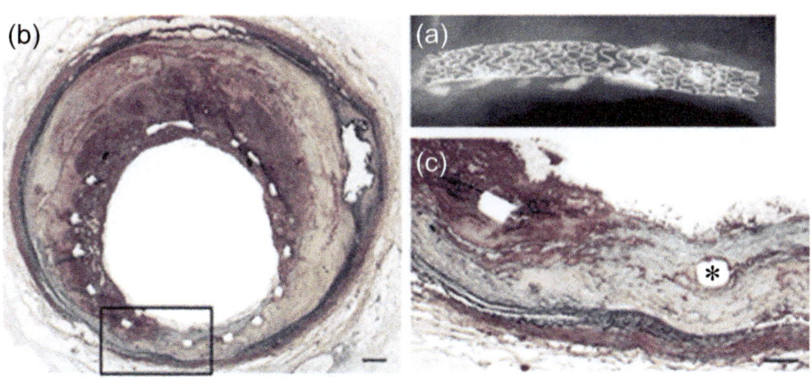

Figure 6.2 A bare-metal stent (a), fibrin-rich nonocclusive mural thrombus (b) focally present between the stent and the underlying vessel (c) (Farb et al., 2003).

of water molecules and counterions from the surface (Andrade and Hlady, 1986). Fibrinogen among these is an important protein from the viewpoint of thrombus formation. It is a precursor for fibrin, an insoluble protein formed by the enzymatic activity of thrombin. Fibrin can bind to activated platelets and enhance aggregation. Fibrin-mediated thrombus formation seems to be more prevalent in the low-shear venous system while the platelet system is dominant in high-shear arterial blood flow.

6.3.2 Passive coatings for blood compatibility

Polymer-based passive coatings seem like a valid approach to circumvent these two problems. Several biosynthetic polymers with good antithrombogenic properties have been studied and reported in the literature.

They seem to broadly follow three mechanisms. These are the minimisation of (1) protein and platelet adsorption, (2) thrombin and fibrin formation or (3) platelet activation and aggregation (Jordan and Chaikof, 2007).

6.3.2.1 Minimisation of protein and platelet adsorption

Coating surfaces can be hydrophilic, hydrophobic or amphiphilic. Those that are highly hydrophilic, like hydrogels; or those that are highly hydrophobic, like silicone and fluoropolymer surfaces, exhibit low levels of thrombus formation because they do not promote protein adsorption (Brash, 1977; Hoffman et al., 1997) . In view of the good thromboresistant properties of extremely hydrophobic surfaces like silicones and fluoropolymers, they are used quite extensively in such blood-contacting devices as covered stent grafts. Attempts have been made to explain the thromboresistant properties of these extremely hydrophobic polymer surfaces on the basis of their low surface-free energies. Being water repellent, they could potentially inhibit protein adsorption; or alternately. they could favour adsorption of inert proteins like albumin (Kim et al., 1974; Eberhart et al., 1987).

Hydrophilic polymer surfaces with very low surface-free energies have also been successfully used in blood-contacting applications. Studies have demonstrated that polyethylene oxide (PEO) has among the lowest levels of protein or cellular adsorption of any known polymer, and the same is attributed to the hydrophilic ether linkage in the structural repeat unit and its property to present a 'liquid-like' surface with highly mobile molecular chains exhibiting no systematic molecular order (Jordan and Chaikof, 2007). Thus, PEO with low interfacial surface energy with water, high surface mobility and steric stabilisation effect is by far one of the most studied in this context (Merril and Salzman, 1983; Lee et al., 1989; Mori et al., 1982). Covalent grafting of PEO to hydrophobic surfaces is expected to be a more efficient method to maintain a hydrophilic character for extended periods of time. Mori et al. (1982) demonstrated that grafting PEO to polyvinyl chloride suppressed protein adsorption and platelet adhesion.

Hydrogels have exhibited excellent resistance to protein adsorption and hence their thromboresistant properties. Hydrogels based on poly(acrylamide), poly(hydroxyethyl methacrylate), poly(*N*-vinyl pyrrlidinone) and poly(vinyl alcohol) have demonstrated resistance to protein adsorption. Attempts to graft hydrophilic polymers onto hydrophobic surfaces like silicones (Ratner et al., 1979) and polyethylene (Hayashi et al., 1985) have remarkably reduced fibrinogen adsorption. Such reduction has been shown to increase with increasing hydrophilic content on the surface.

Passive coatings based on biosynthetic polymers like phosphorylcholine, modified elastin and albumin have been explored to minimise protein and cellular adsorption.

Phosphoryl choline is a member of the phospholipid family. Phospholipids consist of a glyceride backbone with attached zwitterionic choline 'head' group and a long-chain hydrophobic fatty acid 'tail.' Phospholipids, by virtue of their unique amphiphilic structure, tend to self-assemble into membranes that constitute the outer surface of most cells in the body and have been shown to limit protein and cell adhesion (Tegoulia et al., 2001; Lu et al., 2001; Andersson et al., 2003). However, phospholipid films are not very stable in aqueous solutions and tend to delaminate. Attempts have been made to stabilise them and generate thromboresistant coatings by bonding to peptides (Kaladhar and Shrama, 2004, 2006) or heat stabilising at 80 °C (Stine et al., 2005). Modifying phospholipids into polymerisable monomers and subsequent polymerisation has also produced some interesting coatings resistant to protein and cell adhesion (Stine et al., 2005; Marra et al., 1997; Orban et al., 2000; Ross et al., 2003; Kim et al., 2005).

Elastin modification of polymer surfaces: Elastin, a structural protein in the vascular lining, is expected to elicit minimal platelet adsorption and adhesion. Inherent insolubility and difficulties in purifying have led to synthesising polymers with amino acid sequences mimicking those in elastin. Silicone polymers photochemically linked to poly(VPGVG) exhibited reduced fibrinogen and immunoglobulin adsorption *in vitro* and decreased release of proinflammatory cytokines by monocytes (Delfife et al., 1999).

Albumin-treated polymer surfaces: Early studies (Lyman et al., 1970; Kim et al., 1974; Park et al., 1986) have shown that platelets have a considerably lower tendency to adhere to albumin coatings than, for example, fibrinogen or gamma globulin. Hence attempts have been made to modify polymer surfaces with albumin in order to improve thromboresistance. Immobilisation of albumin on polymer surfaces through plasma treatment (Ishikawa et al., 1984; Kang et al., 1993) and gamma radiation (Kamath and Park, 1994) have produced interesting results. Introduction of tethered acyl functionality on polymer surfaces helped binding of albumin from circulating blood selectively (Eberhart, 1987; Frautschi et al., 1996). Gluteraldehyde crosslinked albumin coating on Dacron showed promising results in terms of reduced platelet and leukocyte adhesion and aggregation *in vitro* (Guidoin et al., 1976, 1983; Kottke-Marchant et al., 1989), but in clinical studies the albumin-coated aortic prosthesis behaved no differently than uncoated controls (Al-Kattaf and Chatsworth, 1996; Kudo et al., 2002).

6.3.2.2 Minimisation of thrombin and fibrin formation

Heparin coatings: Heparin has been known as a potent anticoagulant. It is a highly sulphated glycosaminoglycan and has the highest negative charge density of any known biological molecule. It is known to form a complex with antithrombin III and bind with thrombin to produce the non-thrombogenic effect. Non-thrombogenic coatings can be prepared by either immobilising heparin on the surface by strong ionic binding or by chemical grafting. Thus heparin with sulphate groups can bind with cationic polymer surfaces and become immobilised (Hubbell, 1993; Olsson et al., 2000; Tanzi, 2005; Gore et al., 2014). Alternately, a cationic polymer or oligomer can be covalently bound to a polymer surface and then reacted with heparin to promote strong intermolecular ionic bonds (Sperling et al., 2005). The presence of a spacer molecule like flexible PEO between the cationic polymers and heparin seems to enhance the amount of heparin binding several folds (Chen et al., 2005; Wang et al., 2006; Yang et al., 2014). Heparin-loaded silk fibroin coatings and heparin-immobilised nanofibers have also demonstrated a reduced tendency for platelet adhesion (Cestari et al., 2014). Antithrombin–heparin complex immobilisation on a gold surface with a PEG spacer molecule seemed to show reduced platelet adhesion and prolonged clotting times (Sask et al., 2011). Polyether sulphone membranes, upon heparin immobilisation on a surface, demonstrated improved antithrombogenic properties. Santerre et al. (1989) also pointed out based on their studies that the non-thrombogenic effect of sulphonate groups on the surface are a result of their inhibitory effect on the polymerisation of fibrinogen to fibrin.

Hirudin, a polypeptide, is known to exert antithrombin activity. A recombinant version (rHirudin) was crosslinked with gluteraldehyde onto a biodegradable polylactide-co-glycolide (PLGA), and the resulting coating exhibited significantly prolonged periods of nonactivated partial thromboplastin times, and a decreased clot formation rate of whole blood compared to PLGA. rHirudin immobilised on Dacron and polyurethane with albumin base coats exhibited antithrombin activity (Phaneuf et al., 1997, 1998). rHirudin attached to an acrylamide-grafted polytetrafluoroethylene (PTFE) surface showed improved blood compatibility compared to untreated PTFE (Onder et al., 2011). Employing PEG as a spacer during immobilisation of rHirudin seemed to show greater biological activity (thrombin binding and inhibition) despite having a lower density of hirudin (Alibeik et al., 2010). Bivalirudin (BV), derived from hirudin, immobilised on gold with a polydopamine base coat showed prolonged thromboplastin and prothrombin times and significantly inhibited activation of platelets and fibrinogen (Lu et al., 2012).

Thrombomodulin (TM) is an endothelial glycoprotein that binds thrombin, activates protein C and delays clot formation. Thus a sequential and ordered immobilisation of TM and endothelial protein C receptor on a polyurethane surface increased anticoagulant activation and time to clot formation (Kador and Subramanian, 2011). Improvements in the antithrombogenic properties of PTFE were achieved by immobilising TM by various methods (Sperling et al., 1997, 2005; Qu et al., 2014). Multifunctional bilayer polymeric coatings prepared with both controlled nitric oxide (NO) release and surface-bound active TM alone or in combination with immobilised heparin on siloxane-based polyurethane mimic the highly thromboresistant endothelium layer (Wu et al., 2007).

Thromboresistant properties of a group of synthetic polymers that are amphiphilic have also been studied and the results have been encouraging. These polymers, consisting of covalently bonded alternating triblocks or segmented multiblocks of hydrophilic and hydrophobic polymers, have demonstrated good resistance to thrombus build-up. These multiblock copolymers, due to their mutual incompatibility, phase separate and form domains of hydrophobic and hydrophilic character. Depending on the constituent monomers, these domains can exhibit differing surface-free energies, crystallinities and also surface charges. Studies on amphiphilc polymers showed that protein deposition is largely determined by the nature of phase morphology. Thus a triblock copolymer, polyhydroxyethyl methacrylate (HEMA)-styrene (S)-polyhydroxyethyl methacrylate (HEMA), coating on a conventional poly (ester-urethane) with a highly ordered lamellar structure exhibited less protein and platelet adhesion compared to the poly(HEMA)-PDMS-poly(HEMA) triblock copolymer in an arteriovenous (A-V) shunt application (Okano et al., 1978, 1981, 1986). Similarly, block copolymers composed of crystalline and amorphous segments also seem to influence platelet adhesion.

Polyion complexes formed from poly(trimethylammonium)ethyl styrene bromide and poly(sodium styrenesulphonate) seemed to allow platelet adhesion but the degree of deformation was suppressed (Kataoka et al., 1980). Poly(tertieryamine) grafted on poly(HEMA) exhibited a microphase-separated structure and weak cell interaction (Nishimura et al., 1982).

6.3.2.3 Minimisation of platelet activation

Several small molecules have been explored in efforts to minimise platelet activation and adhesion. Among the small molecules, oral thienopyridine-class compounds like clopidogrel and ticlopidine are widely prescribed to patients with stent placement. Along with aspirin, these compounds have proven to be effective in minimising thrombotic risks (Müller et al., 2000).

Local delivery of NO released from polymeric substrates has also been explored to inhibit platelet activation. It is immobilised on a polymer surface containing secondary amine groups by a process known as diazenium diolation. Immobilisation on hydrophobic surfaces does not seem to carry the risk of generating carcinogenic nitrosoamines observed in some hydrophilic substrates (Bohl and West, 2000; Mowery et al., 2000).

Immobilising antiplatelet compounds like prostacyclins and prostaglandins on a wide variety of polymer surfaces, ranging from albuminated polycarbonate to polyesters like polyethylene terephthalate, has resulted in the inhibition of platelet adhesion (Joseph and Sharma, 1987; Chandy and Sharma, 1984).

6.3.2.4 Testing for blood compatibility

Blood compatibility of coatings can be evaluated *in vitro* and *in vivo*. Expectedly, *in vitro* tests tend to be of shorter duration and the results are influenced by the blood source, the manner in which they are handled, and the level of anticoagulants used. They provide adequate information in screening materials for medical applications but are not very valuable in predicting long-term performance as *in vivo* tests.

In a typical *in vitro* test, a coated specimen is immersed in citrated human blood and the platelets adhering to the surface are counted and their morphology examined (Waples et al., 1996). Platelet morphology can be examined at the end of the test by any number of methods, including light microscopy, scanning or transmission electron microscopy or fluorescent methods. Activated platelets are differentiated from unactivated by their morphologies. Non-activated platelets generally appear as discoids, and those activated are dendritic and spread more. In a more relevant method, citrated or heparinised blood is circulated through a tubular device where the tubing is coated with the polymer being tested (Haycox and Ratner, 1993; Kottke-Marchant et al., 1985) and the adhering platelets counted and their morphologies examined.

In vivo tests involve inserting coated tubes or rings in arteries or veins of experimental animals like dogs, pigs, rabbits or baboons for short or long periods of time (Hanson et al., 1980; Sefton et al., 2000). A-V or arterio–arterio (A-A) shunts can be employed where the coated tubing specimen is inserted as a part of the blood loop. Results from studies with baboons are more useful, since they are haematologically similar to humans. At the end of the test period, information gathered – such as the amount of local thrombus accumulation, consumption of circulating platelets and fibrinogen, and plasma levels of factors released by platelets and coagulation proteins during thrombosis and embolisation of microthrombi to downstream circulatory beds – is very valuable in assessing the blood compatibility of coating.

6.3.2.5 Passive coatings on stents: clinical study results

Attempts have been made to improve blood compatibility of stents through a passive coating approach. A few biosynthetic polymer coatings like those based on phosphorylcholine and heparin, and some inorganic coatings like gold, titanium nitride, silicon carbide and diamond-like carbon coatings, have been evaluated in clinical trials. Results from clinical trials are inconclusive, however (Colombo and Airoldi, 2003).

In a 100-patient trial, a phosphorylcholine coating produced no acute or subacute thrombosis, but at six-month follow-up major adverse events added up to 13% and the angiographic restenosis rate was 12% (Galli et al., 2000). In the Italian BiodivYsio 218-patient stent trial, except for one death on day 7 due to subacute occlusion, a majority of patients were asymptomatic. No cases of thrombosis were recorded at the six-month follow-up, suggesting that the coating seemed to be thromboresistant (Galli et al., 2001). However, in a third trial with 425 patients, the six-month death rate was high, at 3.8%, and the restenosis rate was 17.7% (Boland et al., 2000).

Heparin coating has been tried as an alternative to counterbalance intrinsic stent thrombogenicity and to decrease the incidence of stent thrombosis (Mehran et al., 2005). Thus a heparin-coated stent was compared against the bare-metal version of the same design in a total of 3098 patients at high risk for stent thrombosis. At the 30-day end-point, stent thrombosis occurred in 0.6% of the 1417 patients treated with the heparin-coated stent and in 0.9% of the 1681 patients treated with the bare-metal stent (relative risk reduction 33%, $P = 0.41$). The rates of cardiac death, myocardial infarction and target lesion revascularisation did not differ significantly between the groups. In a separate small-vessel study, heparin-coated stents performed similarly to the bare-metal stents, and hence the results were inconclusive.

6.4 Drug-eluting stent coatings

When a stent, whether balloon or self-expandable, is deployed in an artery – as in the case of angioplasty, discussed earlier – the deployment force tends to be quite robust to injure the delicate endothelium. The stent in this case prevents the collapse of the vessel, but a cascade of biological events leads to reblockage known as restenosis. That is, the artery gets stenosed again to block the blood flow. Such blockage in this case is due to the body's response. Platelets get aggregated and activated leading to inflammation. Smooth muscle cells migrate to the injury site and proliferate, and in the process block passage of blood. This restenosis process makes revascularisation(s) inevitable. Passive coatings, despite being biocompatible and potentially non-thrombogenic, have not been able to inhibit restenosis. Local delivery of an anti-proliferative drug from a polymer coating has proven to alleviate to a very large measure the reblockage or restenosis. Indeed, once-common bypass surgeries have given way to the current standard of care: the drug-eluting stent (DES). Target lesion revascularisations are still prevalent, but such incidences have been reduced from about 15 to 20% for earlier modalities like balloon angioplasty and bare-metal stents to single digits. These impressive results are predicated on the controlled but sustained release of drug over an extended period of time.

Two classes of drugs have been successfully employed in this connection: (1) the limus family of antimitotic drugs like sirolimus, everolimus and zotarolimus, among others, which arrest the cell-cycle progression in the G1 phase (Poon et al., 1996) and (2) paclitaxel, a microtubule-stabilising drug that interrupts mitotic division in the late metaphase, which results in arresting the cell-cycle (Axel et al., 1997). Several other drugs have been explored, but with only limited success.

Selecting or designing a polymer for application as a DES coating demands careful consideration (Udipi et al., 2008) (Figure 6.3). First and foremost, the polymer has to

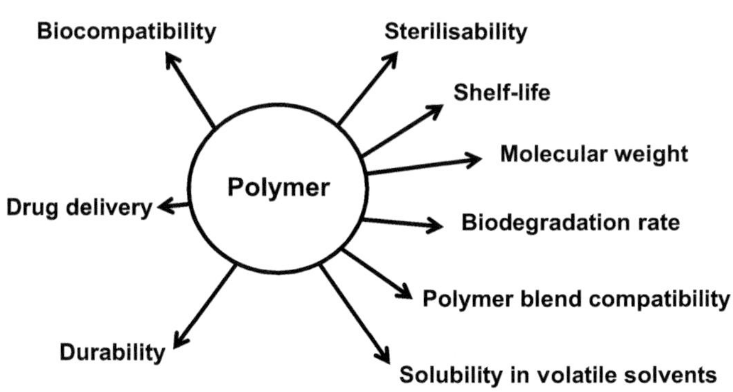

Figure 6.3 Polymer property requirements for a stent coating.

be biocompatible, that is, it should not elicit inflammatory response and minimise the risk of thrombosis. Blood compatibility is an important property for a stent coating, but the injury resulting during the implantation and the sequelae of events leading to restenosis demands that the coating also elute an anti-proliferative drug in a controlled and sustained manner. This feature adds additional constraints on selecting a polymer. It has to be compatible with the drug such that the drug becomes uniformly distributed in the coating to offer controlled elution. Since both of the classes of anti-proliferative drugs mentioned are highly hydrophobic, the polymers necessarily have to be hydrophobic to meet this criterion. But the blood and the environment in the vasculature being hydrophilic, a certain degree of hydrophilicity incorporated into the polymer architecture helps modulate the interfacial tension and the adverse response. The glass transition temperature of the polymer greatly influences the amount of drug eluted at any given instant. The polymer should be adequately elastomeric to withstand the stent crimping and expansion and yet provide a robust coating with excellent adhesion to the metal surface. Poor adhesion leads to delamination (Figure 6.4) and the fragments generated can elicit inflammatory response. If the polymers employed are bioabsorbable, the degradation rate and the nature of the degradation products are important. Degradation products should not react with the drug or lead to a fast rise in local acidity. The latter can cause inflammation. It is also important that the polymer has to be manufactured reproducibly and meet several other criteria.

A large number of DES have gained approval from regulatory bodies in the United States, Europe, Japan and several other countries, and some of them are listed in Table 6.1.

6.4.1 Current drug-eluting stent coatings

Drug-eluting stents have evolved over the past 12 years since their first introduction in the device field both in terms of stent design and the type of polymer used. With regard to drugs, paclitaxel is rarely ever used anymore, relegating the space to sirolimus and its various analogues. First and second-generation stent coatings are based

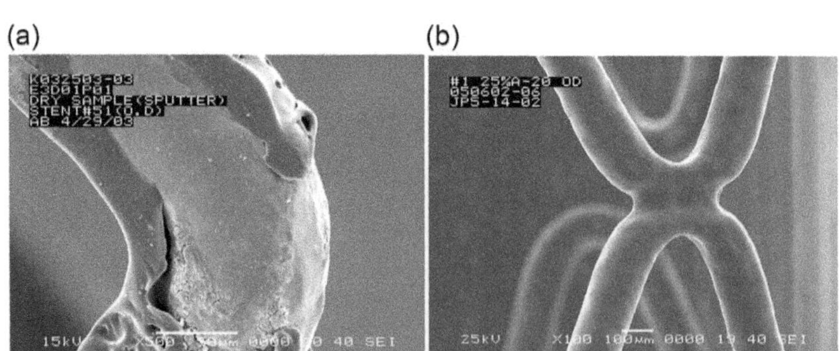

Figure 6.4 Images of (a) delaminating and (b) robust stent coatings.
Courtesy: Medtronic Cardiovascular.

Table 6.1 Various drug-eluting stents marketed around the world

Drug-eluting stent	Company	Drug	Polymer
Cypher	Cordis	Sirolimus	PEVA + PBMA
Taxus	Boston Scientific	Paclitaxel	S-IB-S
Endeavor	Medtronic	Zotarolimus	Phosphorylcholine
Xience	Abbott	Everolimus	Fluoropolymer
Resolute	Medtronic	Zotarolimus	BioLinx®
Biomatrix	Biosensors	Biolimus A-9	PLA
Nobori	Terumo	Biolimus A-9	PLA
Supralimus	Shahajanand	Sirolimus	PLA + PLGA
Infinium	Shahajanand	Paclitaxel	PLA + PLGA
DeSyne	Elixir	Novolimus	PLA
BioMime	Meril Life Sciences	Sirolimus	PLA + PLGA
Excel	JW Medical	Sirolimus	PLA

on biostable polymers, although bioabsorbable polymers are increasingly being used in second- and next-generation DES.

Current stent coatings are mostly limited to DES, which constitute a very large fraction of the stents marketed, with a smaller share captured by bare-metal stents. Stents with only passive coatings such as phosphorylcholine or titanium nitride form a much smaller segment. Some of the salient features of the current stent coatings follow.

6.4.1.1 First-generation stents

Cypher®: This Cordis sirolimus-eluting coronary stent was the first DES introduced in the market, but has since been discontinued. The biostable polymer employed to elute sirolimus was a blend of poly(ethylene-co-vinyl acetate) (PEVA) and poly(*n*-butyl methacrylate) (PBMA). Although both PBMA and PEVA were known to be biocompatible and had a long history of use in medical applications, Cypher application was the first of its kind for a cardiovascular stent. The BX Velocity® stent was coated with Parylene C® to improve the adhesion of the subsequent drug-polymer coating. A PBMA cap-coat was then applied to provide controlled drug elution (Parker et al., 2010; Wolf et al., 2008).

Taxus®: This Boston Scientific DES uses a polystyrene (PS)–polyisobutylene(PIB)–PS triblock thermoplastic elastomer to elute paclitaxel. The metal stents that form the base are either Express® or Liberté® stents. The morphology of these copolymers consists of a microphase-separated structure that exists at the nanoscale (Pinchuk et al., 2008; Ranade et al., 2004, 2005). Relative weight percentages of the soft rubbery PIB and hard PS components determine the morphologies to be spherical, lamellar or cylindrical depending on composition.

It is apparent that the polymers employed both in Cypher® and Taxus® are hydrophobic.

Endeavor®: The polymer used by Medtronic in its first-generation DES, Endeavor® is based on phosphorylcholine. A cobalt chromium modular stent forms the base and employs zotarolimus as the anti-proliferative drug. Zotarolimus is a version of sirolimus, similar in structure but with the hydroxyl group at the C40 position substituted by a tetrazole group. The phosphorylcholine polymer used in Endeavor® is a phospholipid mimic (Hayward and Chapman, 1984; Hunter and Angelini, 1993; Lewis et al., 2001) in that it is synthesised from methacryloyl phopsphorylcholine and lauryl methacrylate along with hydroxypropyl methacrylate and trimethoxysilyl methacrylate.

The phosphorylcholine groups provide the charged hydrophilic 'head' groups and the lauryl chains, the hydrophobic 'tails.' The hydroxypropyl groups confer additional hydrophilic character. The polymer does not exhibit enough strength on its own and requires a high degree of crosslinking to exhibit adequate strength. Hence TMSA is incorporated to form an integral part of the polymer. The coating is crosslinked with heat and gamma radiation. The subsequent drug coating has a high drug load and only about 10% of polymer and an ultrathin over-sprayed protein C coating. As a result, the entire drug load gets released in about 21 days leaving behind a biomimetic coating on the stent surface.

6.4.1.2 Second-generation stents

Xience V®: Abbot Vascular's stent employs a biostable, semicrystalline fluorocopolymer, poly(vinylidene fluoride-co-hexafluoropropylene) (PVDF-HFP), to elute a limus drug, everolimus. Everolimus is similar in structure to sirolimus, but the hydroxyl group at the C40 position is replaced by a hydroxyl ethyl group. The polymer has a molecular weight in the range of 254,000–293,000, and although it has a low degree of crystallinity, it exhibits high elasticity (>600% elongation). The wide-angle X-ray scattering data showed that the bulk PVDF-HFP copolymer in Xience V® has an α-crystalline structure and is similar to that observed for the PVDF-HFP coating (Xu, 2009). Differential scanning calorimetry of the stent coating, without the drug, shows a melting endotherm due to the crystalline phase of the polymer at approximately 100 °C. The presence of everolimus in the polymer does not alter the crystallinity or the melting point of PVDF-HFP. The base stent is multilink, fabricated from a medical-grade L605 cobalt-chromium alloy. The stent is coated first with a ~1 μ thick primer coating of PBMA to improve the adhesion of drug coating to the stent surface.

Resolute®: Medtronic's next DES has a proprietary Biolinx® polymer-based coating on a sinusoidal cobalt chromium Integrity® stent over a Parylene C® primer and employs the same Zotarolimus® drug as in the Endeavor® DES. BioLinx® is comprised of a blend of three different polymers: a 95/5 butyl methacrylate–vinyl acetate copolymer, 77/18/5 hexyl methacrylate-vinyl pyrrolidinone-vinyl acetate terpolymer and polyvinyl pyrrolidinone.

The BioLinx® polymer system was designed to exhibit similar, predominantly hydrophilic properties as Endeavor®'s PC polymer. C19 contains enough vinyl pyrrolidinone units to exhibit a hydrophilic character. C10 is hydrophobic, but the two polymers are compatible with each other in all proportions, thus producing blends devoid of phase separation (Udipi et al., 2008; Hezi-Yamit et al., 2009; Carter et al., 2006; Taniwaki et al., 2014).

6.4.1.3 Drug-eluting stents with bioabsorbable polymer coatings

Currently there are a large number of DES marketed in Europe and elsewhere (Table 6.1) with bioabsorbable polymer coatings (Jain, 2000; Gambhir, 2006; Grube, 2008; Meredith et al., 2012). Most of these coatings are based on polylactic acid (PLLA and PDLA) and/or copolymers of lactic and glycolic acids (PLGA) with various L/G ratios. The incentive to use bioabsorbable polymers appears to be that upon complete polymer degradation, a bare-metal surface is presented in the vasculature. This is believed to shorten the dual antiplatelet therapy predicated on shorter degradation times. PLLA, being a crystalline polymer, invariably takes a long time to completely degrade. PDLA, being an amorphous polymer, appears to be a better choice from the point of view of degradation time. PLGA polymer tends to degrade fast, but higher glycolic acid contents, while speeding up the degradation, can increase the local acid concentration and lead to inflammation and related adverse reactions.

However, cases of thrombosis related to DES remain a concern, and it is imperative that such polymer coatings are blood compatible.

6.4.2 Thrombotic risks related to drug-eluting stents

Gains in reduced revascularisations with DES seem to have come at the cost of higher incidences of stent thrombosis. It is not unique for DES to exhibit stent thrombosis, since bare-metal stents also are prone to this problem albeit to a lesser extent. Stents, being foreign bodies next to the vessel wall, induce platelet adhesion and activation of the coagulation cascade. Also, the high-pressure deployment of stents with noncompliant balloons causes considerable vascular injury, leading to the exposure of thrombogenic molecules of the subintima and media to the bloodstream. Dual antiplatelet therapy with aspirin ($\geq$75 mg) and clopidogrel (75 mg) is therefore recommended for extended periods after the intervention for patients with DES and for shorter periods ($\sim$90 days) for bare-metal stent recipients. Although the incidence of stent thrombosis is observed in about 0.5–2% of patients, the clinical impact is huge due to the high risk of myocardial infarction and high rates ($\sim$45%) of mortality (Iakovou et al., 2005).

Various factors listed in Table 6.2 (Kirtane and Stone, 2011) are believed to cause stent thrombosis in general and in DES in particular. It is a complex process, and polymeric coatings among others play an important role in such critical steps as presenting

Table 6.2 Potential mechanisms of DES thrombosis (Kirtane and Stone, 2011)

Patient-related factors relating to increased thrombogenicity
Smoking
Diabetes mellitus
Chronic kidney disease
Acute coronary syndrome presentation
Thrombocytosis
High posttreatment platelet reactivity
Premature discontinuation or cessation of dual antiplatelet therapy
Surgical procedures (unrelated to the percutaneous coronary intervention (PCI))
Lesion-based factors relating to rheology/thrombogenicity within stents
Diffuse coronary artery disease with long stented segments
Small vessel disease
Bifurcation disease
Thrombus-containing lesions
Significant inflow or outflow lesions proximal or distal to the stented segment
Stent-related factors
Poor stent expansion
Edge dissections limiting inflow or outflow
Delayed or absent endothelialization of stent struts
Hypersensitivity/inflammatory and/or thrombotic reactions to DES polymers
Strut fractures
Late malapposition/aneurysm formation
Development of neoatherosclerosis within stents with new plaque rupture

a noninflammatory surface and promoting a speedy and functional reendothelialization (Lüscher et al., 2007; Cieffo et al., 2004; Finn et al., 2005; Fujii et al., 2005; Kereiakes et al., 2004; Kolandaivelu et al., 2011; Palmerini et al., 2013). Biostable polymers remain in the body well after all of the drug gets eluted and hence play an important role in determining the thrombotic potential. If they tend to be inflammatory, the hypersensitivity reactions that they generate predispose the stents to late and very late stent thrombosis. In the case of bioabsorbable polymers, if they degrade and get metabolised about the time the drug gets exhausted, the stent would then behave more like a bare-metal stent. An underlining feature of a stent coating has to be good blood compatibility in modulating thrombotic potential.

Results from a number of clinical trials and anecdotal reports from clinicians have documented the problem of thrombosis at various stages following stent implantation and of varying severity. In order to compare the true rates of stent thrombosis across different trials and registries, a new standard definition was proposed by an Academic Research Consortium (ARC), which is composed of clinical investigators, industrial representatives and regulators including the Food and Drug Administration (Cutlip et al., 2007). The definition categorises stent thrombosis according to the level of documentation and timing:

- Definite or confirmed event (symptoms suggestive of an acute coronary syndrome and angiographic or pathologic confirmation of stent thrombosis).
- Probable event (unexplained death within 30 days or target vessel myocardial infarction without angiographic confirmation of stent thrombosis).
- Possible event (any unexplained death after 30 days).

Based on the elapsed time since stent implantation, stent thrombosis can be classified as:

- Early (0–30 days post stent implantation)
- Late (>30 days)
- Very late (>12 months)

Often, early stent thrombosis is further subdivided into acute (<24 h) and subacute (1–30 days) events.

It has to be remembered that in clinical studies, patients are selected based on some exclusionary criteria, which can potentially modulate the number of thrombosis cases. 'All-comers trials,' where patients are treated without any such restrictions, perhaps mimic the real-life setting and the results may be more representative.

Early evidence of higher incidents of thrombosis with DES has led to hundreds of clinical trials over the years, and the analyzed data were published widely in the medical literature. Given the complex nature of the patient population, selection protocols, patient disease histories, variability in implantation procedures, deviations from or cessation of prescribed regimens of dual antiplatelet therapy, etc., it is difficult to judge the thrombotic performances of these various coatings. However, it is important to consider some of the thrombosis results of the stents described above and make some comments related to stent coatings.

Mauri et al. (2007) applied a hierarchical classification of stent thrombosis set by the ARC across randomised trials involving 878 patients treated with sirolimus-eluting stents, 1400 treated with paclitaxel-eluting stents, and 2267 treated with bare-metal stents. The incidences of definite or probable events of thrombosis occurring in the DES groups were higher than for the bare-metal stents.

Virmani et al. (2004) reported one of the early cases of stent thrombosis in a 58-year-old patient who had died of acute circumflex vessel blockage with a Cypher® stent 18 months after implantation. Pathological examination revealed the absence of neointimal growth, stent malapposition and aneurismal dilatation in the stented region. Furthermore, they observed signs of coating delamination and inflammatory response near the polymer fragments.

Joner et al. (2006) studied autopsy specimens from 23 patients with Cypher® and Taxus® stents with matched controls of bare-metal stents from a large registry of 484 stent specimens. They observed delayed healing and impaired endothelialization in Cypher® and Taxus® compared to the bare-metal stent implants. Of the 23 patients, 14 showed signs of late stent thrombosis. Although it is difficult to definitely define the contribution of drug or polymer to these cases of delayed healing, in 3 of the 11 cases there was evidence of a full-blown chronic hypersensitivity reaction, which may have been a direct response to the biostable polymer.

Endeavor® stents from the first-generation group, on the other hand, continued to show low thrombosis rates. In a study of 722 patients with Endeavor® stents and 718 patients with Taxus® stents, the definite/probable stent thrombosis rates were only slightly lower in Endeavor® compared to Taxus®, but rates of very late stent thrombosis at a 5-year time point were considerably lower than with Taxus® (Kirtane et al., 2013).

In the case of second-generation stents, Xience® and Resolute®, both with biostable polymers, the thrombosis rates are comparable to each other but lower than for Cypher® and Taxus® (Xu et al., 2013; Mukherjee et al., 2013). Thus in the 130-patient clinical trial, Resolute® showed no signs of thrombosis for up to 2 years, and Xience® in their Spirit II trial had only 0.5% and 0.9% rates at 1- and 2-year time-points. Even in the 2000-patient all-comers trial, where the patients were randomly assigned for treatment with no exclusion criteria, the thrombosis rates at 4 years were low and comparable for Xience® and Resolute®.

From the clinical trial results and field data gathered over the years, although it is neither possible nor prudent to draw some firm and conclusive relationship between stent thrombosis results and polymer coatings in view of the complexities listed earlier in this section, it is possible to associate higher rates of inflammation and thrombosis with the first-generation DES like Cypher® and Taxus® with the hydrophobic nature of their coatings relative to Endeavor® and Resolute®. In the case of Xience®, the fluoropolymer coating is extremely hydrophobic and would be less prone to promote protein deposition and subsequent reactions leading to thrombus formation. Likewise, coatings in the case of Endeavor® and Resolute® are hydrophilic and behave in a similar manner.

In the case of bioabsorbable stent coatings, since they degrade and get metabolised, longer-term thrombosis results would be expected to be similar to those for bare-metal stents.

6.5 Conclusions

It is important that for a stent coating to be blood compatible, the surface should be designed and formulated to be either extremely hydrophobic or hydrophilic, to minimise platelet adhesion and aggregation and thus minimise thrombosis risks.

Acknowledgment

The author is grateful to Dr. J.N. Wilcox for helpful comments.

References

Alibeik, S., Zhu, S., Brash, J.L., December 1, 2010. Surface modification with PEG and hirudin for protein resistance and thrombin neutralization in blood contact. Colloids Surf. B Biointerf. 81 (2), 389. http://dx.doi.org/10.1016/j.colsurfb. 2010.07.024. Epub July 15, 2010.

Al-Kattaf, H., Charlesworth, D., 1996. Albumin coated vascular prostheses: a five year follow-up. J. Vasc. Surg. 23, 686. http://dx.doi.org/10.1016/S0741-5214(96)80050-4.

Andersson, A.S., Glasmästar, K., Sutherland, D., Lidberg, U., Kasemo, B., March 5, 2003. Cell adhesion on supported lipid bilayers. J. Biomed. Mater. Res. A 64 (4), 622. http://dx.doi.org/10.1002/jbm.a.10442.

Andrade, J.D., Hlady, V., 1986. Protein adsorption and material biocompatibility—a tutorial review and suggested hypothgeses. Adv. Polym. Sci. 79, 1. http://dx.doi.org/10.1007/3-540-16422-7_6.

Axel, D.I., Kunert, W., Göggelmann, C., Oberhoff, M., Herdeg, C., Küttner, A., Wild, D.H., Brehm, B.R., Riessen, R., Köveker, G., Karsch, K.R., 1997. Paclitaxel inhibits arterial smooth muscle cell proliferation and migration in vitro and in vivo using local drug delivery. Circulation 96 (2), 636—645. http://dx.doi.org/10.1161/01.CIR.96.2.636.

Bohl, K.S., West, J.L., 2000. Nitric oxide-generating polymers reduce platelet adhesion and smooth muscle cell proliferation. Biomaterials 21 (22), 2273—2278. http://dx.doi.org/10.1016/S0142-9612(00)00153-8.

Boland, J.L., Corbeij, H.A., Van Der Giessen, W., Seabra-Gomes, R., Suryapranata, H., Wijns, W., Hanet, C., Suttorp, M.J., Buller, C., Bonnier, J.J., Colombo, A., Van Birgelen, C., Pieper, M., Mangioni, J.A., Londero, H., Carere, R.G., Hamm, C.W., Bonan, R., Bartorelli, A., Kyriakides, Z.S., Chauhan, A., Rothman, M., Grinfeld, L., Oosterwijk, C., Serruys, P.W., Cumberland, D.C., 2000. Multicenter evaluation of the phosphorylcholine-coated biodivYsio stent in short de novo coronary lesions: the SOPHOS study. Int. J. Cardiovasc. Intervent. 3 (4), 215. http://dx.doi.org/10.1080/14628840050515966.

Bowen, P.K., Drelich, A., Drelich, J., Goldman, J., March 25 , 2014. Rates of in vivo (arterial) and in vitro biocorrosion for pure magnesium. J. Biomed. Mater. Res. A. http://dx.doi.org/10.1002/jbm.a.35179 [Epub ahead of print].

Brash, J.L., 1977. Hydrophobic polymer surface and their interaction with blood. In: Vroman, L., Leonard, E.F. (Eds.), The Behavior of Blood and Its Components at Interfaces, Ann N.Y. Acad. Sci., vol. 283. The New York Academy of Science, New York, p. 356. http://dx.doi.org/10.1111/j.1749-6632.1977.tb41781.x.

Campos, C.M., Muramatsu, T., Iqbal, J., Zhang, Y.J., Onuma, Y., Garcia-Garcia, H.M., Haude, M., Lemos, P.A., Warnack, B., Serruys, P.W., 2013. Bioresorbable drug-eluting magnesium-alloy scaffold for treatment of coronary artery disease. Int. J. Mol. Sci. 14 (12), 24492. http://dx.doi.org/10.3390/ijms141224492.

Carter, A.J., Melder, R.J., Udipi, K., Ozdil, F., Virmani, R., Wilcox, J.N., 2006. In vivo performance of a novel co-polymer system for the extended release of zotarolimus in a next generation durg eluting stent. In: Transcatheter Cardiovascular Therapeutics (TCT), 2006, Washington, DC.

Cestari, M., Muller, V., Rodrigues, J.H., Nakamura, C.V., Rubira, A.F., Muniz, E.C., 2014. Preparing silk fibroin nanofibers through electrospinning: further heparin immobilization toward hemocompatibility improvement. Biomacromolecules 15 (5), 1762. http://dx.doi.org/10.1021/bm500132g.

Chandy, T., Sharma, C.P., 1984. The antithrombotic effect of prostaglandin E1 immobilized on albuminated polymer matrix. J. Biomed. Mater. Res. 18 (9), 1115–1124. http://dx.doi.org/10.1002/jbm.820180913.

Chen, H., Chen, Y., Sheardown, H., Brook, M.A., 2005. Immobilization of heparin on a silicone surface through a heterobifunctional PEG spacer. Biomaterials 26 (35), 7418. http://dx.doi.org/10.1016/j.biomaterials.2005.05.053.

Cieffo, A., Bonizzoni, E., Orlic, D., Stankovic, G., Rogacka, R., Airoldi, F., Mikhail, G.W., Montorfano, M., Michev, I., Carlino, M., Colombo, A., 2004. Intraprocedural stent thrombosis during implantation of sirolimus eluting stents. Circulation 109, 2732. http://dx.doi.org/10.1161/01.CIR.0000131890.83839.5B.

Colombo, A., Airoldi, F., 2003. Passive coating: dream does not come true. J. Invasive Cardiol. 10, 566.

Cutlip, D.E., Windecker, S., Mehran, R., Boam, A., Cohen, D., van Es, G.A., Steg, P.G., Morel, M., Mauri, L., Vranckx, P., McFadden, E., Lansky, A., Hamon, M., Krucoff, M.W., Serruys, P., 2007. On behalf of the Academic Research Consortium, clinical end points in coronary stent trials: a case for standardized definitions. Circulation 115, 2344. http://dx.doi.org/10.1161/CIRCULATIONAHA.106.685313.

Delfife, K.M., Hagen, K.M., Clapper, D.L., Anderson, J.M., 1999. Photochemically immobilized polymer coatrings: effects on protein adsorption, cell adhesion and leukocyte activation. J. Biomater. Sci. Polym. Ed. 10, 1063. http://dx.doi.org/10.1163/156856299X00676.

Eberhart, R.C., Munro, M.S., Frautschi, J.R., Lubin, M., Clubb, F.J., Jr., Miller, C.W., Sevastianov, V.I., 1987. In: Brash, J.L., Horbett, T.A., (Eds.), Proteins at Interfaces. Ann N Y Acad Sci, vol. 516, pp. 78–95. http://dx.doi.org/10.1111/j.1749-6632.1987.tb33032.x.

Farb, A., Burke, A.P., Kolodgie, F.D., Virmani, R., 2003. Pathological mechanisms of fatal late coronary stent thrombosis in humans. Circulation 108, 1701. http://dx.doi.org/10.1161/01.CIR.0000091115.05480.B0.

Finn, A.V., Kolodgie, F.D., Harnek, J., Guerrero, L.J., Acampado, E., Tefera, K., Skorija, K., Weber, D.K., Gold, H.K., Virmani, R., 2005. Differential response of delayed healing and persistent inflammation at sites of overlapping sirolimus- or paclitaxel-eluting stents. Circulation 112 (2), 270. http://dx.doi.org/10.1161/CIRCULATIONAHA.104.508937.

Frautschi, J.R., Eberhart, R.C., Hubbell, J.A., 1996. Alkylated cellulosic membranes with enhanced albumin affinity: influence of competing proteins. J. Biomater. Sci. Polym. Ed. 7 (7), 563. http://dx.doi.org/10.1163/156856295X00481.

Fujii, K., Carlier, S.G., Mintz, G.S., Yang, Y.M., Moussa, I., Weisz, G., Dangas, G., Mehran, R., Lansky, A.J., Kreps, E.M., Collins, M., Stone, G.W., Moses, J.W., Leon, M.B., April 5, 2005. Stent underexpansion and residual reference segment stenosis are related to stent thrombosis after sirolimus-eluting stent implantation: an intravascular ultrasound study. J. Am. Coll. Cardiol. 45 (7), 995. http://dx.doi.org/10.1016/j.jacc.2004.12.066.

Galli, M., Bartorelli, A., Bedogni, F., DeCesare, N., Klugmann, S., Maiello, L., Miccoli, F., Moccetti, T., Onofri, M., Paolillo, V., Pirisi, R., Presbitero, P., Sganzerla, P., Viecca, M., Zerboni, S., Lanteri, G., 2000. Italian BiodivYsio open registry (BiodivYsio PC-coated stent): study of clinical outcomes of the implant of a PC-coated coronary stent. J. Invasive Cardiol. 12 (9), 452.

Galli, M., Sommariva, L., Prati, F., Zerboni, S., Politi, A., Bonatti, R., Mameli, S., Butti, E., Pagano, A., Ferrari, G., 2001. Acute and mid-term results of phosphorylcholine-coated stents in primary coronary stenting for acute myocardial infarction. Catheter Cardiovasc. Interv. 53 (2), 182. http://dx.doi.org/10.1002/ccd.1145.

Gambhir, D., 2006. The Sahajanand Infinnium bioabsorbable paclitaxel eluting stent. In: Transcatheter Cardiovascular Therapeutics (TCT) Conference, Washington, DC, 2006.

Gomez-Lara, J., Garcia-Garcia, H.M., Onuma, Y., Garg, S., Regar, E., De Bruyne, B., Windecker, S., McClean, D., Thuesen, L., Dudek, D., Koolen, J., Whitbourn, R., Smits, P.C., Chevalier, B., Dorange, C., Veldhof, S., Morel, M.A., de Vries, T., Ormiston, J.A., Serruys, P.W., 2010. A comparison of the conformability of everolimus-eluting bioresorbable vascular scaffolds to metal platform coronary stents. JACC Cardiovasc. Interv. 3 (11), 1190. http://dx.doi.org/10.1016/j.jcin.2010.07.016.

Gonzalo, N., Macaya, C., 2012. Absorbable stent: focus on clinical applications and benefits. Vasc. Health Risk Manage. 8, 125. http://dx.doi.org/10.2147/VHRM.S22551.

Gore, S., Andersson, J., Biran, R., Underwood, C., Riesenfeld, J., April 8, 2014. Heparin surfaces: impact of immobilization chemistry on hemocompatibility and protein adsorption. J. Biomed. Mater. Res. B Appl. Biomater. http://dx.doi.org/10.1002/jbm.b.33154.

Gruentzig, A.R., 1978. Transluminal dilatation of coronary arterystenosis [letter]. Lancet 311, 263. http://dx.doi.org/10.1016/S0140-6736(78)90500-7.

Grube, E., 2008. JACTAX clinical Trial: Interim 9 Month Results. In: Transcatheter Cardiovascular Therapeutics (TCT) Conference, Washington, DC.

Guidoin, R.G., Awad, J., Brassard, A., Domurado, D., Lawny, F., Barbotin, J.N., Calvor, C., Broun, G., 1976. Blood compatibility of silicone rubber chemically coated with cross-linked albumin. Biomater. Med. Devices Artif. Organs 4 (2), 205.

Guidoin, R.G., King, M.W., Awad, J., Martin, L., Domurado, D., Marois, M., Sigot-Luizard, M.F., Gosselin, C., Gunasekera, K., Gagnon, D., 1983. Albumin coated and critical point dried polyester prostheses as substitutes in the thoracic aorta of dogs. Trans. Am. Soc. Artif. Intern. Organs 29, 290.

Hanson, S.R., Tucker, E.I., 2013. Blood coagulation and blood −materials interaction, Chapter II.2.6. In: Ratner, B.D., Hoffman, A.S., Schoen, F.J., Lemons, J.E. (Eds.), Biomaterials Science.

Hanson, S.R., Harker, L.A., Ratner, B.D., Hoffman, A.S., 1980. In vivo evaluation of artificial surfaces with a nonhuman primate model of arterial thrombosis. J. Lab. Clin. Med. 95 (2), 289.

Haude, M., Erbel, R., Erne, P., Verheye, S., Degen, H., Böse, D., Vermeersch, P., Wijnbergen, I., Weissman, N., Prati, F., Waksman, R., Koolen, J., March 9, 2013. Safety and performance of the drug-eluting absorbable metal scaffold (DREAMS) in patients with de-novo coronary lesions: 12 month results of the prospective, multicentre, first-in-man BIOSOLVE-I trial. Lancet 381 (9869), 836. http://dx.doi.org/10.1016/S0140-6736(12)61765-6.

Hayward, J.A., Chapman, D., 1984. Biomembrane surfaces as models for polymer design: the potential for haemocompatibility. Biomaterials 5 (3), 135. http://dx.doi.org/10.1016/0142-9612(84)90047-4.

Hezi-Yamit, A., Sullivan, C., Wong, J., David, L., Chen, M., Cheng, P., Shumaker, D., Wilcox, J.N., Udipi, K., 2009. Impact of polymer hydrophilicity on biocompatibility: Implication for DES polymer design. J. Biomed. Mater. Res. Part A 90A (1), 133. http://dx.doi.org/10.1002/jbm.a.32057.

Hunter, S., Angelini, G.D., 1993. Phosphatidylcholine-coated chest tubes improve drainage after open heart operation. Ann. Thorac. Surg. 56 (6), 139. http://dx.doi.org/10.1016/0003-4957(93)90678B.

Hayashi, K., Murata, K., Yamamoto, N., Yamashita, I., 1985. Antithrombogenicity of polyethylene radiation-graftcopolymerized with hydrophilic monomers. Kobunshi Ronbunshu 42, 77 in Japanese.

Haycox, C.L., Ratner, B.D., 1993. In vitro platelet interactions in whole human blood exposed to biomaterial surfaces: insights on blood compatibility. J. Biomed. Mater. Res. 27 (9), 1181. http://dx.doi.org/10.1002/jbm.820270909.

Hoffman, A.S., Horbett, T.A., Ratner, B.D., 1997. Interaction of blood and blood components at interfaces. In: Vroman, L., Leonard, E.F. (Eds.), Ann N.Y. Acad. Sci., vol. 283. The New York Academy of Science, New York, p. 372.

Hubbell, J.A., 1993. Pharmacological modification of materials. Cardiovasc. Pathol. 2, S121.

Hulander, M., Lundgren, A., Faxälv, L., Lindahl, T.L., Palmquist, A., Berglin, M., Elwing, H., 2013. Gradients in surface nanotopography used to study platelet adhesion and activation. Colloids Surf. B Biointerfaces 110, 261. http://dx.doi.org/10.1016/j.colsurfb.2013.04.010.

Iakovou, I., Schmidt, T., Bonizzoni, E., Ge, L., Sangiorgi, G.M., Stankovic, G., Airoldi, F., Chieffo, A., Montorfano, M., Carlino, M., Michev, I., Corvaja, N., Briguori, C., Gerckens, U., Grube, E., Colombo, A., 2005. Incidence, predictors, and outcome of thrombosis after successful implantation of drug-eluting stents. JAMA 293 (17), 2126. http://dx.doi.org/10.1001/jama.293.17.2126.

Ishikawa, Y., Sasakawa, S., Takase, M., Osada, Y., July 15, 1984. Effect of albumin immobilization by plasma polymerization on platelet reactivity. Thromb. Res. 35 (2), 193. http://dx.doi.org/10.1016/0049-3848(84)90214-7.

Jain, R.A., 2000. The manufacturing techniques of various drug loaded biodegradable poly(lactide-co-glycolide) (PLGA) devices. Biomaterials 21 (23), 2475. http://dx.doi.org/10.1016/S0142-9612(00)00115-0.

Joner, M., Finn, A.V., Farb, A., Mont, E.K., Kolodgie, F.D., Ladich, E., Kutys, R., Skorija, K., Gold, H.K., Virmani, R., 2006. Pathology of drug-eluting stents in humans: delayed healing and late thrombotic risk. J. Am. Coll. Cardiol. 48 (1), 193. http://dx.doi.org/10.1016/j.jacc.2006.03.042.

Jordan, S.W., Chaikof, E.I., 2007. Novel thromboresistant materials. J. Vasc. Surg. 45, 104A. http://dx.doi.org/10.1016/j.jvs.2007.02.048.

Joseph, G., Sharma, C.P., 1987. Prostacyclin immobilized albuminated surfaces. J. Biomed. Mater. Res. 21 (7), 937–945. http://dx.doi.org/10.1002/jbm.820210709.

Kaladhar, K., Sharma, C.P., 2004. Supported cell mimetic monolayers and their interaction with blood. Langmuir 20 (25), 11115. http://dx.doi.org/10.1021/la048644y.

Kaladhar, K., Sharma, C.P., 2006. Cell mimetic lateral stabilization of outer cell mimetic bilayer on polymer surfaces by peptide bonding and their blood compatibility. J. Biomed. Mater. Res. A 79 (1), 23. http://dx.doi.org/10.1002/jbm.a.30681.

Kador, K.E., Subramanian, A., 2011. Surface modification of biomedical grade polyurethane to enable the ordered co-immobilization of two proteins. J. Biomater. Sci. Polym. Ed. 22 (15), 1983. http://dx.doi.org/10.1163/092050610X529191.

Kalynych, A.M., King, S.P., 1995. PTCA versus CABG for angina pectoris: a look at the randomized trials. Coron. Artery Dis. 6, 788.

Kamath, K.R., Park, K., 1994. Surface modification of polymeric biomaterials by albumin grafting using h-irradiation. J. Appl. Biomater. 5 (2), 163.

Kang, I.K., Kwon, B.K., Lee, J.H., Lee, H.B., 1993. Immobilization of proteins on poly(methyl methacrylate) films. Biomaterials 14 (10), 787. http://dx.doi.org/10.1016/0142-9612(93)90045-4.

Kataoka, K., Tsuruta, T., Akaike, T., Sakurai, Y., 1980. Biomedical behavior of synthetic polyion complexes toward blood platelets. Makromol. Chem. 181, 1363. http://dx.doi.org/10.1002/macp.1980.021810701.

Kereiakes, D.J., Choo, J.K., Young, J.J., Broderick, T.M., 2004. Thrombosis and drug-eluting stents: a critical appraisal. Rev. Cardiovasc. Med. Winter 5 (1), 9–15. Review.

Kim, H.K., Kim, K., Byun, Y., 2005. Preparation of a chemically anchored phospholipid monolayer on an acrylated polymer substrate. Biomaterials 26, 3435. http://dx.doi.org/10.1016/j.biomaterials.2004.09.066.

Kim, S.W., Lee, R.G., Oster, H., Coleman, D., Andrade, J.D., Lentz, D.J., Olsen, D., 1974. Platelet adhesion to polymer surfaces. Trans. Am. Soc. Artif. Intern. Organs 20 B, 449.

King III, S.B., Lambo, N.J., Weintraub, W.S., et al., 1994. A randomized trial comparing coronary angioplasty with coronary bypass surgery. N. England J. Med. 331, 1044. http://dx.doi.org/10.1056/NEJM199410203311603.

Kirtane, A.J., Stone, G.W., 2011. How to minimize stent thrombosis. Circulation 124, 1283. http://dx.doi.org/10.1161/CIRCULATIONAHA.110.976829.

Kirtane, A.J., Leon, M.B., Ball, M.W., Bajwa, H.S., Sketch Jr., M.H., Coleman, P.S., Stoler, R.C., Papadakos, S., Cutlip, D.E., Mauri, L., Kandzari, D.E., 2013. The "final" 5-year follow-up from the ENDEAVOR IV trial comparing a zotarolimus-eluting stent with a paclitaxel-eluting stent. JACC Cardiovasc. Interv. 325–333. http://dx.doi.org/10.1016/j.jcin.2012.12.123.

Kolandaivelu, K., Swaminathan, R., Gibson, W.J., Kolachalama, V.B., Nguyen-Ehrenreich, K.L., Giddings, V.L., Coleman, L., Wong, G.K., Edelman, E.R., 2011. Stent thrombogenicity early in high-risk interventional settings is driven by stent design and deployment and protected by polymer-drug coatings. Circulation 123 (13), 1400. http://dx.doi.org/10.1161/CIRCULATIONAHA.110.003210.

Kottke-Marchant, K., Anderson, J.M., Rabinovitch, A., Huskey, R.A., Herzig, R., 1985. The effect of heparin vs. citrate on the interaction of platelets with vascular graft materials. Thromb. Haemost. 54 (4), 842.

Kottke-Marchant, K., Anderson, J.M., Umemura, Y., Marchant, R.E., 1989. Effect of albumin coating on the in vitro blood compatibility of Dacron arterial prostheses. Biomaterials 10 (3), 147. http://dx.doi.org/10.1016/0142-9612(89)90017-3.

Kudo, F.A., Nishibe, T., Miyazaki, K., Flores, J., Yasuda, K., 2002. Albumin-coated knitted Dacron aortic prosthses. Study of postoperative inflammatory reactions. Int. Angiol. 21 (3), 214.

Lee, J.H., Kopecek, J., Andrade, J.D., 1989. Protein-resistant surfaces prepared by PEO-containing block copolymer surfactants. J. Biomed. Mater. Res. 23 (3), 351. http://dx.doi.org/10.1002/jbm.820230306.

Lewis, A.L., Cumming, Z.L., Goreish, H.H., Kirkwood, L.C., Tolhurst, L.A., Stratford, P.W., 2001. Crosslinkable coatings from phosphorylcholine-based polymers. Biomaterials 22 (2), 99. http://dx.doi.org/10.1016/S0142-9612(00)00083-1.

Lloyd-Jones, D., 2009. Heart disease and stroke statistics. Circulation 119 (3), 480. http://dx.doi.org/10.1161/CIRCULATIONAHA.109.192667.

Lu, L., Li, Q.L., Maitz, M.F., Chen, J.L., Huang, N., 2012. Immobilization of the direct thrombin inhibitor-bivalirudin on 316L stainless steel via polydopamine and the resulting effects on hemocompatibility in vitro. J. Biomed. Mater. Res. A 100 (9), 2421. http://dx.doi.org/10.1002/jbm.a.34143.

Lu, J.R., Murphy, E.F., Su, T.J., Lewis, A.L., Stratford, P.W., Satija, S.K., 2001. Reduced protein adsorption on the surface of a phospholipid monolayer. Langmuir 17, 3382. http://dx.doi.org/10.1021/la0017429.

Lüscher, T.F., Steffel, J., Eberli, F.R., Joner, M., Nakazawa, G., Tanner, F.C., Virmani, R., 2007. Drug-eluting stent and coronary thrombosis: biological mechanisms and clinical implications. Circulation 115 (8), 1051. http://dx.doi.org/10.1161/CIRCULATIONAHA.106.675934.

Lyman, D.J., Klein, K.G., Brash, J.L., Fritzinger, B.K., 1970. The interaction of platelets with polymer surfaces. I. Uncharged hydrophobic polymer surfaces. Thromb. Diath. Haemorrh. 23 (1), 120. http://dx.doi.org/10.1177/088532829100600105.

Marra, K.G., Winger, T.M., Hanson, S.R., Chaikof, E.I., 1997. Cytomimetic biomaterials I, in situ polymerization of phospholipids on an alkylated surface. Macromolecules 30, 6483. http://dx.doi.org/10.1021/ma970481f.

Mauri, L., Hsieh, W.H., Massaro, J.M., Ho, K.K., D'Agostino, R., Cutlip, D.E., 2007. Stent thrombosis in randomized clinical trials of drug-eluting stents. N. Engl. J. Med. 356 (10), 1020. http://dx.doi.org/10.1056/NEJMMoa067731.

Mehran, R., Nikolsky, E., Camenzind, E., Zelizko, M., Kranjec, I., Seabra-Gomes, R., Negoita, M., Slack, S., Lotan, C., 2005. An internet-based registry examining the efficacy of heparin coating in patients undergoing coronary stent implantation. Am. Heart J. 150 (6), 1171. http://dx.doi.org/10.1016/j.ahj.2005.01.027.

Meredith, I.T., Verheye, S., Dubois, C.L., Dens, J., Fajadet, J., Carri, D., Walsh, S., Oldroyd, K.G., Varenne, O., El-Jack, S., Moreno, R., Joshi, A.A., Allocco, D.J., Dawkins, K.D., 2012. Primary endpoint results of the EVOLVE trial: a randomized evaluation of a novel bioabsorbable polymer-coated, everolimus-eluting coronary stent. J. Am. Coll. Cardiol. 59 (15), 1362. http://dx.doi.org/10.1016/j.jacc.2011.12.016.

Merrill, E.W., Salzman, E.W., 1983. Polyethylene oxide as a biomaterial. ASIO J. 6, 60.

Mori, Y., Nagaoka, S., Takiuchi, H., Kikuchi, T., Noguchi, N., Tanzawa, H., Noishiki, Y., 1982. A new antithrombogenic material with long polyethyleneoxide chains. Trans. Am. Soc. Artif. Intern. Organs 28, 459.

Mowery, K.A., Schoenfisch, M.H., Saavedra, J.E., Keefer, L.K., Meyerhoff, M.E., 2000. Preparation and characterization of hydrophobic polymeric films that are thromboresistant via nitric oxide release. Biomaterials 21 (1), 9–21. http://dx.doi.org/10.1016/S0142-9612(99)00127-1.

Mukherjee, D., Burgos, J.D., Farrag, S., 2013. Clin. Cardiol. 4, 23–37. http://dx.doi.org/10.2147/RRCC.S31012.

Müller, C., Büttner, H.J., Petersen, J., Roskamm, H., 2000. A randomized comparison of clopidogrel and aspirin versus ticlopidine and aspirin after the placement of coronary-artery stents. Circulation 101 (6), 590–593. http://dx.doi.org/10.1161/01.CIR.101.6.590.

Nishimura, T., Maeda, M., Nitadori, N., Tsuruta, T., 1982. Synthesis and copolymerization of polyamine macromer: molecular design of a new functional graft copolymer. Makromol. Chem. 183, 29. http://dx.doi.org/10.1295/polymj.19.593.

Oberhauser, J.P., Hossainy, S., Rapoza, R.J., 2009. Design principles and performance of bioresorbable polymeric vascular scaffolds. EuroIntervention 15 (5 Suppl. F), F15.

Okano, T., Nishiyama, S., Shinohara, I., Akaike, T., Sakurai, Y., 1978. Interaction between plasma protein and microphase separated structure of copolymers. Polym. J. 10, 233. http://dx.doi.org/10.1295/polymj.10.223.

Okano, T., Nishiyama, S., Shinohara, I., Akaike, T., Sakurai, Y., Kataoka, K., Tsuruta, T., May 1981. J. Biomed. Mater. Res. 15 (3), 393–402.

Okano, T., Aoyagi, T., Kataoka, K., Abe, K., Sakurai, Y., Shimada, M., Shinohara, I., 1986. Hydrophilic-hydrophobic microdomain surfaces having an ability to suppress platelet aggregation and their in vitro antithrombogenicity. J. Biomed. Mater. Res. 20 (7), 919. http://dx.doi.org/10.1002/jbm.820200707.

Olsson, P., Sanchez, J., Mollnes, T.E., Riesenfeld, J., 2000. On the blood compatibility of end point immobilized heparin. J. Biomater. Sci. Polym. Ed. 11, 1261. http://dx.doi.org/10.1163/156856200744192.

Onder, S., Kazmanli, K., Kok, F.N., 2011. Alteration of PTFE surface to increase its blood compatibility. J. Biomater. Sci. Polym. Ed. 22 (11), 1443. http://dx.doi.org/10.1163/092050610X510551.

Onuma, Y., Piazza, N., Ormiston, J.A., Serruys, P.W., 2009. EuroIntervention. Suppl 5F, F98–F102. http://dx.doi.org/10.4244/EIJV5IFA17.

Onuma, Y., Serruys, P.W., 2011. Bioresorbable scaffold: the advent of a new era in percutaneous coronary and peripheral revascularization? Circulation 123 (7), 779. http://dx.doi.org/10.1161/CIRCULATIONAHA.110.971606.

Orban, J.M., Faucher, K.M., Dluhy, R.A., Chaikof, E.I., 2000. Cytomimetic biomaterials 4. In-situ polymerization of phospholipids on an alkylated surface. Macromolecules 33, 4205. http://dx.doi.org/10.1021/ma9915780.

Ormiston, J.A., Serruys, P.W., 2009. Bioabsorbable coronary stents. Circ. Cardiovasc. Interv. 2 (3), 255. http://dx.doi.org/10.1161/CIRCINTERVENTIONS.109.859173.

Palmerini, T., Biondi-Zoccai, G., Della Riva, D., Mariani, A., Genereux, P., Branzi, A., Stone, G.W., 2013. Stent thrombosis with drug-eluting stents: is the paradigm shifting? J. Am. Coll. Cardiol. 62 (21), 1915. http://dx.doi.org/10.1016/j.jacc.2013.08.725.

Park, K., Mosher, D.F., Cooper, S.L., 1986. Acute surface-induced thrombosis in the canine ex vivo model: importance of protein composition of the initial monolayer and platelet activation. J. Biomed. Mater. Res. 20 (5), 589. http://dx.doi.org/10.1002/jbm.820200506.

Parker, T., Dave, V., Falotico, R., 2010. Polymers for drug eluting stents. Curr. Pharm. Des. 16 (36), 3978. http://dx.doi.org/10.2174/138161210794454897.

Patel, N., Banning, A.P., 2013. Bioabsorbable scaffolds for the treatment of obstructive coronary artery disease: the next revolution in coronary intervention? Heart 99 (17), 1236. http://dx.doi.org/10.1136/heartjnl-2012-303346.

Phaneuf, M.D., Berceli, S.A., Bide, M.J., Quist, W.C., LoGerfo, F.W., 1997. Covalent linkage of recombinant hirudin to poly(ethylene terephthalate) (Dacron): creation of a novel antithrombin surface. Biomaterials 18 (10), 755. http://dx.doi.org/10.1016/S0142-9612(96)00193-7.

Phaneuf, M.D., Dempsey, D.J., Bide, M.J., Szycher, M., Quist, W.C., LoGerfo, F.W., 1998. Bioengineering of a novel small diameter polyurethane vascular graft with covalently bound recombinant hirudin. ASAIO J. 44 (5), M653.

Pinchuk, L., Wilson, G.J., Barry, J.J., Schoephoerster, R.T., Parel, J.M., Kennedy, J.P., 2008. Medical applications of poly(styrene-block-isobutylene-block-styrene) ("SIBS"). Biomaterials 29 (4), 448. http://dx.doi.org/10.1016/j.biomaterials.2007.09.041.

Poon, M., Marx, S.O., Gallo, R., Badimon, J.J., Taubman, M.B., Marks, A.R., 1996. Rapamycin inhibits vascular smooth muscle cell migration. J. Clin. Invest. 98 (10), 2277–2283. http://dx.doi.org/10.1172/JCI119038.

Qu, Z., Krishnamurthy, V., Haller, C.A., Dorr, B.M., Marzec, U.M., Hurst, S., Hinds, M.T., Hanson, S.R., Liu, D.R., Chaikof, E.L., 2014. Immobilization of actively thromboresistant assemblies on sterile blood-contacting surfaces. Adv. Health Mater. 3 (1), 30. http://dx.doi.org/10.1002/adhm.201300110.

Ranade, S.V., Miller, K.M., Richard, R.E., Chan, A.K., Allen, M.J., Helmus, M.N., 2004. Physical characterization of controlled release of paclitaxel from the TAXUS Express2 drug-eluting stent. J. Biomed. Mater. Res. A 71 (4), 625. http://dx.doi.org/10.1002/jbm.a.30188.

Ranade, S.V., Richard, R., Helmus, M.N., 2005. Styrenic block copolymers for biomaterial and drug delivery applications. Acta Biomater. 1 (1), 137. http://dx.doi.org/10.1016/j.actbio.2004.09.004.

Ratner, B.D., Hoffman, A.S., Hanson, S.R., Harker, L.A., Whiffen, J.D., 1979. Blood-compatibility-water content relationship for radiation grafted hydrogels. J. Polym. Sci. Polym. Symp. 66, 363. http://dx.doi.org/10.1002/polc.5070660134.

Ross, E.E., Rozanski, L.J., Spratt, T., Liu, S.C., O'Brien, D.F., Saavedra, S.S., 2003. Planar supported lipid bilayer polymers formed by vescicle fusion. 1. Influence of diene monomeer structure and polymerization method on film properties. Langmuir 19, 1752. http://dx.doi.org/10.1021/la0261491.

Santerre, J.P., van der Kamp, N.H., Brash, J.L., 1989. Effect of sulfonation of segmented polyurethanes on the transient adsorption of fibrinogen from plasma: possible correlation with anticoagulant behavior. Trans. Soc. Biomater. 12, 113.

Sask, K.N., McClung, W.G., Berry, L.R., Chan, A.K., Brash, J.L., 2011. Immobilization of an antithrombin-heparin complex on gold: anticoagulant properties and platelet interactions. Acta Biomater. 7 (5), 2029. http://dx.doi.org/10.1016/j.actbio.2011.01.031.

Sefton, M.V., Gemmell, C.H., Gorbet, M.B., 2000. What really is blood compatibility? J. Biomater. Sci. Polym. Ed. 11 (11), 1165. http://dx.doi.org/10.1163/156856200744255. Review.

Serruys, P.W., Ormiston, J.A., Onuma, Y., Regar, E., Gonzalo, N., Garcia-Garcia, H.M., Nieman, K., Bruining, N., Dorange, C., Miquel-Hébert, K., Veldhof, S., Webster, M., Thuesen, L., Dudek, D., 2009. A bioabsorbable everolimus-eluting coronary stent system (ABSORB): 2-year outcomes and results from multiple imaging methods. Lancet 373 (9667), 897. http://dx.doi.org/10.1016/S0140-6736(09)60325-1.

Sperling, C., König, U., Hermel, G., Werner, C., Müller, M., Simon, F., Grundke, K., Jacobasch, H.J., Vasilets, V.N., Ikada, Y., 1997. Immobilization of human thrombomodulin onto PTFE. J. Mater. Sci. Mater. Med. 8 (12), 789. http://dx.doi.org/10.1023/A:1018572931351.

Sperling, C., Schweiss, R.B., Streller, U., Werner, C., 2005. In vitro hemocompatibility of self-assembled monolayers displaying various functional groups. Biomaterials 26 (33), 6547. http://dx.doi.org/10.1016/j.biomaterials.2005.04.042.

Stine, R., Pishko, M.V., Hampton, J.R., Dameron, A.A., Weiss, P.S., 2005. Heat-stabilized phospholipid films: film characterization and the production of protein-resistant surfaces. Langmuir 21 (24), 11352. http://dx.doi.org/10.1021/la051150w.

Taniwaki, M., Stefanini, G.G., Silber, S., Richardt, G., Vranckx, P., Serruys, P.W., Buszman, P.E., Kelbaek, H., Windecker, S., April 29, 2014. Four year clinical outcomes and predictors of repeat revascularization in patients treated with new generation drug-eluting stents in the RESOLUTE all comers randomized trial. J. Am. Coll. Cardiol. 63 (16), 1617−1625. http://dx.doi.org/10.1016/j.jacc.2013.12.036.

Tanzi, M.C., 2005. Bioactive technologies for hemocompatibility. Expert Rev. Med. Devices 2 (4), 473. http://dx.doi.org/10.1586/17434440.2.4.473.

Tegoulia, A., Rao, W.S., Kalambur, A.T., Rabolt, J.R., Cooper, S.L., 2001. Surface properties, fibrinogen adsorption and cellular interactions of a novel phosphorylcholine-containing self-assembled monolayer on gold. Langmuir 17, 4396. http://dx.doi.org/10.1021/la001790t.

Udipi, K., Chen, M., Cheng, P., Jiang, K., Judd, D., Caceres, A., Melder, R., Wilcox, J.N., 2008. Development of A Novel biocompatible polymer system for extended drug release in a second generation drug eluting stent. J. Biomed. Mater. Res. 85A, 1064. http://dx.doi.org/10.1002/jbm.a.31664.

Virmani, R., Guagliumi, G., Farb, A., Musumeci, G., Grieco, N., Motta, T., Mihalcsik, L., Tespili, M., Valsecchi, O., Kolodgie, F.D., 2004. Localized hypersensitivity and late coronary thrombosis secondary to a sirolimus-eluting stent: should we be cautious? Circulation 109 (6), 701. http://dx.doi.org/10.1161/01.CIR.0000116202.41966.D4.

Vroman, L., 1988. The life of an artificial device in contact with blood: initial evenys and their effect on its final state. Bull. N.Y. Acad. Med. 64 (4), 352.

Wang, A.F., Cao, T., Tang, H.Y., Lianf, X.M., Black, C., Salley, S.O., 2006. Immobilization of polysaccharides on a fluorinated silicon surface. Colloid Surf. B-Biointerfaces 47, 57. http://dx.doi.org/10.1016/jcolsurfb.2005.11.016.

Waples, L.M., Olorundare, O.E., Goodman, S.L., Lai, Q.J., Albrecht, R.M., 1996. Platelet-polymer interactions: morphologic and intracellular free calcium studies of individual human platelets. J. Biomed. Mater. Res. 32 (1), 65. http://dx.doi.org/10.1002/(SICI)1097-4636(199609)32:1<65::AID-JBM8>3.0.CO;2-N.

Wolf, K.V., Zong, Z., Meng, J., Orana, A., Rahbar, N., Balss, K.M., Papandreou, G., Maryanoff, C.A., Soboyejo, W., 2008. An investigation of adhesion in drug-eluting stent layers. J. Biomed. Mater. Res. Part A 87A (1), 272. http://dx.doi.org/10.1002/jbm.a.31860.

Wu, B., Gerlitz, B., Grinnell, B.W., Meyerhoff, M.E., 2007. Polymeric coatings that mimic the endothelium: combining nitric oxide release with surface-bound active thrombomodulin and heparin. Biomaterials 28 (28), 4047. http://dx.doi.org/10.1016/j.biomaterials.2007.06.002.

Xu, B., Yang, Y., Yuan, Z., Du, Z., Wong, S.C., Généreux, P., Lu, S., July 2013. Zotarolimus- and paclitaxel-eluting stents in an all-comer population in China: the RESOLUTE China randomized controlled trial. JACC Cardiovasc. Interv. 6 (7), 664–670. http://dx.doi.org/10.1016/j.jcin.2013.03.001.

Xu, X., 2009. Characterization of PVDF-HFP copolymer and the model coating of Xience V drug eluting stent by synchrotron. In: SFB (Ed.), Society for Biomaterials 2009 Annual Meeting and Exposition. San Antonio, TX, Paper # 137.

Yang, Y.J., Kwon, Y., Choi, B.H., Jung, D., Seo, J.H., Lee, K.H., Cha, H.J., 2014. Multi-functional adhesive silk fibroin with blending of RGD-bioconjugated mussel adhesive protein. Biomacromolecules 15 (4), 1390–1398. http://dx.doi.org/10.1021/bm500001n.

Yu, X.H., Cooper, S.L., 1991. Physical and blood contacting characteristics of propyl sulphonate grafted Biomer. Biomaterials 12 (1), 3. http://dx.doi.org/10.1016/0142-9612(91)90123-R.

Part Three

Biosynthetic hydrogels

Degradable hydrogel systems for biomedical applications

7

B. Ozcelik
Commonwealth Scientific and Industrial Research Organisation (CSIRO), Clayton, VIC, Australia

7.1 Introduction

Hydrogels have been of significant interest in biomedical and biomaterials research as a result of their appealing characteristics. A hydrogel can be defined as a high water absorbing, chemically or physically bonded insoluble three-dimensional (3D) network.[1,2] The attractiveness of hydrogels for various biomedical applications comes from their high water absorption capability ($\geq$10–99.9 wt%) and similar physicochemical characteristics to that of many tissues.[1,2] Additionally, the mechanical strength and degradation properties of hydrogels can be tailored by tuning parameters such as the type and molecular weight of polymers used, crosslinking densities, porosity and synthesis conditions.[1–5] As a result, these combined versatile properties allow the utilisation of hydrogels for many biomedical applications, such as scaffolds for hard or soft tissues, carriers for cells and therapeutics, or as complete tissue substitutes.

This chapter will focus on polymer-based hydrogels for various biomedical applications. Hydrogel precursors with their advantages and disadvantages, and the desired hydrogel physicochemical properties for biomedical applications will be covered. Degradation requirements of hydrogel materials are application-dependent, hence hydrogels with various degradation mechanisms for therapeutic and tissue regeneration applications will be discussed in detail.

7.2 Hydrogel precursors

Hydrogels can be synthesised from a wide variety of materials, both synthetic and naturally-derived (Figure 7.1). Hydrogels derived from natural polymers can display desirable properties such as biocompatibility, biodegradability and inherent cell–surface interactions as a result of their similarity to the ECM.[6,7] Natural polymers, including collagen, alginate and chitosan, have been utilised to prepare hydrogels for biomedical applications including tissue engineering.[8–11] Regardless of the many advantages, there are certain issues attached to the use of naturally derived materials, such as batch-to-batch variation, risk of disease transmission and immunogenicity.[12–16] In addition, the processing methods required to obtain these

Biosynthetic Polymers for Medical Applications. http://dx.doi.org/10.1016/B978-1-78242-105-4.00007-9

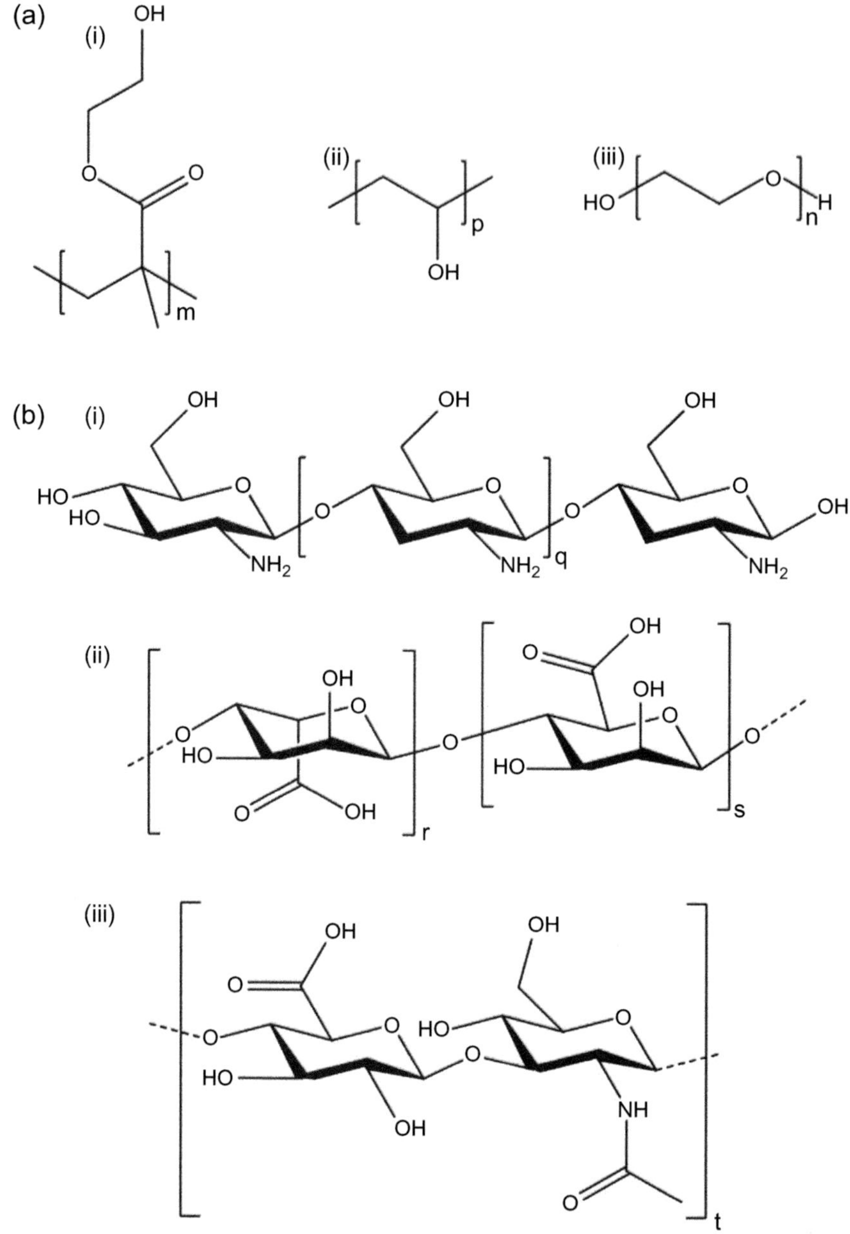

Figure 7.1 Some common precursors used for hydrogel fabrication: (a) synthetic precursors (i) poly(2-hydroxyethyl methacrylate), (ii) poly(vinyl alcohol) and (iii) poly(ethylene glycol) and (b) natural precursors (i) chitosan, (ii) alginate and (iii) hyaluronan.

natural materials can affect their mechanical properties. For example, even though collagen demonstrates high mechanical strength *in vivo*, the process of harvesting, isolation and purification negatively impacts its mechanical properties through the loss of natural crosslinks.[17]

Use of synthetic polymers offers certain advantages over natural polymers, including improved batch-to-batch consistency and a high degree of control during the fabrication processes.[18] However, there are certain shortcomings, such as the need for organic solvents during synthesis.[19] In addition, challenges in regard to cellular interactions arise since synthetic polymers lack the biological moieties that are present within the ECM.[6,20] Various hydrophilic synthetic polymers; i.e. poly(vinyl alcohol), poly(2-hydroxyethyl methacrylate), and poly(ethylene glycol) (PEG) have been used in the synthesis of hydrogels.[21–34] Synthetic hydrophilic polymers, such as PEG, have been explored for biomedical applications due to their low-toxicity, minimal immunogenicity and anti-protein fouling properties.[35–38] The hydrophilic nature of hydrogels and low-protein fouling properties are also beneficial when trying to minimise inflammatory responses.[39,40] As a result of their low-protein fouling properties, coatings from materials such as PEG also prevent nonspecific protein and bacterial binding on implantable material surfaces.[41] Specifically, PEG-based polymers have been widely investigated for biomedical and tissue engineering applications, as their United States Food and Drug Administration approval for certain applications make them additionally appealing.[35]

7.3 Desired hydrogel properties

Biomaterials, including hydrogels, need to possess certain physicochemical properties to be successful in their diverse applications[6,42–44] including (1) 3D structural support; (2) a permeable/interconnected porous structure; (3) suitable and controllable biodegradation rates; (4) low toxicity and immunogenicity of both the hydrogel and its degradation products; and (5) good mechanical properties for maintenance of the 3D shape during degradation and function.[6,42–44]

A 3D permeable structure is required for the diffusion of nutrients, cellular waste or therapeutic compounds depending on the application, while an interconnected porous structure may be required for penetration and proliferation of tissue for regeneration purposes. Appropriate and controllable biodegradation rate is highly desirable to allow the hydrogel to degrade at a rate similar to tissue growth or for controlled release of conjugated/loaded bioactive molecules. Mechanical robustness of the hydrogel scaffold is important for structural integrity of the construct during its function. No toxicity and low immunogenicity are essential to minimise any adverse effects in biological systems.

7.4 Degradable hydrogel systems

Resulting from the ease and versatility of the synthesis of hydrogel materials, it is possible to incorporate various functionalities into hydrogel networks. Depending on the target application it may or may not be desirable to incorporate degradation capabilities into the fabricated hydrogel. Applications involving tissue regeneration and targeted delivery of cells or therapeutics may require that the hydrogel support degrades and does not persist once it delivers its load or the tissue function has been restored.

Various degradation mechanisms can be utilised in the preparation of hydrogels for biomedical applications. The material used in the synthesis of the hydrogels can be inherently degradable (natural or synthetic) or degradation mechanisms can be introduced to provide biodegradability to the final hydrogel construct.

Hydrogel systems based on synthetic polymers may often lack degradable properties. To provide degradability to such systems, modification or functionalisation of the polymers may be necessary. For example, copolymerisation of degradable polymers or insertion of degradable sequences into the backbone of nondegradable polymers can provide biodegradability to the hydrogels employing such modified polymers.

The following sections will cover hydrogel materials that possess various degradation mechanisms. Furthermore, how each degradation mechanism provides benefits for the target application will be discussed.

7.4.1 Hydrolytically degraded hydrogels

Functional groups such as esters, anhydrides and thioesters among others are susceptible to hydrolysis (Figure 7.2). When such groups are present in polymer backbones or crosslinks they can lead to the cleavage of the polymer chain or the crosslinks. Various studies have taken advantage of these hydrolysable groups to prepare biodegradable hydrogels.

Hydrolytic degradation can occur in the presence of water or actively through enzymes; hence it can be difficult to directly control degradation rates. Certain strategies have been adopted to slow or accelerate degradation of hydrogels. Zhang et al. have synthesised ultraviolet (UV)-curable polyurethane-based hydrogels with variable

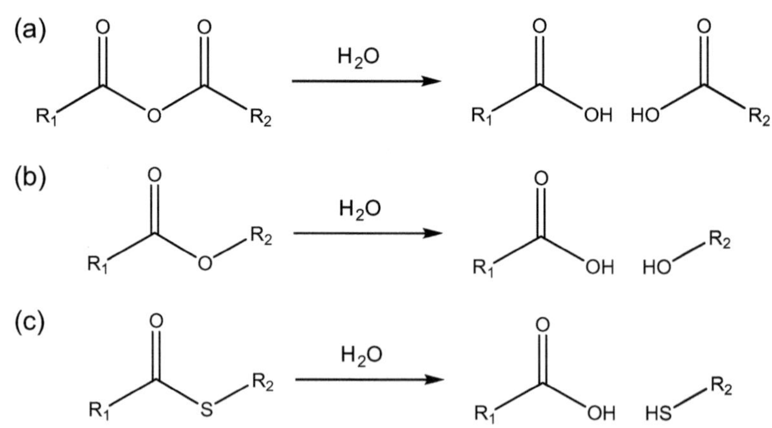

Figure 7.2 Hydrolysis of (a) anhdyrides, (b) esters and (c) thioesters.

PEG and polycaprolactone (PCL) ratios.[45] The study found that by increasing the PEG content of the hydrogels, the swelling and degradation rate could be increased as a result of the increasing hydrophilicity while increasing the PCL content eventuated in the opposite. Similarly, novel polyester PEG-based hydrogel films were previously synthesised for the regeneration of corneal endothelial cells.[46] The crosslinking between three-arm PEGs and sebacoyl chloride (a diacid chloride) that were utilised leads to the formation of ester crosslinks. Tensile strength and the degradation rate of the hydrogel films were also controlled by varying the cocrosslinked PCL amount in the transparent films. Controlling the degradation rate of hydrogels allows the tuning of the degradation rate to suit each patient, as treatment and evaluation duration of patients can vary depending on the surgical procedure undertaken.

Hydrolytically degraded hydrogels can also be employed for use in the delivery of drugs. Ulbrich et al. synthesised *N*-(2-hydroxyl propyl)-methacrylamide-based hydrogels with cleavable amide and ester bonds.[47] The hydrogels were loaded with or copolymerised with doxorubicin during synthesis. The two methods of drug incorporation into the hydrogel carrier allowed the release of doxorubicin via two mechanisms; in the case of direct loading, the drug was released via diffusion simultaneously with hydrogel degradation, while copolymerisation allowed release only following degradation of the hydrogels, providing a level of control over the release. This is advantageous where dosing requirements vary with the type of drug, and control over its release may be necessary to minimise side effects.

Certain polymers possess excellent biocompatible properties both *in vitro* and *in vivo* but lack biodegradability which is required for many biomedical applications. For example, even though PEG is nontoxic and widely used for many applications, the polymer itself is nondegradable at any desirable timescale. In such cases, incorporation of a degradable polymer into the backbone can impart the required degradability (Figure 7.3). Metters et al. have described the synthesis of block copolymer; PEG and the degradable α-hydroxy acid poly(lactic acid) to produce photo-cross-linkable biodegradable hydrogels.[48] The poly(lactic acid) block of the block-copolymer is susceptible to hydrolytic cleavage allowing the crosslinked hydrogel to degrade, making these hydrogels more attractive for biomedical applications.

In addition to the type of polymer and the type of crosslinking that play major roles in hydrogel degradation, physical properties such as porosity can also contribute significantly. Wachiralarpphaithoon et al. have synthesised poly(2-methacryloyloxyethyl phosphorylcholine) hydrogels crosslinked with polyphosphoesters that are susceptible to hydrolytic and enzymatic degradation.[49] Hydrogels were prepared using a gas foaming method utilising potassium hydrogen carbonate as a porogen salt to introduce highly interconnected pores. This study demonstrated the significant contribution the presence of pores can have on the degradation of the hydrogels, with the porous hydrogels degrading significantly faster than the nonporous counterparts. Introduction of pores, especially interconnected pores, into hydrogel networks allows enhanced diffusion of fluid, enzymes and hydrolytic agents which increase the degradation rate of these networks. The effect of porosity on the degradation rate is not limited to hydrolysable hydrogels, for example Hamid et al. have described the synthesis of degradable PEG porous hydrogels with disulfide degradable crosslinks, with small and large pores

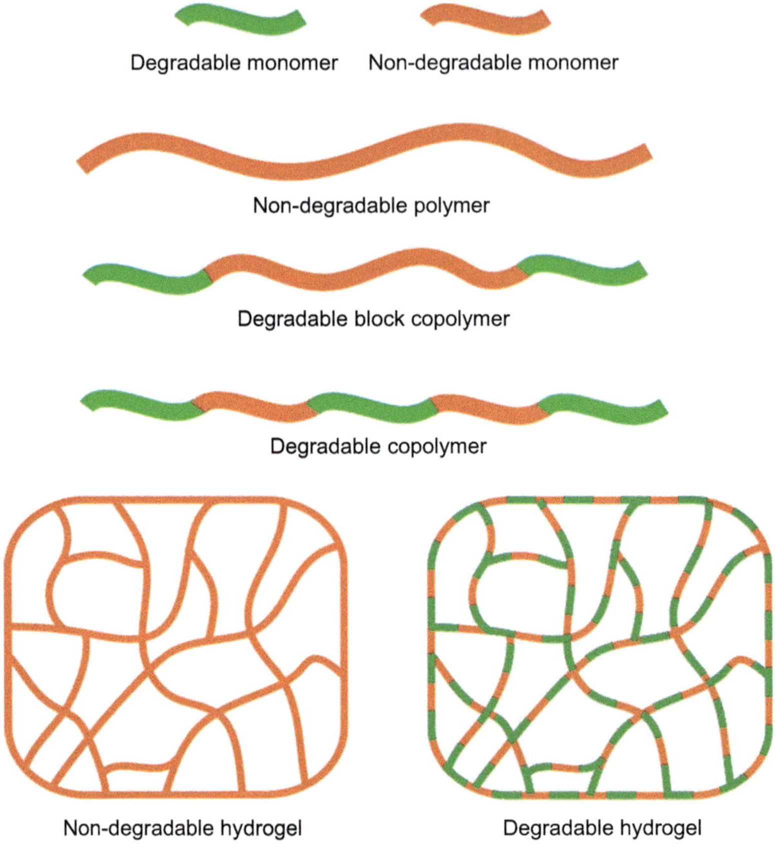

Figure 7.3 Copolymerisation of degradable and nondegradable polymers to produce degradable hydrogels.

for soft tissue engineering applications.[50] *In vitro* and *in vivo* studies with the porous and nonporous versions of the hydrogels demonstrated the effect of both the presence and size of the pores on the hydrogel degradation. While *in vitro*, hydrogels with larger pore sizes degraded quickly (i.e. 14 days), those with smaller pores still remained after 8 weeks. *In vivo*, a similar result was observed whereby histology revealed that nonporous hydrogels were largely unchanged while degradation was evident in both small- and large-sized pore hydrogels. Interconnected pores are often required for tissue engineering applications, and especially in these cases where pores are required to allow infiltration of cells and vascularisation, it is important to take into consideration the effect of porosity and pore size in fine tuning the degradation rate of hydrogels for specific applications. Although varying parameters such as the type and molecular weight of polymers or the degree of crosslinking can allow regulation of degradation, *in vivo* cellular and enzymatic processes can significantly affect these degradation rates. For applications where strict degradation rates are not required, hydrolysable hydrogels may be suitable, in contrast complex applications may require more precisely controlled mechanisms such as cell-mediated hydrogel degradation, which will be discussed in the next section.

7.4.2 Cell-mediated degradation in hydrogel systems

Cells remodel their environment by secreting certain enzymes for the degradation of ECM and its components *in vivo*. Especially in tissue engineering applications, it is important that the degradation of the scaffold occurs simultaneously with the regeneration of tissue and proliferation of cells. Taking advantage of the remodelling ability of cells *in vivo* is a good strategy to achieve such controlled degradation of scaffolds whereby the material is able to provide 3D support to the cells, but also provide expanding space to the cells as needed.

With this strategy in mind, hydrogel materials have been synthesised that degrade upon exposure to cell-secreted enzymes. West and Hubbell have described the synthesis of PEG-based hydrogels with incorporated peptide sequences that are specifically susceptible to cleavage by collagenase and plasmin proteases.[51] *In vitro* studies showed degradation of the synthesised hydrogels in the presence of the specific enzyme but stability in the presence of the nonspecific protease. The use of specific peptide sequences not only allows degradation by the enzyme-secreting cells but also specificity to the type of enzyme that can degrade the material.

If a tissue engineering scaffold allows cells to remodel their surroundings, it would provide a more biomimetic environment for them to proliferate. Feng et al. have demonstrated that human mesenchymal stem cells (hMSCs) can be encapsulated in a methacrylated hyaluronic acid hydrogel crosslinked with matrix metalloproteinase (MMP) degradable crosslinkers.[52] When compared to MMP-insensitive hydrogels, the hMSCs displayed chondrocytic morphology and expressed a higher level of chondrogenic marker genes. While the hMSCs in the insensitive hydrogel remained round, the hMSCs encapsulated in the MMP-sensitive hydrogels took on a more natural, spread profile as a result of degradation and remodelling during culture.

The use of peptides sensitive to cell-secreted enzymes in preparing degradable hydrogels not only allows cells to remodel their surroundings but also can be used in releasing bioactive molecules in assisting tissue regeneration *in vivo*. Angiogenesis is essential for tissue regeneration and survival of growing tissue.[53] In a study by Zisch et al. MMP degradable peptides are crosslinked within a vinyl sulfone functionalised PEG matrix to prepare degradable hydrogels.[54] Vascular endothelial growth factor (VEGF), an angiogenic factor, was covalently incorporated into the synthesised hydrogels, and as a result would only be released during the MMP-mediated degradation. *In vivo* studies in rats resulted in neovascularisation within the hydrogel and the tissue interface especially. On the other hand, hydrogels loaded with nonconjugated soluble VEGF only resulted in an increase of capillary density surrounding the hydrogel implants. The hydrogels were integrated into the implant sites leading to the formation of vascular native tissue. The degradation and controlled release of covalently bound VEGF via MMP-mediated mechanisms are also advantageous in the dosing of such bioactive molecules. When carriers are noncovalently loaded with the bioactive molecule, it is very difficult to control the amount released which is of concern regarding adverse side effects, whereas release via cell-demanded actions would provide a slow release mechanism dependent on cellular remodelling and proliferation.

Scaffolds fabricated for tissue engineering applications are often designed to possess interconnected porous structures to allow cellular infiltration and formation of uniform tissue. These pores are produced using a variety of methods but pore morphology and structure may not be ideal for certain cell types. On the other hand, the use of proteolytically degradable supports may allow these cells to form their own interconnected networks and pores through the scaffold material. Almany and Seliktar prepared fibrinogen–PEG hydrogels which provide biocompatible and cell adhesive hydrogels which also possess proteolytic sensitivity.[55] The proteolytic properties imparted by the fibrinogen component of the hydrogel allowed bovine aortic smooth muscle cells to 'tunnel' and migrate through the bulk of the hydrogel via the secreted proteolytic enzymes, whereby cells were able to form more natural networks (Figure 7.4).

Cell-mediated degradation of hydrogels is not only limited to mammalian cells and can also be achieved by bacteria. Certain parts of the human body, such as the colon, have a natural microbial flora. Brønsted and Kopeček aimed to exploit the presence of these microbes in the colon for the site-specific delivery of drugs.[56] *N*, *N*-dimethylacrylamide, *N*-tert-butylacrylamide and acrylic acid-based hydrogels crosslinked with azoaromatic compounds were synthesised for this application. The crosslinks present in the hydrogels are designed to be susceptible to degradation by microbial azoreductases, which in turn would allow the release of selected drugs. In the study, it was found that the degradation rate of the hydrogels was significantly affected by the crosslinking density which in turn determined the swelling capability of the hydrogels. The length of the azoaromatic crosslinkers determined the crosslinking density, with the longer crosslinkers reducing this density. The swelling and the crosslinking density of the hydrogels were inversely correlated, whereby the lower crosslinking densities increased hydrogel swelling. The increased swelling of the hydrogel also allows enhanced permeation of the enzymes that degrade the crosslinks (Figure 7.5).

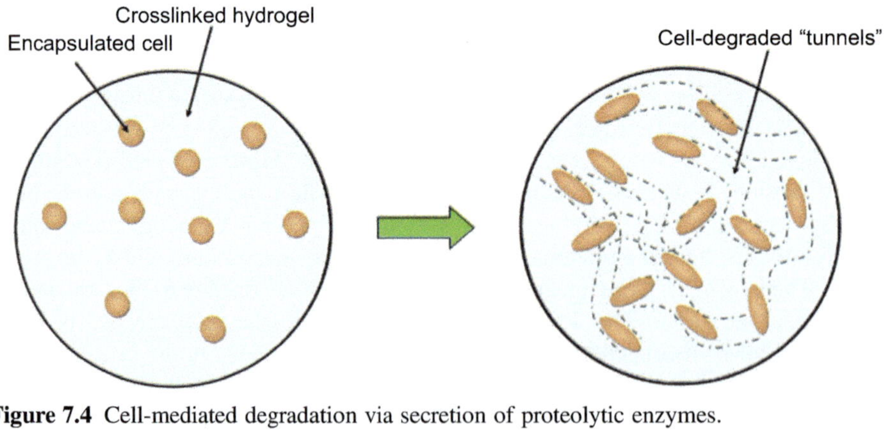

Figure 7.4 Cell-mediated degradation via secretion of proteolytic enzymes.

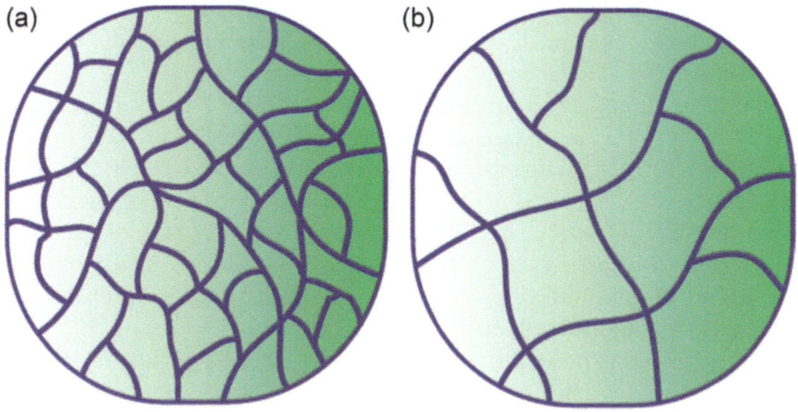

Figure 7.5 Demonstration of hydrogels with (a) high and (b) low crosslink densities. The higher crosslinking density acts like a filter minimising permeation while low crosslinking density allows easier permeation of fluid and other molecules.

7.4.3 Degradable hydrogels based on natural polymers

As mentioned in the previous sections, hydrogels can be synthesised from polymers derived from natural sources. Alginate, chitosan, collagen, hyaluronan and fibrin are such polymers. Naturally derived polymers can be abundantly available, and in addition to possessing functionalities that can interact with cells, these polymers can be degraded by oxidative processes or enzymes (hyaluronidases, collagenases and lysozyme to name a few) naturally present *in vivo*. As a result of their permeable nature, hydrogels are able to provide protection and support to cells while allowing the diffusion of nutrients and metabolites through their structure.[57] The cell and hydrogel types can be matched according to the method of cell encapsulation that is required.[21–23] This section will be discussing degradable hydrogels derived from natural polymers.

Photopolymerisable hyaluronic acid hydrogels have been utilised for the delivery of satellite, and muscle progenitor cells for muscle tissue repair.[58] These hyaluronic acid-based hydrogels were designed for *in situ* curing of the hydrogel–cell combination *in vivo* in the injury site. *In situ* photopolymerisation offers the advantage of delivery of cells in a hydrogel network that would be able to take the shape of the defect site prior to curing. Use of the hyaluronic acid hydrogels in injured mice muscles showed muscle regeneration while providing improved function. Liu et al. on the other hand developed microbeads encased in an alginate hydrogel and Arg–Gly–Asp (RGD).[59] The alginate and fibrin microbeads were designed as biodegradable carriers for human umbilical cord mesenchymal stem cells (hUCMSCs) that would be released while creating macropores within the hydrogel matrix. Hence the alginate–RGD hydrogel would be able to act as a porous scaffold following microbead degradation to provide the support for the hUCMSCs.

A significant loss of adipose tissue can take place as a result of trauma, disease and surgery.[60] A wide range of techniques have been investigated for adipose tissue reconstruction. A method that has been explored is the delivery of adipogenic cells via encapsulation with hydrogels. Collagen- and alginate-based hydrogels have been employed for the fabrication of cell/hydrogel vehicles to promote the formation of fat tissue in the target area where loss of adipose tissue occurred.[60,61]

Myocardial infarction can lead to cardiac tissue death. To repair such damaged tissues grafts of regenerated tissue may be necessary. Giraud et al. have investigated skeletal muscle grafts for the treatment of infarcted cardiac tissue by regenerating myoblasts in a collagenous hydrogel *in vitro*.[62] On the other hand regeneration of smooth muscle for intestinal and blood vessel tissue engineering have garnered interest via the use of degradable hydrogels also. Culture of smooth muscle cells in a fibrin hydrogel and their seeding onto hybrid chitosan/collagen scaffolds has shown growth of smooth muscle for intestinal tissue engineering applications.[63]

Even though natural polymers offer advantages regarding biocompatibility and biodegradability, it may be difficult to tune the degradation and other properties of resultant hydrogels. It may be necessary to use chemical modification or other strategies to provide control over such properties. Alginate for example, even though biocompatible, possesses slow and uncontrolled degradation properties. Boonetheekul et al. described the chemical modification and the use of low-molecular-weight alginates to control the degradation of produced hydrogels.[64] Boontheekul et al. found that partial oxidation of the alginate created more hydrolysis-susceptible acetal groups which increased the degradation rate of the hydrogels. Further to the partial oxidation, combination of low-molecular-weight (M_w) alginate with high M_w alginate also improved the degradation of the produced hydrogels. The incorporation of lower M_w alginate reduces the number of degradable groups per polymer chain allowing more rapid degradation of individual polymer chains and ultimately the hydrogel.

Natural polymers offer desirable properties and functionalities for biomedical applications including in the synthesis of hydrogels. If the shortcomings (see Section 7.2) associated with naturally derived polymers could be minimised or if such materials are utilised for applications where these drawbacks have a minimal impact, then it would be possible to apply such natural hydrogels for a wide array of biomedical purposes.

7.4.4 Photodegradable hydrogels

Direct manipulation of hydrogel degradation can be highly advantageous for biomedical applications where temporal and stimuli-responsive control over cell or therapeutic delivery is necessary. Photodegradation is one way such control could be achieved. A source of light can be employed to degrade hydrogels where light-sensitive functionalities are incorporated into the polymer networks. Photodegradable groups can be directly incorporated into polymer backbones or photodegradable crosslinks can be utilised for various hydrogel systems to achieve a stimulus-responsive degradation.

Photoresponsive degradation of hydrogels can be exploited to influence cell behaviour and phenotype. Kirschner et al. have synthesised clickable hydrogels using PEG-star macromers that are crosslinked via an azide-functionalised photodegradable crosslinker.[65] The degradation of the synthesised hydrogels via the use of UV light allowed control over the hydrogel modulus, which in turn affected the activation of porcine valvular interstitial cells (VICs). Seeded VICs displayed fibroblast-to-myofibroblast phenotype switching depending on the stiffness of the hydrogels with and without UV degradation (Figure 7.6). Initial VIC activation to myofibroblasts were partially reversed when the modulus of the hydrogels were significantly reduced following irradiation with UV light. Similar hydrogel systems are also very attractive for biomedical applications where the direction of cell migration or network formation is significant. For example McKinnon et al. utilised similarly photodegradable PEG hydrogels to modulate extension of motor axons in embryonic stem cell-derived motor neurons.[66] Such systems not only allow control over cell phenotype, but also allow investigation of the effect of the surface and environment on cell behaviour.

Targeted delivery is highly attractive in reducing side effects of such therapeutics by minimising the nonspecific release of drugs or other bioactive molecules. Not only is the delivery of the therapeutic to its destination but its controlled release is also desired. Photodegradation in hydrogels is not only beneficial for degradation of the hydrogel but also in allowing the temporal release of bioactive molecules. Hydrogels utilising photodegradable macromers with different functionalities that can conjugate to various therapeutic agents have been synthesised in previous studies.[67] Such hydrogels allow the release of the conjugated therapeutic following exposure to UV light at the exact desired time. Griffin et al. has demonstrated as examples successful release of cell adhesive peptide bovine serum albumin, and transforming growth factor-β1 and confirmed that the released molecules maintained their bioactivity (Figure 7.7).

Isolating specific cells for diagnosis and identification of diseases or infections can be highly advantageous. Selective capture of specific cells and their subsequent release have been demonstrated using photodegradable hydrogels. Shin et al. have employed antibody-functionalised PEG-based hydrogels with photolabile crosslinkers that can

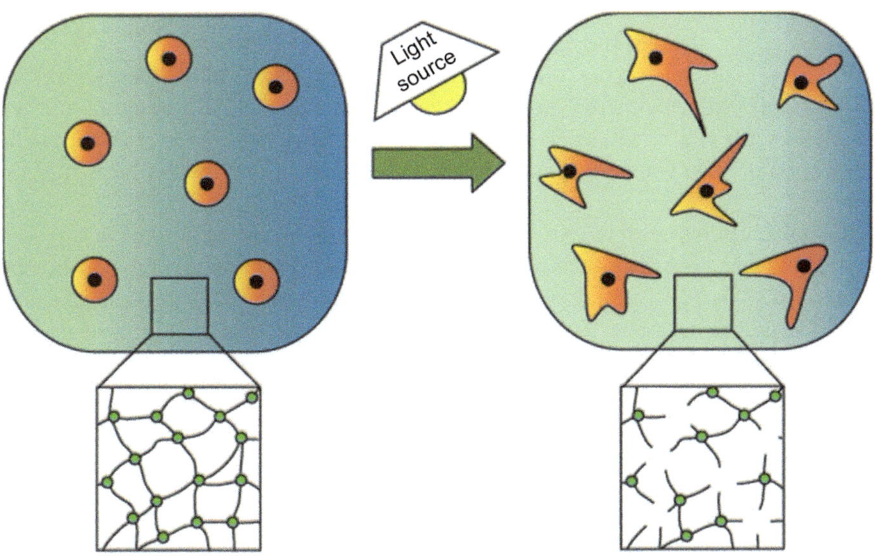

Figure 7.6 Modulation of the cell phenotype/morphology of cells through photodegradation of crosslinks.

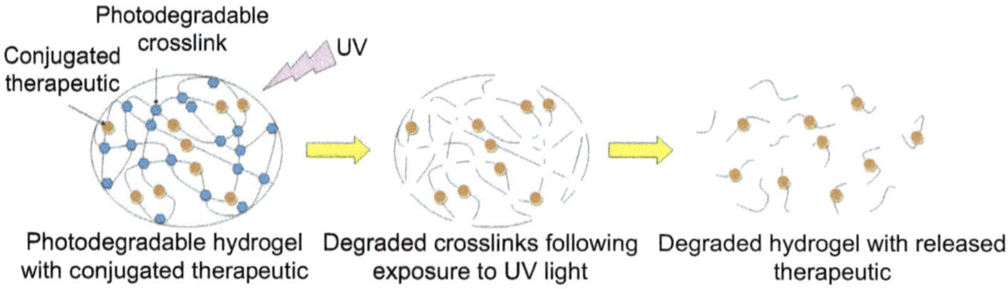

Figure 7.7 Release of conjugated therapeutic via photodegradation of crosslinks in a hydrogel carrier.

capture CD4 and CD8 T cells through their surface markers and subsequently release them via the photodegradation of the underlying hydrogel.[68] Such use of degradable hydrogels may provide more efficient, selective and high-throughput methods for pathological analyses.

7.5 Where to? – degradable hydrogels

Biological systems are highly complex, and the use of current biomaterials for biomedical applications in therapeutic and tissue repair applications is lacking. Even though researchers have developed breakthrough materials that show promise both *in vitro* and *in vivo*, only a very small fraction of these materials ever make it to an applied clinical level. To accommodate these complexities, versatility and customisation are the key to obtain positive, individually tailored results. Hydrogel-based biomaterials are of particular interest as a result of their tunable physicochemical characteristics. As discussed in this chapter, the ability to tailor all of these properties from a molecular level makes hydrogels highly versatile. Being able to control all of the properties of hydrophilicity/hydrophobicity, swelling capability, mechanical strength, stiffness, morphology, elasticity, cellular interactions, functionality, degradation rates and permeability, among many others, demonstrates the extent of flexibility these materials possess.

Degradable materials have always been attractive for biomedical applications, since the need to retrieve or dispose of the materials once they have completed their function is eliminated. Especially for applications where implantation is required, surgical and other invasive procedures to remove the implanted material would no longer be required. Similarly for hydrogels, due to their potential use in many biomedical applications, the ability to impart biodegradability remains highly desirable. As demonstrated in this chapter, degradable hydrogels not only allow the facile removal of a 'foreign' material, but as a carrier for the delivery of therapeutics and cells. Even though there are many degradation mechanisms available for exploitation in hydrogel systems, often a single method is not sufficient when considering the vastly complex biological systems. Even though difficult, the combination of multiple mechanisms of degradation would produce hydrogels that are adaptable to many more applications.

Investigation of degradable hydrogel materials for biomedical applications is highly extensive. The amount of techniques, precursors, functionalities and degradation mechanisms available for synthesis of hydrogels and the variety of applications for these materials are immense. With all of this knowledge at hand, future research on degradable hydrogel materials needs to focus on taking advantage of this available knowledge to produce complex materials that can mimic biology as closely as possible for relevant applications. It is after millions of years of evolution that biological systems have reached this level of complexity. For practicality and applicability purposes, 'simple' is always more attractive. Even though finding the simplest methods to synthesise the required biomaterials should be sought, the necessary complexities should not be sacrificed. As a result of this, within the bounds of limitations, it is important that any possibility of combining different polymers, techniques and degradation mechanisms should be explored. Regardless of the large amount of current research in regard to hydrogels, because of their extensively tailorable and desirable properties, hydrogels will continue to be at the forefront of biomedical research for many years to come, and only with more biomimetic structures will it be possible to produce constructs that satisfy the needs of clinical applications.

References

1. Drury JL, Mooney DJ. Hydrogels for tissue engineering: scaffold design variables and applications. *Biomaterials* 2003;**24**:4337–51.
2. Hoffman AS. Hydrogels for biomedical applications. *Adv Drug Deliv Rev* 2012;**64**: 18–23.
3. Hoare TR, Kohane DS. Hydrogels in drug delivery: progress and challenges. *Polymer* 2008;**49**:1993–2007.
4. Kopecek J, Yang J. Hydrogels as smart biomaterials. *Polym Int* 2007;**56**:1078–98.
5. Lee KY, Mooney DJ. Hydrogels for tissue engineering. *Chem Rev* 2001;**101**(7):1869–77.
6. Liu X, Holzwarth JM, Ma PX. Functionalized synthetic biodegradable polymer scaffolds for tissue engineering. *Macromol Biosci* 2012;**12**:911–9.
7. Hoffman AS. Hydrogels for biomedical applications. *Anns NY Acad Sci* 2001;**944**:62–73.
8. Kawazoe N, Inoue C, Tateishi T, Chen G. A cell leakproof PLGA-collagen hybrid scaffold for cartilage tissue engineering. *Biotechnol Prog* 2010;**26**(3):819–26.
9. Valente JFA, Valente TAM, Alves P, Ferreira P, Silva A, Correia IJ. Alginate based scaffolds for bone tissue engineering. *Mat Sci Eng C* 2012;**32**:2596–603.
10. Wen P, Gao J, Zhang Y, Li X, Long Y, Wu X, et al. Fabrication of chitosan scaffolds with tunable porous orientation structure for tissue engineering. *J Biomater Sci Polym Ed* 2011; **22**:19–40.
11. Gervaso F, Scalera F, Padmanabhan SK, Sannino A, Licciulli A. High-performance hydroxyapatite scaffolds for bone tissue engineering applications. *Int J Appl Ceram Technol* 2012;**9**(3):507–16.
12. Kim S, Healy KE. Synthesis and characterisation of injectable poly(*N*-isopropylacrylamide-co-acyrlic acid) hydrogels with proteolytically degradable cross-links. *Biomacromolecules* 2003;**4**:1214–23.
13. Adds PJ, Hunt CJ, Dart JKG. Amniotic membrane grafts, "fresh" or frozen? A clinical and in vitro comparison. *Br J Ophthalmol* 2001;**85**:905–7.

14. Angelova N, Hunkeler D. Rationalising the design of polymeric biomaterials. *Trends Biotechnol* 1999;**17**:409–21.
15. Zhu H, Ji J, Shen J. Surface engineering of poly(DL-lactic acid) by entrapment of biomacromolecules. *Macromol Rapid Commun* 2002;**23**:819–23.
16. Ko HF, Sfeir C, Kumta PN. Novel synthesis strategies for natural polymer and composite biomaterials as potential scaffolds for tissue engineering. *Phil Trans R Soc A* 2010;**368**: 1981–97.
17. Liang Y, Liu W, Han B, yang C, Ma Q, Zhao W, et al. Fabrication and characters of a corneal endothelial cells scaffold based on chitosan. *J Mater Sci Mater Med* 2011;**22**: 175–83.
18. Lu DR, Xiao CM, Xu SJ. Starch-based completely biodegradable polymer materials. *Express Polym Lett* 2009;**3**(6):366–75.
19. Sachlos E, Czerbuszka JT. Making tissue engineering scaffolds work: review on the application of solid freeform fabrication technology to the production of tissue engineering scaffolds. *Eur Cell Mater* 2003;**5**:29–40.
20. Sadr N, Pippenger BE, Scherberich A, Wendt D, Mantero S, Martin I, et al. Enhancing the biological performance of synthetic polymeric materials by decoration with engineered, decellularized extracellular matrix. *Biomaterials* 2012;**33**:5085–93.
21. Jen AC, Wake MC, Mikos AG. Hydrogels for cell immobilisation. *Biotechnol Bioeng* 1996;**50**(4):357–64.
22. Alsberg E, Anderson KW, Albeiruti A, Franceschi RT, Mooney DJ. Cell-interactive alginate hydrogels for bone tissue engineering. *J Dent Res* 2001;**80**(11):2025–9.
23. De Chalain T, Phillips JH, Hinek A. Bioengineering of elastic cartilage with aggregated porcine and human auricular chondrocytes and hydrogels containing alginate, collagen and K-elastin. *J Biomed Mater Res A* 1999;**44**(3):280–8.
24. Kim W, Mooney D, Arany P, Lee K, Huebsch N, Kim J. Adipose tissue engineering using injectable, oxidized alginate hydrogels. *Tissue Eng A* 2012;**18**(7–8):737–43.
25. Li Z, Guan J. Hydrogels for cardiac tissue engineering. *Polymers* 2011;**3**(2):740–61.
26. Reis L, Chiu L, Liang Y, Hyunh K, Momen A, Radisic M. A peptide-modified chitosan-collagen hydrogel for cardiac cell culture and delivery. *Acta Biomater* 2012;**8**(3): 1022–36.
27. Chiu L, Janic K, Radisic M. Engineering of oriented myocardium on three-dimensional micropatterned collagen-chitosan hydrogel. *Int J Artif Organs* 2012;**35**(4):237–50.
28. Guarino V, Gloria A, Raucci M, Ambrosio L. Hydrogel-based platforms for the regeneration of osteochondral tissue and intervertebral disc. *Polymers* 2012;**4**(3): 1590–612.
29. Li F, Ba QJ, Niu SM, Guo Y, Duan YK, Zhao P, et al. In-situ forming biodegradable glycol chitosan-based hydrogels: synthesis, characterization, and chondrocyte culture. *Mater Sci Eng C Mater Biol Appl* 2012;**32**(7):2017–25.
30. Lind M, Larsen A, Clausen C, Osther K, Everland H. Cartilage repair with chondrocytes in fibrin hydrogel and MPEG polylactide scaffold: an in vivo study in goats. *Knee Surg Sport Tr A* 2008;**16**(7):690–8.
31. Strange D, Oyen M. Composite hydrogels for nucleus pulposus tissue engineering. *J Mech Behav Biomed* 2012;**11**:16–26.
32. Hu JG, Chen B, Guo F, Du JY, Gu PC, Lin XJ, et al. Injectable silk fibroin/polyurethane composite hydrogel for nucleus pulposus replacement. *J Mater Sci Mater Med* 2012; **23**(3):711–22.
33. Gong JP, Katsuyama Y, Kurokawa T, Osada Y. Double network hydrogels with extremely high mechanical strength. *Adv Mater* 2003;**15**(14):1155–8.

34. Merchant RE, Zhu J. Design properties of hydrogel tissue engineering scaffolds. *Exp Rev Med Dev* 2011;**8**(5):607–26.
35. Ronda L, Bruno S, Abbruzzetti S, Viappiani C, Bettati S. Ligand reactivity and allosteric regulation of haemoglobin based oxygen carriers. *Biochim Biophys Acta* 2008;**1784**: 1365–77.
36. Bailon P, Berhtold W. Polyethylene glycol-conjugated pharmaceutical proteins. *Pharm Sci Technol Today* 1998;**1**(8):352–6.
37. Kim DN, Lee W, Koh WG. Preparation of protein microarrays on non-fouling and hydrated poly(ethylene glycol) hydrogel substrates using photochemical surface modification. *J Chem Technol Biotechnol* 2009;**84**:279–84.
38. Quirk RA, Davies MC, Tendler SJB, Chan WC, Shakesheff KM. Controlling biological interactions with poly(lactic acid) by surface entrapment modification. *Langmuir* 2001;**17**: 2817–20.
39. Ma Z, Mao Z, Gao C. Surface modification and property analysis of biomedical polymers used for tissue engineering. *Colloids Surf B* 2007;**60**:137–57.
40. Shen M, Pan YV, Wagner MS, Hauch KD, Castner DG, Ratner BD, et al. Inhibition of monocyte adhesion and fibrinogen adsorption on glow discharge plasma deposited tetraethylene glycol dimethyl ether. *J Biomat Sci Polym Ed* 2001;**12**(9):961–78.
41. Dalton PD, Hostert C, Albrecht K, Moeller M, Groll J. Structure and properties of urea-crosslinked star poly(ethylene oxide)-ran-(proplyene oxide) hydrogels. *Macromol Biosci* 2008;**8**:923–31.
42. Freed LE, Vunjack-Novakovic G, Biron RJ, Eagles DB, Lesnoy DC, Barlow SK, et al. Biodegradable polymer scaffolds for tissue engineering. *Biotechnol* 1994;**12**(7):680–93.
43. Hutmacher DW. Scaffold design and fabrication technologies for engineering tissues – state of the art and future perspectives. *J Biomater Sci Polym Ed* 2001;**12**(1):107–24.
44. Marler JJ, Upton J, Langer R, Vacanti JP. Transplantation of cells in matrices for tissue regeneration. *Adv Drug Deliv Rev* 1998;**33**:165–82.
45. Zhang C, Zhang N, Wen X. Synthesis and characterization of biocompatible, degradable, light-curable, polyurethane-based elastic hydrogels. *J Biomed Mater Res A* 2007;**82**: 637–50.
46. Ozcelik B, Brown KD, Blencowe A, Ladewig K, Stevens GW, Scheerlinck JPY, et al. Biodegradable and biocompatible poly(ethylene glycol)-based hydrogel films for the regeneration of corneal endothelium. *Adv Healthcare Mater* 2014;**3**:1496–507.
47. Ulbrich K, Subr V, Podperova P, Buresova M. Synthesis of novel hydrolytically degradable hydrogels for controlled drug release. *J Control Release* 1995;**34**: 155–65.
48. Metters AT, Anseth KS, Bowman CN. Fundamental studies of a novel, biodegradable PEG-*b*-PLA hydrogel. *Polymer* 2000;**41**:3993–4004.
49. Wachiralarpphaithoon C, Iwasaki Y, Akiyoshi K. Enzyme-degradable phosphorylcholine porous hydrogels cross-linked with polyphosphoesters for cell matrices. *Biomaterials* 2007;**28**:984–93.
50. Hamid ZAA, Blencowe A, Ozcelik B, Palmer JA, Stevenes GW, Abberton KM, et al. Epoxy-amine synthesised hydrogel scaffolds for soft-tissue engineering. *Biomaterials* 2010;**31**:6454–67.
51. West JL, Hubbell JA. Polymeric biomaterials with degradation sites for proteases involved in cell migration. *Macromolecules* 1999;**32**:241–4.
52. Feng Q, Zhu M, Wei K, Bian L. Cell-mediated degradation regulates human mesenchymal stem cell chondrogenesis and hypertrophy in MMP-sensitive hyaluronic acid hydrogels. *PLoS One* 2014;**9**:e99587.

53. Guan J, Stankus JJ, Wagner WR. Biodegradable elastomeric scaffolds with basic fibroblast growth factor release. *J Control Release* 2007;**120**:70–8.
54. Zisch AH, Lutolf MP, Ehrbar M, Raeber GP, Rizzi SC, Davies N, et al. Cell-demanded release of VEGF from synthetic, biointeractive cell ingrowth matrices for vascularised tissue growth. *FASEB J* 2003;**17**:2260–2.
55. Almany L, Seliktar D. Biosynthetic hydrogel scaffolds made from fibrinogen and polyethylene glycol for 3D cell cultures. *Biomaterials* 2005;**26**:2467–77.
56. Brønsted H, Kopeček J. Hydrogels for site-specific drug delivery to the colon: *in vitro* and *in vivo* degradation. *Pharm Res* 1992;**9**:1540–5.
57. Cavalieri F, Miano F, D'Antona P, Paradossi G. Study of gelling behavior of poly(vinyl alcohol)-methacrylate for potential utilizations in tissue replacement and drug delivery. *Biomacromolecules* 2004;**5**:2439–46.
58. Rossi CA, Flaibani M, Blaauw B, Pozzobon M, Figallo E, Reggiani C, et al. In vivo tissue engineering of functional skeletal muscle by freshly isolated satellite cells embedded in a photopolymerizable hydrogel. *FASEB J* 2011;**25**:2296–304.
59. Liu J, Zhou H, Weir MD, Xu HHK, Chen Q, Trotman CA. Fast-degradable microbeads encapsulating human umbilical cord stem cells in alginate for muscle tissue engineering. *Tissue Eng A* 2012;**18**(21–22):2303–14.
60. Yao R, Zhang RJ, Lin F, Luan J. Injectable cell/hydrogel microspheres induce the formation of fat lobule-like microtissues and vascularized adipose tissue regeneration. *Biofabrication* 2012;**4**:1–10.
61. Galateanu B, Dimonie D, Vasile E, Nae S, Cimpean A, Costache M. Layer-shaped alginate hydrogels enhance the biological performance of human adipose-derived stem cells. *BMC Biotechnol* 2012;**12**:35–48.
62. Giraud MN, Ayuni E, Cook S, Siepe M, Carrel TP, Tevaearai HT. Hydrogel-based engineered skeletal muscle grafts normalize heart function early after myocardial infarction. *Artif Organs* 2008;**32**(9):692–700.
63. Zakhem E, Raghavan S, Gilmont RR, Bitar KN. Chitosan-based scaffolds for the support of smooth muscle constructs in intestinal tissue engineering. *Biomaterials* 2012;**33**: 4810–7.
64. Boontheekul T, Kong HJ, Mooney DJ. Controlling alginate gel degradation utilizing partial oxidation and bimodal molecular weight distribution. *Biomaterials* 2005;**26**: 2455–65.
65. Kirschner CM, Alge DL, Gould ST, Anseth KS. Clickable, photodegradable hydrogels to dynamically modulate valvular interstitial cell phenotype. *Adv Healthcare Mater* 2014;**3**: 649–57.
66. McKinnon DD, Brown TE, Kyburz KA, Kiyotake E, Anseth KS. Design and characterization of synthetically accessible photodegradable hydrogel for user-directed formation of neural networks. *Biomacromol* 2014;**15**:2808–16.
67. Griffin DR, Schlosser JL, Lam SF, Nguyen TH, Maynard HD, Kasko AM. Synthesis of photodegradable macromers for conjugation and release of bioactive molecules. *Biomacromol* 2013;**14**:1199–207.
68. Shin SA, You J, Rahimian A, Vu T, Siltanen C, Ehsanipour A, et al. Photodegradable hydrogels for capture, detection and release of live cells. *Angew Chem Int Ed* 2014;**53**: 8221–4.

Angiogenesis in hydrogel biomaterials

8

B.A. Nsiah, E.M. Moore, L.C. Roudsari, N.K. Virdone, J.L. West
Duke University, Durham, NC, USA

8.1 Introduction

Angiogenesis, the sprouting of new vasculature from existing vasculature, or related vasculogenesis, de novo formation of vessels, is an important biological process across a number of biomedical applications such as cancer, ischemic diseases, some types of implantable biosensors, and tissue engineering and regenerative medicine. Many cancer therapies seek to prevent or inhibit angiogenesis in order to cut off the blood, nutrient and oxygen supply to tumours. Conversely, in ischemic diseases, therapies seek to restore blood flow to dying tissues. In some biosensor applications, promoting growth of microvasculature adjacent to the sensor is critical for efficient transport of analytes to the sensor. In tissue engineering and regenerative medicine, formation of functional microvasculature is critical to the survival and efficacy of most types of tissue constructs.

To date, many of the engineered tissues that have been used successfully in the clinic have been limited to thin and avascular tissues such as skin (Falanga and Sabolinski, 1999) and cartilage (Fulco et al., 2013). Even in tissue-engineered bladder wall, a quite thin tissue, an omental wrap was required for tissue vascularisation to quickly supply the new tissue with adequate oxygen, nutrients and waste transport (Atala et al., 2006). The need for functional microvasculature in engineered tissues remains a major barrier to the success of tissue engineering and regenerative medicine technologies. For either tissue engineering applications or the generation of vessels within host tissue to treat ischemia or near a biosensor, hydrogel materials that can support and promote establishment of functional vasculature are attractive due to hydrogel mechanical properties, which can often be 'tuned' to match tissue properties, the excellent biocompatibility of many hydrogel materials and the ability to spatially localise angiogenic activity. In order to address the need for functional vasculature, tissue engineers and biomaterials scientists are taking clues from the biology of the angiogenesis process and developing methods to mimic nature when designing pro-angiogenic hydrogel materials.

8.2 Biology of angiogenesis

Angiogenesis in vivo occurs during embryogenesis, wound healing and during disease states such as intraocular neovascular disorders and cancer. Angiogenesis

Biosynthetic Polymers for Medical Applications. http://dx.doi.org/10.1016/B978-1-78242-105-4.00008-0

is a highly coordinated process that is mediated by several angiogenic signalling factors, extracellular matrix components and cells resulting in the formation of new blood vessels.

Embryonic angiogenesis occurs after the initial elements of the cardiovascular system have been established and the embryo reaches a critical size where passive nutrient transport can no longer adequately support the tissue, with new blood vessels sprouting from the existing nascent vessels. Similar angiogenesis occurs in the adult during wound repair and in tissues undergoing different disease pathologies such as tumour formation or hypoxia. This process is initiated by hypoxia-inducible factors HIF-1 and HIF-2 at sites of low oxygen tension, leading to the expression of vascular endothelial growth factors VEGF-A, VEGF-B, VEGF-C and VEGF-D as well as fibroblast growth factor-2 (FGF-2) (Marti, 2005). These growth factors are frequently targeted for therapeutic angiogenesis and design of pro-angiogenic materials.

Vascular cells migrate, proliferate and remodel surrounding the tissue to form new vasculature in response to the soluble factors released from ischemic tissue. Vessels sprout towards angiogenic factor gradients mediating disruption of the connections between endothelial cells and the surrounding mural pericytes of existing vasculature. Sprouting is initiated by the tip endothelial cell detaching from the basement membrane, followed by endothelial cell migration. Next, vacuoles form and fuse to create tubule lumen, and pericytes, supportive mural cells that stabilise vessels, are recruited in response to platelet-derived growth factor-BB (PDGF-BB) secreted by endothelial cells (Zhang et al., 2009; Lindahl et al., 1997). Finally, the resulting vasculature stabilises, remodels and matures, with the endothelial cells returning to a nonmigratory, quiescent state (Madeddu, 2005). This process is depicted in the diagram in Figure 8.1.

8.3 Protein hydrogels to support angiogenic activity

An approach to optimal formation of vessel networks in a material has been to provide a substitute for the normal tissue extracellular matrix (ECM). A relatively straightforward way to accomplish this goal is to employ hydrogels formed from matrix proteins such as collagen gels (Nicossia and Ottinetti, 1990) or gels formed from the reconstituted basement membrane (i.e. Matrigel™, Kubota et al., 1988). Fibrin gels can also be used (Nicossia and Ottinetti, 1990), mimicking the provisional matrix during wound healing. These materials provide ligands for adhesive receptors such as the integrin receptor, and can be degraded by cellular proteases as cells migrate and form tissue. These biological properties allow cells encapsulated in or seeded on such materials to adhere and migrate in order to organise themselves into vascular structures and networks, as demonstrated in Figure 8.2.

In pioneering work, Rakesh Jain's group was able to form stable, functional vessel networks by encapsulating human umbilical vein endothelial cells (HUVECs) and pericyte precursor cells (10T 1/2 cells) in three-dimensional fibronectin and collagen gels (Koike et al., 2004). Upon implantation, the HUVECs quickly formed interconnecting tubule networks. Over the first two weeks, these neovessels connected to

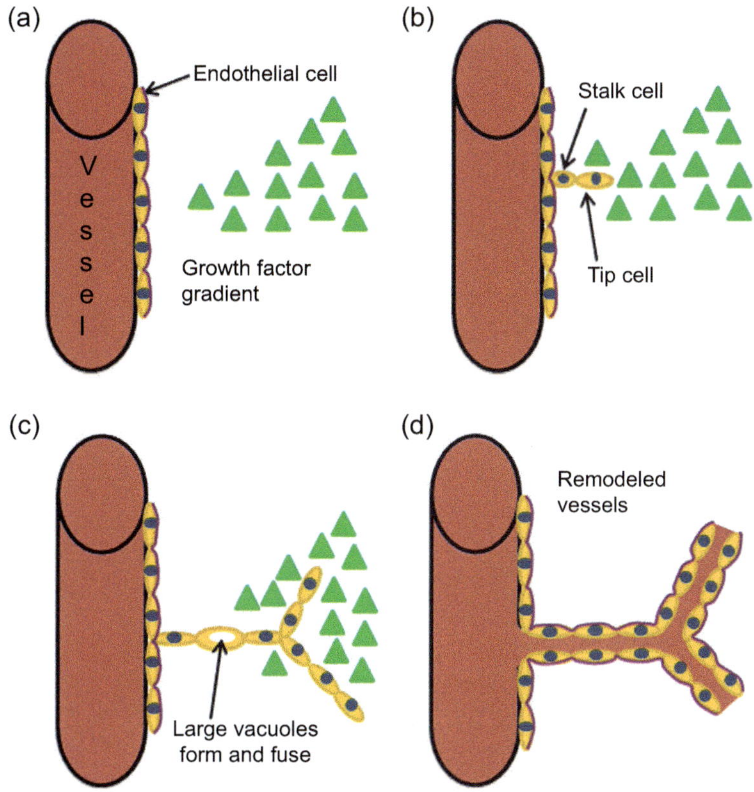

Figure 8.1 The process of angiogenesis. (a) Endothelial cells associated with an existing vessel sense and respond to a gradient of an angiogenic factor. (b) The leading tip endothelial cell degrades the basement membrane in order to migrate along the gradient; the tip cell is followed by additional cells. (c) Large vacuoles form into tubule lumens. (d) Pericytes stabilise newly formed vessels with deposition of basement membrane.

the mouse's vasculature and supported blood flow, remaining stable and functional for at least a year. Interestingly, when HUVECs alone were implanted, vessel structures quickly regressed, indicating the critical role of the mural pericytes in vessel stabilisation.

8.4 Synthetic hydrogels to support angiogenic activity

Synthetic hydrogels have been widely used as scaffolds for tissue engineering because they can provide mechanical properties similar to many soft tissues, often provide excellent biocompatibility, and can be designed to support a variety of cell types, behaviours and phenoytpes. Compared to protein-based hydrogels, tuning of mechanical properties is usually easier and can be accomplished over a broader range,

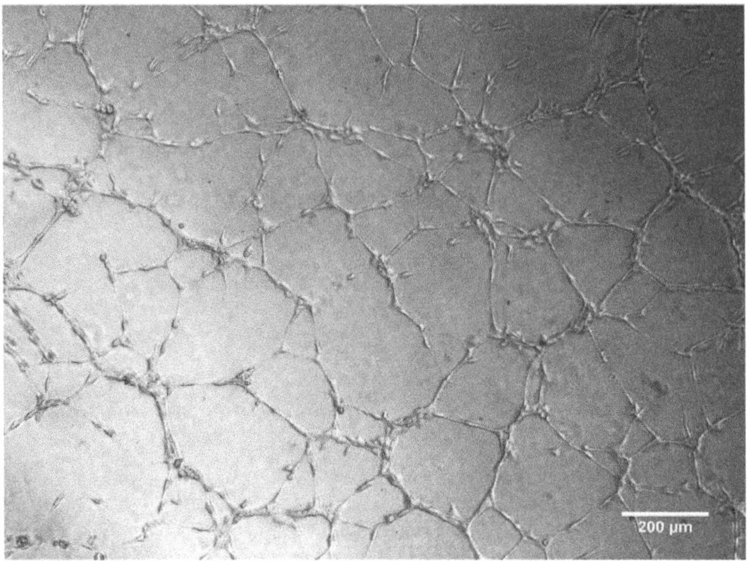

Figure 8.2 Endothelial cells spontaneously assemble into interconnecting tubule networks when cultured in appropriate protein-based hydrogels. This example shows the use of Matrigel™ as the hydrogel material.

cell–material interactions can be controlled and intentionally manipulated, and issues associated with proteins isolated from blood or tissue are avoided. When hydrogels are employed as scaffolds, cells are usually homogeneously encapsulated within the hydrogel network during the hydrogel formation process, though it is also possible to fabricate porous hydrogel scaffolds to seed cells following fabrication to allow tissue ingrowth. While outstanding results have been accomplished in protein-based gels (Nicosia and Ottinetti, 1990; Koike et al., 2004), synthetic hydrogels provide engineers with the opportunity to intentionally design materials to promote or control angiogenesis. This chapter thus primarily focuses on the intentional design of hydrogel materials to support and guide angiogenic activity. The most common strategy in the design of such materials has been to select a relatively inert synthetic hydrogel material and then to modify it with bioactive factors to support and promote angiogenesis, as depicted in Figure 8.3.

For angiogenesis-like activity to occur in synthetic hydrogels, the most basic prerequisite is that vascular cells must be able to migrate in the material to allow vessel assembly. Cell-adhesive interactions are thus required to permit cells to develop the traction forces required for migration. Most synthetic hydrogels, such as poly(ethylene glycol), poly(vinyl alcohol) or poly(hydroxyethylmethacrylate), are inherently cell nonadhesive or at least minimally cell adhesive, due to their highly hydrophilic nature and lack of interaction with cell surface receptors. Polysaccharides such as alginate have also been utilised as the inert base material. The chemical structures of these inert hydrogel base materials are shown in Figure 8.4. To render these types of hydrogels

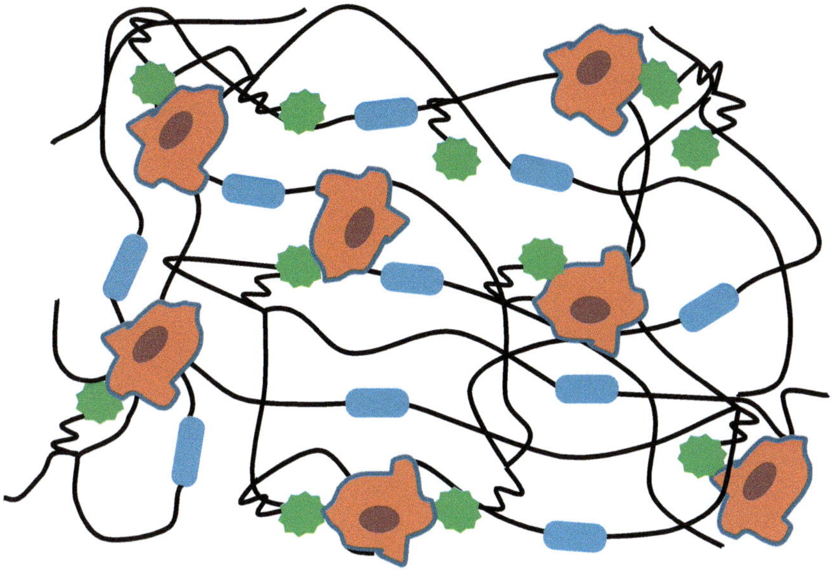

Figure 8.3 Cells (red) can be encapsulated within bioactive hydrogels formed from a bio-inert base polymer (black lines) modified with protease-sensitive peptides (blue) and cell adhesion ligands (green).

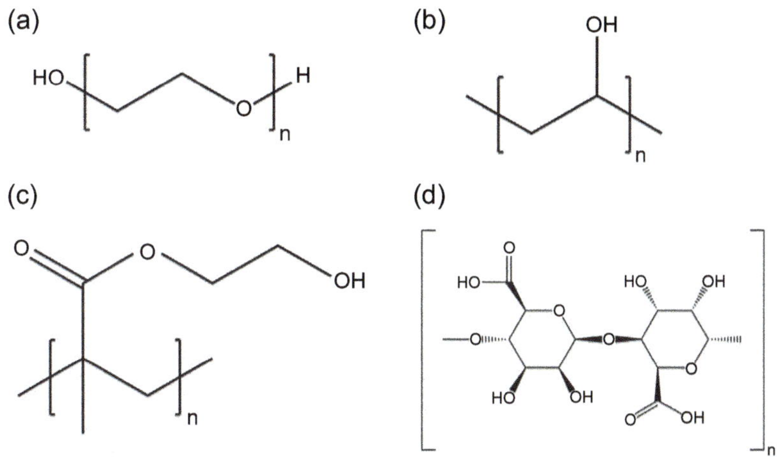

Figure 8.4 Chemical structures of PEG (a), PVA (b), PHEMA (c) and alginate (d). Crosslinked networks of these polymers form relatively bio-inert hydrogels.

cell-adhesive, short peptides representing the adhesion domains of ECM proteins such as collagen, laminin or fibronectin have been incorporated into hydrogels. The most commonly used adhesive sequence for promotion of angiogenesis in hydrogels has been the fibronectin-derived arg-gly-asp-ser (RGDS) sequence, which binds to several

Table 8.1 Endothelial cell-adhesive peptides that can be utilised in hydrogel modification to promote angiogenic-like activity

Peptide sequence	Source protein
RGDS	Fibronectin
Cyclic RGD	Fibronectin
PHSRN	Fibronectin
REDV	Fibronectin
YIGSR	Laminin
IKVAV	Laminin
QHREDGS	Angiopoietin-1
CRRETAWAC	Identified via phage display

integrin receptors including $\alpha_v\beta_3$. Table 8.1 lists a variety of adhesive peptides that have been investigated for mediating vascular cell adhesion to hydrogel biomaterials. As an example, RGDS has frequently been incorporated into poly(ethylene glycol) diacrylate-based (PEGDA) hydrogels by attaching either the carboxyl or amino terminus of the peptide sequence to a bifunctional PEG-acrylate molecule, with a reactive group such as an acrylate available to crosslink into the hydrogel to covalently immobilise the peptide (Hern and Hubbell, 1998). This allows for facile control of cell-adhesive properties independent of the hydrogel mechanical properties, which depend primarily on the length and concentration of the PEGDA component of the formulation (Nemir et al., 2010). In the absence of the immobilised peptide, the PEG hydrogels were cell nonadhesive, whereas with covalent immobilisation of RGDS, cell adhesion and spreading were robust (Hern and Hubbell, 1998). Additionally, hydrogels with acrylate or methacrylate crosslink sites can be easily fabricated using photochemical processes, even in the presence of cells (Sawhney et al., 1993). This provides the opportunity for spatiotemporal control over hydrogel formation and peptide immobilisation (Hahn et al., 2006).

Migration in three-dimensional hydrogels also requires the presence of pathways that are conducive to cell movement. One approach is to fabricate porous hydrogel scaffolds, with continuous, interconnected pore networks of sufficient diameter to allow cell movements. One way to create such pore structures in hydrogels has been to use a sacrificial porogen to define the pore network (Madden et al., 2010; Scott et al., 2010; Miller et al., 2012; Shepard et al., 2012). Using 3D printed carbohydrate glass filaments as the sacrificial porogen, Miller et al. were able to form precisely patterned tubular voids that could then be lined with endothelial cells and ultimately even perfused with culture media. This technique was compatible with a variety of pro-angiogenic hydrogels, including fibrin, Matrigel™ and photopolymerised PEG hydrogels. Another interesting strategy has been the assembly of scaffolds from fusion of hydrogel microspheres, where gaps between fused microspheres form an interconnected pore network; this technique potentially allows a modular approach to scaffold design where different sets of microspheres with differing compositions (such as types of encapsulated cells or releasable factors) could be combined at will to create customised scaffold environments (Nguyen et al., 2013).

As an alternative to porous scaffolds, hydrogels can be designed to be degraded by cellular proteases involved in migration (West and Hubbell, 1999; Gobin and West, 2002; Lee et al., 2005), so that cells migrate using similar processes as they would during migration in tissue or in protein-based gels. This has been accomplished in synthetic hydrogels by incorporating short peptides that are substrates for targeted proteolytic enzymes into the polymer structures used to form hydrogels (see Figure 8.3). This approach allows cells to essentially create their own pathways through an otherwise solid hydrogel material via localised degradation, and ties material degradation rates to cellular activity. PEGDA-based hydrogels modified with the cell-adhesive peptide RGDS and designed to be degraded by matrix metalloproteinase-2 (MMP2), a key protease in angiogenesis, are able to support angiogenesis-like activity in vitro when endothelial cells and pericytes are encapsulated within them (Moon et al., 2010). Figure 8.5 shows the capillary-like tubules that spontaneously assemble in the

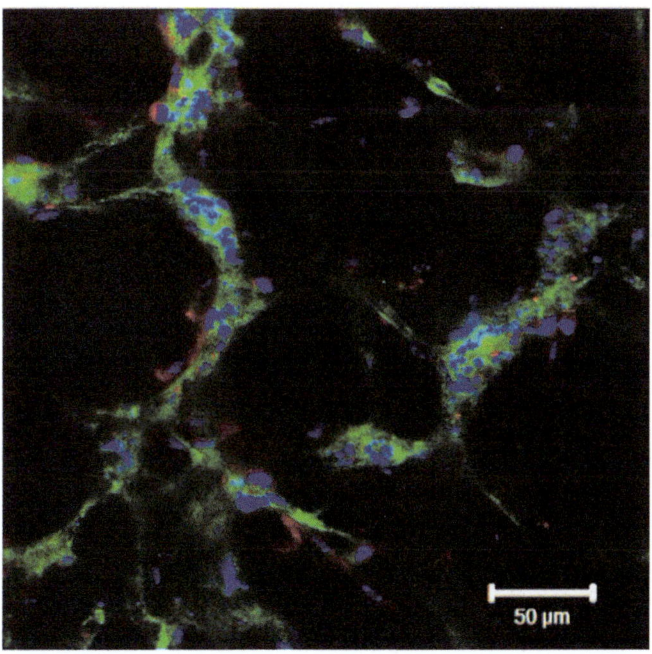

Figure 8.5 When endothelial cells (green) and pericytes (red) are encapsulated in MMP-degradable PEG hydrogels modified with RGDS adhesion peptides, the cells spontaneously organise into extensive tubule networks.

hydrogel materials. While RGDS is sufficient, combinations of adhesive peptides can provide enhanced tubulogenesis (Ali et al., 2013).

Several alternate strategies have been developed for intentional design of pro-angiogenic hydrogel biomaterials, but with omission of a synthetic polymer component. One of these has been the formation of hydrogels from self-assembling peptides (Narmoneva et al., 2005; Sieminski et al., 2008). Self-assembling peptide gels can be easily designed to incorporate cell-adhesive domains, proteolytically degradable domains and/or cell signalling domains (Malkar et al., 2003; Jun et al., 2008; Webber et al., 2011). Protein engineering has also been utilised to design highly controlled bioactive hydrogel precursors that present cell adhesion ligands and signalling domains (Foo et al., 2009). Such materials retain the requirements to support vascular cell adhesion and migration.

8.5 In vitro culture of vascular networks

When endothelial and mural cells such as pericytes are seeded into appropriate hydrogel materials, they will spontaneously assemble into interconnecting vascular networks (refer to Figures 8.2 and 8.5). Endothelial cells seeded alone will often form tubular structures early after seeding, but the tubules will usually quickly regress in the absence of supportive mural cells (Koike et al., 2004; Moon et al., 2010). Pericyte-containing vessel structures have been shown to remain stable long term when cultured in three-dimensional hydrogels (Moon et al., 2010).

Stable ex vivo vessel formation requires both endothelial cells and pericytes, and there are several sources for each cell type. When selecting from these sources it is important to consider ex vivo culturing conditions, homogeneity of the population, functional retention of each cell type when in co-culture conditions, requirements of harvesting or accessibility of the cells, and clinical translation potential in terms of availability, culturing/differentiation time and immunological competency. For endothelial cells, primary, differentiated endothelial cells offer appropriate cellular functionality (Morin and Tranquillo, 2013), and are somewhat available from autologous tissue sources. While primary endothelial cells are functionally defined and capable of vessel formation within hydrogels, there are several restrictions associated with their continued use such as limited passaging before morphological and phenotypic losses occur as well as immunological recognition of non-self (Novosel et al., 2011). Harvesting endothelial cells can also lead to donor site morbidity, thus limiting potential for autologous use. An alternative cell source is endothelial progenitor cells (EPCs). These cells are isolated from peripheral blood or bone marrow and can be differentiated into endothelial cells under specific culturing conditions (Hofer-Warbinek, 2014; Tura et al., 2013; Asahara et al., 1997). EPC-derived endothelial cells have been shown to form vessel structures and organised lumen within gelatin hydrogels (Hanjay-Putra et al., 2012). However, the culturing time for EPCs can be prolonged; it can take as many as four weeks to generate a substantial number of EPCs (Tura et al., 2013; Asahara et al., 1997) and endothelial functionality can be variable (Hofer-Warbinek, 2014). Induced pluripotent stem cells (iPSCs) are also a cell source that can be used to generate endothelial cells. iPSCs can be obtained from a variety of tissues and then differentiated into endothelial cells through exposure to specific cytokines such as vascular endothelial growth factor (VEGF-A) and bone morphogenetic protein-4 (BMP-4) (Rufaihah et al., 2013). Endothelial cells (ECs) derived from iPSCs demonstrate the phenotype and functionality of primary endothelial cells (Rufaihah et al., 2013; Adams et al., 2013). iPSC-derived ECs have recently been shown to form vessel structures within collagen—fibronectin hydrogels (Samuel et al., 2013). Limitations of iPSC-derived ECs include possible reprogramming of cells after differentiation, efficiency of differentiation and prolonged culture times required to obtain functional endothelial cells.

Primary pericytes can be obtained from a variety of tissues. However, markers for pericyte differentiation and function are poorly defined, making cell isolation and characterisation more problematic than for endothelial cells. Nonetheless, primary pericytes co-cultured with endothelial cells have been shown to stabilise neo-vessels within hydrogel materials (Saik et al., 2011a; Zheng et al., 2012). Mesenchymal stem cells (MSCs; Koike et al., 2004) and adipose-derived stem cells (ADSCs; Hutton et al., 2012) can be used as an alternative source of pericyte-like cells, stabilising vessel structures in hydrogels during culture (Moon et al., 2010). A recently uncovered source of pericyte-like cells is macrophages. In the process of wound repair and inflammation, macrophages are known to play a major role in mediating repair and regeneration of the tissue. To that end, macrophages have been shown to interact with endothelial cells of sprouting vessels and guide the formation and stabilisation of vessels in a manner similar to pericytes (Nucera et al., 2011). The harvesting and culturing processes of macrophages are typically less invasive than other harvesting methods as the cells can be isolated from whole blood, though their use as a pericyte source for tissue engineering has not yet been explored.

Blood flow, and the related shear stress experienced by vascular endothelial cells, has also been shown to play a critical role in the formation and maintenance of vessels in vivo. It is hypothesised that this could be an important mechanism to regulate or improve angiogenesis in vitro as well, and perfusion may also improve cell survival and tissue formation through enhanced mass transport. Several groups are developing strategies to incorporate hydrogel biomaterials into microfluidic devices and perfuse microvascular networks in culture (Cuchiara et al., 2012; Morgan et al., 2013; Hasan et al., 2014). Microfluidic systems possess several advantages when considering in vitro angiogenesis, including low cost, small working volumes, optical transparency, oxygen permeability, high reproducibility and scale-up potential, and minute spatial and temporal control over fluid dynamics and solute delivery achievable through the vast flexibility in design. This could enable more controlled studies of the effects of shear on angiogenesis than what has been possible in vivo and also enable culture of larger tissue-engineered constructs through the addition of convective transport. These systems are also being utilised as in vitro models to study processes such as tumour metastasis (Chen et al., 2013).

8.6 Inducing angiogenesis in host tissue

Depending on the application, it may be desirable to form vessels ex vivo, implanting relatively mature vascular networks, seed cells in a hydrogel and allow vessel assembly to proceed in vivo; or to implant a pro-angiogenic material that becomes vascularised through host tissue invasion. In all of these scenarios, it will likely be necessary to induce an angiogenic response in the tissue surrounding the implanted hydrogel. Even when preformed vascular networks are implanted, angiogenic activity in the surrounding tissue facilitates anastomosis of the implanted vessel to host vasculature so that perfusion can be attained. Thus, hydrogels have often been used as delivery vehicles and reservoirs for factors involved in stimulating and promoting angiogenesis such as VEGF, PDGF and FGF, or even combinations of such factors (Jiang et al., 2014; Kim et al., 2014; Oliviero et al., 2012). Localised delivery can alleviate challenges associated with delivering angiogenic factors systemically, such as unwanted offsite angiogenic effects, while stimulating angiogenesis at a local tissue site. In the context of stimulating angiogenesis *within* a hydrogel material, growth factor release upon implantation of a hydrogel may be required in order to recruit vascular cells resident in the surrounding tissue to migrate towards, and ultimately into, the implanted hydrogel material. Figure 8.6 shows an example of functional microvessels that have invaded a PEGDA-based hydrogel susceptible to degradation by MMP2 and modified with RGDS for cell adhesion in response to release of PDGF-BB.

Many angiogenic factors can also be immobilised in hydrogels for more localised and sustained effects (Leslie-Barbick et al., 2011a,b; Porter et al., 2011; Saik et al., 2011a,b). In some cases, peptide fragments can be employed in place of full growth factors (Leslie-Barbick et al., 2011a). For in vivo studies, a releasable factor may still be required to generate a chemotactic gradient and recruit local tissue-derived vascular

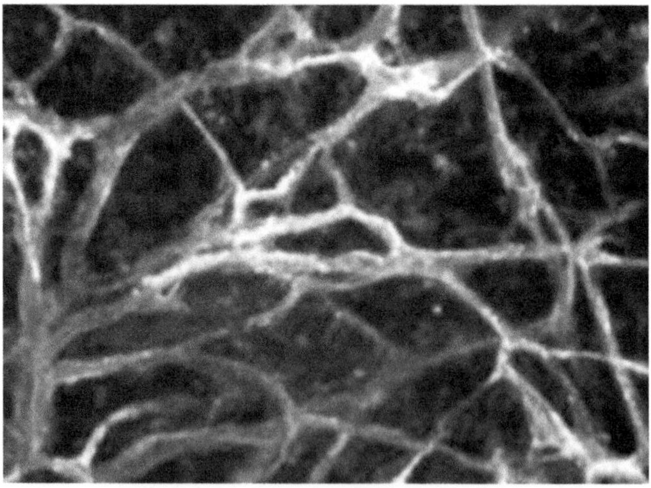

Figure 8.6 Microvessels invaded into an MMP-degradable hydrogel modified with RGDS cell-adhesion peptides in response to PDGF-BB release. These vessels supported blood flow.

cells, but the immobilised factors within the hydrogel assure that the environment within the biomaterial is actively pro-angiogenic when the cells arrive and invade into the hydrogel. In addition to traditional growth factors, ephrins have also been immobilised in hydrogels to influence angiogenesis (Moon et al., 2007; Saik et al., 2011b). Immobilisation also allows one to employ patterning strategies, such as photolithography, to localise regions with heightened angiogenic activity or to establish stable chemotactic gradients (DeLong et al., 2005; Leslie-Barbick et al., 2011b; Culver et al., 2012).

Alternatively, cells can be included within the hydrogel matrix as a source of angiogenic factors. Encapsulated cells can be transduced to express angiogenic factors for prolonged, local production to influence angiogenesis within a hydrogel or tissue (Olabisi et al., 2010; Orive et al., 2009). Some stromal cells will produce relatively high levels of angiogenic factors without the need for transduction (Hunt et al., 2013). Modification of materials with signalling molecules that upregulate expression of angiogenic factors by stromal cells can further optimise this response (Jose et al., 2014).

8.7 Conclusions

Our ever-improving understanding of the cellular and molecular processes involved in angiogenesis will enable increasingly sophisticated design of pro-angiogenic biomaterials. More complex interactions may be required for formation of optimally functional vasculature. For example, in recent years, a critical role of macrophages in angiogenesis has started to be elucidated (Chen et al., 2011), and materials that can manipulate the macrophage phenotype may aid in promotion or stabilisation of angiogenesis. Engineered microvasculature in hydrogel biomaterials may also have far-reaching impacts on the development of optimised culture systems for a variety of stem cells. In vivo, many stem cell niches are closely associated with microvasculature, and these associations have been shown to be critical to the maintenance of stem cells in the niche microenvironment (Culver et al., 2013; Kunisaki et al., 2013). Recapitulating key cellular and molecular interactions that occur in the stem cell niche in vivo may enable significant improvements in stem cell culture.

References

Adams, W.J., Zhang, Y., Cloutier, J., Kuchimanchi, P., Newton, G., Sehrawat, S., Aird, W.C., Mayadas, T.N., Luscinskas, F.W., Garcia-Cardena, G., 2013. Functional vascular endothelium derived from human induced pluripotent stem cells. Stem Cell Rep. 1, 105–113.

Ali, S., Saik, J.E., Gould, D.J., Dickinson, M.E., West, J.L., 2013. Immobilization of cell-adhesive laminin peptides in degradable PEGDA hydrogels influences endothelial cell tubulogenesis. BioResearch 2, 241–249.

Asahara, T., Murohara, T., Sullivan, A., Silver, M., van der Zee, R., Li, T., Witzenbichler, B., Schatteman, G., Isner, J.M., 1997. Isolation of putative progenitor endothelial cells for angiogenesis. Science 275, 964–966.

Atala, A., Bauer, S.B., Soker, S., Yoo, J.J., Retik, A.B., 2006. Tissue-engineered autologous bladders for patients needing cystoplasty. Lancet 15, 1241–1246.

Chen, M.B., Whisler, J.A., Jeon, J.S., Kamm, R.D., 2013. Mechanisms of tumor cell extravasation in an in vitro microvascular network platform. Integr. Biol. 5, 1262–1271.

Chen, P., Huang, Y., Bong, R., Ding, Y., Song, N., Wang, X., Song, X., Luo, Y., 2011. Tumor-associated macrophages promote angiogenesis and melanoma growth via adrenomedullin in a paracrine and autocrine manner. Clin. Cancer Res. 17, 7230–7239.

Cuchiara, M.P., Gould, D.J., McHale, M.K., Dickinson, M.E., West, J.L., 2012. Integration of self-assembled microvascular networks with microfabricated PEG-based hydrogels. Adv. Func. Mater. 22, 4511–4518.

Culver, J.C., Hoffmann, J.C., Poche, R.A., Slater, J.H., West, J.L., Dickinson, M.E., 2012. Three-dimensional biomimetic patterning in hydrogels to guide cellular organization. Adv. Mater. 24, 2344–2348.

Culver, J.C., Vadakkan, T.J., Dickinson, M.E., 2013. A specialized microvascular domain in the mouse neural stem cell niche. PLoS One 8, e53546.

DeLong, S.A., Moon, J.J., West, J.L., 2005. Covalently immobilized gradients of bFGF on hydrogel scaffolds for directed cell migration. Biomaterials 26, 3227–3234.

Falanga, V., Sabolinski, M., 1999. A bilayered living skin construct (APLIGRAF) accelerates complete closure of hard-to-heal venous ulcers. Wound Repair Regen. 7, 201–207.

Foo, C.T.S.W.P., Lee, J.S., Mulyasasmita, W., Parisi-Amon, A., Heilshorn, S.C., 2009. Two-component protein-engineered physical hydrogels for cell encapsulations. Proc. Natl. Acad. Sci. U.S.A. 106, 22067–22072.

Fulco, I., Largo, R.D., Miot, S., Wixmerten, A., Martin, I., Schaefer, D.J., Haug, M.D., 2013. Toward clinical application of tissue-engineered cartilage. Facial Plast. Surg. 29, 99–105.

Gobin, A.S., West, J.L., 2002. Cell migration through defined, synthetic ECM analogs. FASEB J. 16, 751–753.

Hahn, M.S., Taite, L.J., Moon, J.J., Rowland, M.C., Ruffino, K.A., West, J.L., 2006. Photolithographic patterning of polyethylene glycol hydrogels. Biomaterials 27, 190–200.

Hanjaya-Putra, D., Wong, K.T., Hirotsu, K., Khetan, S., Burdick, J.A., Gerecht, S., 2012. Spatial control of cell-mediated degradation to regulate vasculogenesis and angiogenesis in hyluronan hydrogels. Biomaterials 33, 6123–6131.

Hasan, A., Paul, A., Vrana, N.E., Zhao, X., Memic, A., Hwang, Y.S., Dokmeci, M.R., Khademhosseini, A., 2014. Microfluidic techniques for development of 3D vascularized tissue. Biomaterials 35, 7308–7325.

Hern, D.L., Hubbell, J.A., 1998. Incorporation of adhesion peptides into nonadhesive hydrogels useful for tissue resurfacing. J. Biomed. Mater. Res. 39, 266–276.

Hofer-Warbinek, R., 2014. Endothelial progenitor cells derived from cord or peripheral blood and their potential for regenerative therapies. In: Adult and Pluripotent Stem Cells. Springer, Netherlands.

Hunt, N.C., Shelton, R.M., Henderson, D.J., Grover, L.M., 2013. Calcium-alginate hydrogel-encapsulated fibroblasts provide sustained release of vascular endothelial growth factor. Tissue Eng. Part A 19, 905–914.

Hutton, D.L., Logsdon, E.A., Moore, E.M., Mac Gabhann, F., Gimble, J.M., Grayson, W.L., 2012. Vascular morphogenesis of adipose-derived stem cells is mediated by heterotypic cell-cell interactions. Tissue Eng. Part A 18, 1729–1740.

Jiang, B., Akar, B., Waller, T.M., Larson, J.C., Appel, A.A., Brey, E.M., 2014. Design of a composite biomaterial system for tissue engineering applications. Acta Biomater. 10, 1177–1186.

Jose, S., Hughbanks, M.L., Binder, B.Y., Ingavle, G.C., Leach, K., 2014. Enhanced trophic factor production by mesenchymal stem/stromal cells with glycine-histidine-lysine (GHK)-modified alginate hydrogels. Acta Biomater. 10, 1955–1964.

Jun, H.W., Paramonov, S.E., Dong, H., Forraz, N., McGuckin, C., Hartgerink, J.D., 2008. Tuning the mechanical and bioresponsive properties of peptide-amphiphile nanofiber networks. J. Biomater. Sci. Polym. Ed. 19, 665–676.

Kim, D.W., Lee, C.M., Kim, N.H., Lee, S.Y., Lee, M.Y., Choi, E.S., Park, S.A., Kim, C.G., Seok, H.H., Lim, S.T., Sohn, M.H., Jeong, H.J., 2014. Radiolabeled chitosan hydrogel containing VEGF enhances angiogenesis in a rodent model of acute myocardial infarction. Macromol. Res. 22, 272–278.

Koike, N., Fukumura, D., Gralla, O., Au, P., Schechner, J.S., Jain, R.K., 2004. Tissue engineering: creation of long-lasting blood vessels. Nature 428, 138–139.

Kubota, Y., Kleinman, H.K., Martin, G.R., Lawley, T.J., 1988. Role of laminin and basement membrane in the morphological differentiation of human endothelial cells into capillary-like structures. J. Cell Bio. 107, 1589–1598.

Kunisaki, Y., Bruns, I., Scheiermann, C., Ahmed, J., Pinho, S., Zhang, D., Mizoguchi, T., Wei, Q., Lucas, D., Ito, K., Mar, J.C., Bergman, A., Frenette, P.S., 2013. Arteriolar niches maintain haematopoietic stem cell quiescence. Nature 502, 637–643.

Lee, S.H., Mill, J.S., Moon, J.J., West, J.L., 2005. Proteolytically degradable hydrogels with a flurogenic substrate for studies of cellular proteolytic activity and migration. Biotechnol. Prog. 21, 1736–1741.

Leslie-Barbick, J.E., Saik, J.E., Gould, D.J., Dickinson, M.E., West, J.L., 2011a. The promotion of microvasculature formation in poly(ethylene glycol) diacrylate hydrogels by an immobilized VEGF-mimetic peptide. Biomaterials 32, 5782–5789.

Leslie-Barbick, J.E., Shen, C., Chen, C., West, J.L., 2011b. Micron-scale spatially patterned, covalently immobilized vascular endothelial growth factor on hydrogels accelerates endothelial tubulogenesis and increases cellular angiogenic responses. Tissue Eng. Part A 17, 221–229.

Lindahl, P., Johnasson, B.R., Leveen, P., Betsholtz, C., 1997. Pericyte loss and microaneurysm formation in PDGF-B-deficient mice. Science 277, 242–245.

Madden, L.R., Mortisen, D.J., Sussman, E.M., Dupras, S.K., Fugate, J.A., Cuy, J.L., Hauch, K.D., Laflamme, M.A., Murry, C.E., Ratner, B.D., 2010. Proangiogenic scaffolds as functional templates for cardiac tissue engineering. Proc. Natl. Acad. Sci. U.S.A. 107, 15211–15216.

Madeddu, P., 2005. Therapeutic angiogenesis and vascularization for tissue regeneration. Exp. Physiol. 90, 315–326.

Malkar, N.B., Lauer-Fields, J.L., Juska, D., Fields, G.B., 2003. Characterization of peptide-amphiphiles possessing cellular activation sequences. Biomacromolecules 4, 518–528.

Marti, H.H., 2005. Angiogenesis – a self adapting principle in hypoxia. EXS 94, 163–180.

Miller, J.S., Stevens, K.R., Yang, M.T., Baker, B.M., Nguyen, D.H., Cohen, D.M., Toro, E., Chen, A.A., Galie, P.A., Yu, X., Chaturvedi, R., Bhatia, S.N., Chen, C.S., 2012. Rapid casting of patterned vascular networks for perfusable engineered three-dimensional tissues. Nat. Mater. 11, 768–774.

Moon, J.J., Lee, S.H., West, J.L., 2007. Synthetic biomimetic hydrogels incorporated with ephrin-A1 for therapeutic angiogenesis. Biomacromolecules 8, 42–49.

Moon, J.J., Saik, J.E., Poche, R.A., Leslie-Barbick, J.E., Lee, S.H., Smith, A.A., Dickinson, M.E., West, J.L., 2010. Biomimetic hydrogels with pro-angiogenic activities. Biomaterials 31, 3840–3847.

Morgan, J.P., Delnero, P.F., Zheng, Y., Verbridge, S.S., Chen, J., Craven, M., Choi, N.W., Diaz-Santana, A., Kermani, P., Hempstead, B., Lopez, J.A., Corso, T.N., Fischbach, C., Stroock, A.D., 2013. Formation of microvascular networks in vitro. Nat. Protoc. 8, 1820–1836.

Morin, K.T., Tranquillo, R.T., 2013. In vitro models of angiogenesis and vasculogenesis in fibrin gel. Exp. Cell Res. 319, 2409–2417.

Narmoneva, D.A., Oni, O., Sieminski, A.L., Zhang, S., Gertier, J.P., Kamm, R.D., Lee, R.T., 2005. Self-assembling short oligopeptides and the promotion of angiogenesis. Biomaterials 26, 4837–4846.

Nemir, S., Hayenga, H.N., West, J.L., 2010. PEGDA hydrogels with patterned elasticity: novel tools for the study of cell responses to substrate rigidity. Biotech. Bioeng. 105, 636–644.

Nguyen, P.K., Snyder, C.G., Shields, J.D., Smith, A.W., Elbert, D.L., 2013. Clickable poly (ethylene glycol)-microsphere-based cell scaffolds. Macromol. Chem. Phys. 214, 948–956.

Nicosia, R.F., Ottinetti, A., 1990. Growth of microvessels in serum-free matrix culture of rat aorta. A quantitative assay of angiogenesis in vitro. Lab. Invest. 63, 115–122.

Novosel, E.C., Kleinhans, C., Kluger, P.J., 2011. Vascularization is the key challenge in tissue engineering. Adv. Drug Del. Rev. 63, 300–311.

Nucera, S., Biziato, D., De Palma, M., 2011. The interplay between macrophages and angiogenesis in development, tissue injury and regeneration. Int. J. Dev. Biol. 55, 495–503.

Olabisi, R.M., Lazard, Z.W., Franco, C.L., Hall, M.A., Kwon, S.K., Sevick-Muraca, E.M., Hipp, J.A., Davis, A.R., Olmsted-Davis, E.A., West, J.L., 2010. Hydrogel microsphere encapsulation of a cell-based gene therapy system increases cell survival of injected cells, transgene expression, and bone volume in a model of heterotopic ossification. Tissue Eng. Part A 16, 3727–3736.

Oliviero, O., Ventre, M., Netti, P.A., 2012. Functional porous hydrogels to study angiogenesis under the effect of controlled release of vascular endothelial growth factor. Acta Biomater. 8, 3294–3301.

Orive, G., De Castro, M., Kong, H.J., Hernandez, R.M., Ponce, S., Mooney, D.J., Pedraz, J.L., 2009. Bioactive cell-hydrogel microcapsules for cell-based drug delivery. J. Control. Rel. 135, 203–210.

Porter, A.M., Klinge, C.M., Gobin, A.S., 2011. Covalently grafted VEGF(165) in hydrogel models upregulates the cellular pathways associated with angiogenesis. Am. J. Physiol. Cell Physiol. 301, 1086–1092.

Rufaihah, A.J., Huang, N.F., Kim, J., Herold, J., Volz, K.S., Park, T.S., Lee, J.C., Zambidis, E.T., Reijo-Pera, R., Cooke, J.P., 2013. Human induced pluripotent stem cell-derived endothelial cells exhibit functional heterogeneity. Am. J. Trans. Res. 5, 21.

Saik, J.E., Gould, D.J., Watkins, E.M., Dickinson, M.E., West, J.L., 2011a. Covalently immobilized platelet-derived growth factor-BB promotes angiogenesis in biomimetic poly(ethylene glycol) hydrogels. Acta Biomater. 7, 133–143.

Saik, J.E., Gould, D.J., Keswani, A.H., Dickinson, M.E., West, J.L., 2011b. Biomimetic hydrogels with immobilized ephrin A1 for therapeutic angiogenesis. Biomacromolecules 11, 2715–2722.

Samuel, R., Daheron, L., Liao, S., Vardam, T., Kamoun, W.S., Batista, A., Buecker, C., Schafer, R., Han, X., Au, P., Scadden, D.T., Duda, D.G., Fukumura, D., Jain, R.K., 2013. Generation of functionally competent and durable engineered blood vessels from human induced pluripotent stem cells. Proc. Natl. Acad. Sci. U.S.A. 110, 12774–12779.

Sawhney, A.S., Pathak, C.P., Hubbell, J.A., 1993. Bioerodible hydrogels based on photopolymerized poly(ethylene glycol)-co-poly(alpha-hydroxy acid) diacrylate macromers. Macromolecules 26, 581–587.

Scott, E.A., Nichols, M.D., Kuntz-Willits, R., Elbert, D.L., 2010. Modular scaffolds assembled around living cells using poly(ethylene glycol) microspheres with macroporation via a non-cytotoxic porogen. Acta Biomater. 6, 29–38.

Shepard, J.A., Virani, F.R., Goodman, A.G., Gossett, T.D., Shin, S., Shea, L.D., 2012. Hydrogel macroporosity and the prolongation of transgene expression and the enhancement of angiogenesis. Biomaterials 33, 7412–7421.

Sieminski, A.L., Semino, C.E., Gong, H., Kamm, R.D., 2008. Primary sequence of ionic self-assembling peptide gels affects endothelial cell adhesion and capillary morphogenesis. J. Biomed. Mater. Res. A 87, 494–504.

Tura, O., Skinner, E.M., Barclay, G.R., Samuel, K., Gallagher, R.C., Brittan, M., Hadoke, P.W., Newby, D.E., Turner, M.L., Mills, N.L., 2013. Late outgrowth endothelial cells resemble mature endothelial cells and are not derived from bone marrow. Stem Cells 31, 338–348.

Webber, M.J., Tongers, J., Newcomb, C.J., Marquardt, K.T., Bauersachs, J., Losordo, D.W., Stupp, S.I., 2011. Supramolecular nanostructures that mimic VEGF as a strategy for ischemic tissue repair. Proc. Natl. Acad. Sci. U.S.A. 108, 13438–13443.

West, J.L., Hubbell, J.A., 1999. Polymeric biomaterials with degradation sites for proteases involved in cell migration. Macromolecules 12, 241–244.

Zhang, J., Cao, R., Zhang, Y., Jia, T., Cao, Y., Wahlberg, E., 2009. Differential roles of PDGFR-alpha and PDGFR-beta in angiogenesis and vessel stability. FASEB J. 23, 153–163.

Zheng, Y., Chen, J., Craven, M., Choi, N.W., Totorica, S., Diaz-Santana, A., Kermani, P., Hempstead, B., Fischbach-Teschi, C., Lopez, J.A., Stroock, A.D., 2012. In vitro microvessels for the study of angiogenesis and thrombosis. Proc. Natl. Acad. Sci. U.S.A. 109, 9342–9347.

Engineering biosynthetic cell encapsulation systems

9

J.J. Roberts, P.J. Martens
Graduate School of Biomedical Engineering, University of New South Wales, Sydney, NSW, Australia

9.1 Introduction

Polymeric hydrogels have been a rapidly developing group of biomedical materials since the 1960s. Traditionally, hydrogels were utilised for applications *adjacent* to cells, such as contact lenses and absorbable sutures (Langer and Peppas, 2003), and used synthetic polymeric materials such as polyhydroxyethyl methacrylate (e.g. contact lenses). Natural hydrogels were also explored in addition to synthetic hydrogel materials. For example, Yannas et al. designed natural hydrogels based on collagen and glycosaminoglycans for burn dressings (Yannas and Burke, 1980). These simple, preliminary biomedical polymers were hydrophilic (i.e. water soluble), nontoxic, and could be tailored for biodegradability or stability depending on the application.

As the advantages of polymer hydrogels for biomedical applications became recognised, more advanced chemistries and applications have been explored. It was soon realised that there was great potential if cells could be encapsulated *within* the hydrogel materials. The delivery of cells as newly engineered tissues and organs is often necessary clinically due to insufficient organ donors and the inability of any transplanted organs to function adequately. The first use of hydrogels for cell encapsulation was pioneered by Lim and Sun. They created calcium alginate microspheres for the encapsulation of islet cells as an approach to treat diabetes and were able to correct the diabetic state of rats for several weeks (Lim and Sun, 1980). This work truly demonstrated the potential for cell encapsulation within hydrogel biomaterials for the first time and has ongoing contributions to the development of advanced hydrogels for the transplantation of therapeutic cells. As a result, researchers around the world have focused on using natural, synthetic and biosynthetic hydrogels for the local and controlled delivery of therapeutic products and cells for a variety of defects and diseases. Examples of areas of research include treatment of diabetes, liver disease (Maguire et al., 2006), myocardial infarction (Yu et al., 2010), cancer (Hao et al., 2005) and numerous diseases of the central nervous system (e.g. Parkinson's disease, glioma, Huntington's disease) (Kim et al., 2005; Read et al., 2001; Emerich et al., 1997).

Despite the groundbreaking work from Lim and Sun in the 1980s, cell encapsulation within biomaterials still poses many challenges for researchers today. If the

Biosynthetic Polymers for Medical Applications. http://dx.doi.org/10.1016/B978-1-78242-105-4.00009-2

application requires the materials to be degradable, then the materials need to be not only cytocompatible but also capable of renal filtration for removal from the body, which limits the available chemistries and molecular weights. In addition, there can be no small molecules remaining from hydrogel synthesis (e.g. unreacted monomer, initiator, crosslinkers) or resulting from the biomaterial crosslinking or degradation, as these molecules can be toxic to cells. Macromers have to undergo mild, cytocompatible polymerisation reactions in aqueous solution that will not damage encapsulated cells, which limits temperature, pH, and/or initiator type and concentration (see Figure 9.1 for example). Ideally, crosslinking reactions should be able to occur in situ and on a clinically relevant timescale, which is generally on the order of minutes. Once formed, there needs to be oxygen, nutrient, and waste diffusion to and from the cells and the surrounding tissue. Some cell types may also require localised biological molecules to promote viability, attachment, proliferation, migration and differentiation for tissue engineering applications. Additionally, the

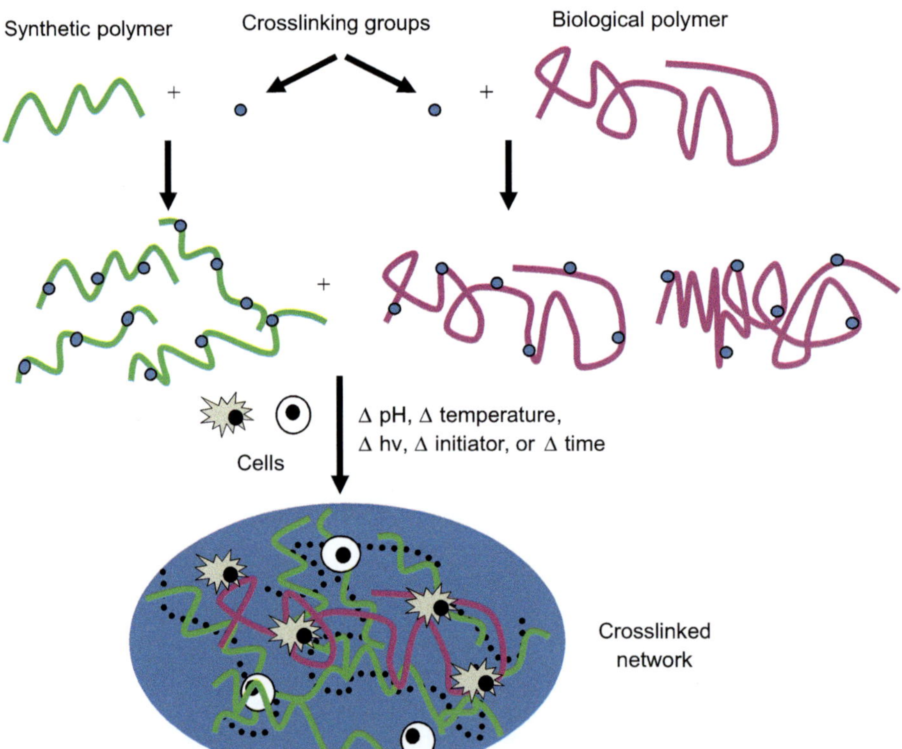

Figure 9.1 Schematic of one method of creating a biosynthetic hydrogel for cell encapsulation. Cytocompatible polymers are synthesised or purchased commercially, modified with crosslinkable functional groups (if desired), dissolved in aqueous solution with cells and polymerised via changes in pH, temperature, light, initiators or time.

hydrogels need to be capable of mechanical tuning to be robust enough to withstand manipulations associated with implantation and in vivo existence, but also to mimic the mechanical integrity of the tissue of interest and avoid mechanical mismatch that may result in fibrotic encapsulation of the biomaterial. For some applications, such as immunoisolation of pancreatic beta cells, hydrogel degradation may not be desirable and so chemistries that are nondegradable will be selected. However, for many tissue engineering applications, hydrogel degradation is often desired so that the hydrogel degrades in sync with tissue development. The timing of hydrogel degradation is critical so that it is not so fast that major defects may develop, but not so slow as to hinder developing tissue. Hydrolytic and enzymatic hydrogel degradation have been explored extensively (Sahoo et al., 2008; Roberts et al., 2011b; Rice and Anseth, 2007), as well as new approaches such as photodegradation (Kharkar et al., 2013).

Hydrogels have many advantages for cell encapsulation (Peppas et al., 2006). Hydrogels are hydrophilic networks that consist of water-insoluble polymers. They have characteristics that are similar to those of soft tissue, with water content that ranges from a few percent to over 99%. Their ability to swell in biological mediums, without polymer dissolution, makes hydrogels ideal for many biomedical applications, such as drug delivery and cell encapsulation. The water in hydrogels provides for a moist environment that is important for applications such as wound healing and ocular lenses. The mesh size of swollen, crosslinked polymer networks allows for diffusion of oxygen, nutrients and waste and can be tailored to provide controlled diffusion of larger, soluble factors such as proteins and polysaccharides. Hydrogels can allow for homogenous encapsulation of cells in three dimensions (3D), which is important because it better mimics the in vivo environment as compared to two-dimensional (2D) cell culture.

This ability to match the mechanics, permeability, hydration and 3D structure of tissue makes hydrogels very attractive for cell encapsulation. However, the extracellular matrix (ECM) is a very complex environment and researchers are finding that it is also important to incorporate cell-interactive signals into hydrogels. It is well established that cellular phenotypic activity is regulated by the ECM, soluble factors (e.g. growth factors) and neighbouring cells. Cells interact with these signals via receptors, such as integrins and cadherins, which can then orchestrate cell signalling pathways that lead to diverse cellular activities involved in tissue homoeostasis, repair and regeneration. This suggests that when developing hydrogels for cell encapsulation it may not only be important to have the advantages of synthetic polymers, which include a high degree of tailorability and robust mechanical properties, but also to incorporate natural biologic polymers, which better mimic the native ECM and can drive cellular signalling cascades. Designing biosynthetic hydrogels, which combine biological and synthetic polymers, is a process of trying to join the best features of both types of polymers. Understanding the best attributes and advantages of the base polymers is crucial to this design process. Therefore, this chapter reviews the strengths and limitations of commonly used biological hydrogels and synthetic hydrogels, and discusses recent strategies to develop biosynthetic hydrogels for cell encapsulation that guide and control specific cell functions.

9.2 Natural polymers

Natural, biological polymers that are used in the design of hydrogels for cell encapsulation are generally composed of proteins, glycosaminoglycans and/or their combinations (e.g. Matrigel™, Cardiogel (VanWinkle et al., 1996), Adipogel (Sharma et al., 2010), decellularised matrix (Hoshiba et al., 2010)). These polymers are derived from both non-mammalian and mammalian sources, and are advantageous because they generally have low toxicity and are cytocompatible. Natural polymers often assemble in vitro into higher-order nanofibrous structures through ionic interactions, hydrogen bonding and Van der Waals forces in a manner similar to the native ECM. In the body, the ECM is the 3D microenvironment surrounding the cells of each tissue. It acts as a complex and dynamic network that provides the physical structure, mechanical integrity and biochemical activity of a cell's environment. Natural polymers serve as ideal building blocks to mimic the structure and biological properties of the cell microenvironment because many natural polymers, such as collagen and fibrin, contain cellular binding and signalling domains that allow for cell adhesion and phenotypic regulation. Moreover, many of these natural polymers regulate cellular phenotypic activities in combination with soluble signalling factors. For example, hyaluronan and fibronectin modulate angiogenic activities when stimulated by angiogenic growth factors and cytokines (Kim et al., 2000; Lokeshwar and Selzer, 2000). Collagen will enhance stem cell differentiation when placed in an osteogenic medium (Salasznyk et al., 2004). Additionally, these natural polymers may be able to be degraded by naturally occurring cell-secreted enzymes in the cellular microenvironment, mimicking the dynamic nature of the ECM by supporting localised, cell-mediated degradation.

Natural polymers also have several limitations (Langer and Tirrell, 2004; Drury and Mooney, 2003). They can be degraded by enzymes, and as a result they may be degraded uncontrollably by soluble enzymes diffusing throughout the body. This limited tunability of degradation kinetics makes it difficult to retain controlled chemical and physical properties of natural hydrogels over extended culture times. Additionally, the small-molecule degradation products of these natural polymer hydrogels may affect encapsulated cells. For example, different molecular-weight fragments of hyaluronan hydrogels have been shown to regulate ECM production (Nuttelman et al., 2008), and low-molecular-weight hyaluronan oligomers can shift hyaluronan from being noninflammatory to pro-inflammatory (Noble, 2002). Because of limited supplies and costly extraction procedures, isolation and purification of natural polymers can be expensive. Batch-to-batch variations often occur and depend on the manufacturing procedure and the natural polymer's derived source, and may decrease the reproducibility of a material's properties and functions. Moreover, any contamination during processing and/or cross-species variations in structure may lead to immunological issues. For example, pure alginate has relatively little immune response; however, the purity of commercially available alginate is a problem (Zhang et al., 2001). Another challenge with cell encapsulation in natural hydrogels is decoupling biological responses. In most studies comparing gel stiffness, the protein concentration in the gel precursor solution is varied. This variation makes it impossible to orthogonally control mechanics and ligand density, which is problematic because ligand density is known to influence integrin-dependent signalling (Ingber, 1990). Stupp and co-workers developed self-assembling peptide materials that allow for varying stiffness by varying the number of valines and alanines (Pashuck et al., 2010). However, this changes the chemical structure, thereby influencing folding and the availability of ligands. Recently non-enzymatic collagen glycation has been used to control stiffness while maintaining collagen density; however, the variation in stiffness was over a narrow range from 175 to 730 Pa (Mason et al., 2013). In vivo, different tissues can range in stiffness from a few Pa to GPa, and the obtainable stiffness range of these natural hydrogels is often inadequate compared to native tissue. In order to improve mechanical properties of natural polymers, chemical crosslinking has been employed. Chemical crosslinking methods include glutaraldehyde, carbodiimide, succinic anhydride, and hexamethylene diisocyanate treatment or photochemical crosslinking (Rault et al., 1996). However, many chemical crosslinkers are toxic, resulting in a limited capacity for in situ cellular encapsulation and long-term 3D cell culture. When crosslinking techniques that are cytocompatible (e.g. Micheal addition or radical crosslinking) are selected, care has to be taken to ensure that the crosslinked proteins are not damaged, which is highly dependent on the crosslinking method and initiator concentration (Bryant et al., 2000; McCall and Anseth, 2012). Despite the limitations of natural polymers, their many advantages have led to their widespread use for cell encapsulation. The following is an overview of commonly utilised natural hydrogel materials for cell encapsulation.

9.2.1 Non-mammalian natural hydrogel materials

Of the many non-mammalian materials that exist, the most commonly used non-mammalian natural polymers that are used for biomedical application are outlined below and in Table 9.1.

9.2.1.1 Agarose

Agarose is a polysaccharide derived from seaweed and used as a matrix to encapsulate cells (Iwata et al., 1992). Agarose is comprised of a basic repeat unit consisting of 1,3-linked-D-galactopyranose and 1,4-linked 3,6-anhydro-α-L-galactopyranose (Normand et al., 2000) that undergoes thermal crosslinking. Agarose is an attractive platform for cell encapsulation because it undergoes mild gelation through the formation of extensive intermolecular hydrogen bonds resulting in double helical structures that aggregate into thick bundles (Xiong et al., 2005). These hydrogen bonds create hydrogels that have time-dependent mechanical properties, leading to stress relaxation similar to native tissue (Buschmann et al., 1992). Agarose has been used extensively for the encapsulation of cells for cartilage tissue engineering. When compressive bioreactors were employed, tissue-engineered cartilage in an agarose hydrogel has approached the sulphated glycosaminoglycan content and mechanical properties of native articular cartilage (Lima et al., 2007). However, a

Table 9.1 Examples of common nonmammalian natural polymers used for cell encapsulation and their method of crosslinking with a variety of cell types

Polymer	Crosslinking groups	Cell type	References
Agarose	Hydrogen bonding	Islets	Iwata et al. (1992)
	Hydrogen bonding	Chondrocyte	Lima et al. (2007)
Alginate	Ionic bonding	Islets	Lim and Sun (1980)
	Ionic bonding	Fibroblast	Smidsrod and Skjak-Braek (1990)
	Ionic bonding	Lymphoma	Smidsrod and Skjak-Braek (1990)
Chitosan	Hydrogen bonding	Chondrocyte	Suh and Matthew (2000), Chenite et al. (2000)
Dextran	Tyramine	Chondrocyte	Jin et al. (2010)
	Acrylate	Embryonic stem cell	Ferreira et al. (2007)
Silk	Methacrylate	Fibroblast	Lim et al. (2012)
	Hydrogen bonding	Mesenchymal stem cell	Bini et al. (2006)
	Hydrogen bonding	Fibroblast, carcinoma, osteoblast, bone marrow stromal cell	Altman et al. (2003)

drawback of agarose is that it forms stable hydrogels that have no in vitro or in vivo basis for degradation. Also, mammalian cells do not have receptors that bind to the agarose polysaccharide, and therefore agarose does not interact with encapsulated cells.

9.2.1.2 Alginate

Alginate is a hydrophilic, linear polysaccharide copolymer of 1,4-linked β-D-mannuronic acid and α-L-guluronic acid monomers that is derived from brown seaweed and bacterial sources. Alginate has been applied to a variety of medical applications including cell encapsulation and drug delivery, because it is readily available and has low toxicity in vivo. It is attractive for cell encapsulation because of its mild ionic gelation between divalent cations (e.g. Ca^{2+}, Ba^{2+} or Sr^{2+}) and the guluronic acid monomers to form ionic bridges (Smidsrod and Skjak-Braek, 1990). However, depending on the species, location and age of the seaweed that the alginate is isolated from, there is variability in the amount and distribution of each monomer within the alginate polymer (Smidsrod and Skjak-Braek, 1990). The longevity of alginate gels within the body can be an issue due to leaching of ions from the hydrogel, resulting in a loss of mechanical stiffness over time (LeRoux et al., 1999). If the alginate has a high-molecular weight, hydrogel degradation products are too large for renal clearance, and since mammalian cells do not have receptors to interact with the alginate, it will not break down in the body (Alshamkhani and Duncan, 1995). However, alginate gels can be tailored to have different size byproducts and mechanical properties by changing the monomer ratios, concentration of alginate in solution and the molecular weight of the alginate polymer.

9.2.1.3 Chitosan

Chitosan, derived from chitin, is a linear polysaccharide utilised for cell encapsulation and is composed of 1,4-linked D-glucosamine and *N*-acetyl-D-glucosamine residues. Chitosan has been investigated for a variety of tissue engineering applications because of its biocompatibility and low immunogenicity. Unlike alginate and agarose, chitosan can be enzymatically degraded in humans by lysosome (Lee et al., 1995). Chitosan derivatives have been gelled via photo-crosslinking (Ishihara et al., 2002), glutaraldehyde crosslinking (Mi et al., 2000) and thermal variations (Zhang and Zhang, 2001), giving a more diverse range of mechanical properties. However, the applications of unmodified chitosan as an injectable cell carrier are limited because its strong intermolecular hydrogen bonds mean that it can only be dissolved under acidic solutions. Unmodified chitosan hydrogels undergo gelation when chitosan is dissolved in dilute acid to protonate the free amino groups, and then the pH is increased or a nonsolvent is added (Suh and Matthew, 2000; Chenite et al., 2000; Lee and Mooney, 2001).

9.2.1.4 Dextran

Dextran is a polysaccharide derived from bacteria that is largely composed of linear α-1,6-linked D-glucopyranose residues. Dextran has found popularity for tissue engineering because it can be enzymatically degraded by dextranase, which is found in mammalian tissue. Additionally, the large number of chemically reactive hydroxyl groups allow dextran to be modified to form a variety of unique spherical, tubular and 3D network structures (Sun and Mao, 2012). Dextran has been modified with functional groups such as tyramine (Jin et al., 2010), ethylamine (Sun and Mao, 2012), vinylsulphones (Hiemstra et al., 2007), thiols (Hiemstra et al., 2007) and acrylates (Baldwin and Kiick, 2010) to form hydrogels. Dextran hydrogels have been utilised to promote vascularisation (Sun et al., 2011), wound healing (Sun et al., 2011) and cartilage development (Jin et al., 2010). However, dextran does not contain any native cell-binding domains for encapsulated cells, and so affinity binding sites have to be incorporated via chemical modification (Ferreira et al., 2007).

9.2.1.5 Silk

Silk is composed of fibrous proteins produced by a variety of insects and spiders, such as silkworm cocoons and spider orb webs. Silk is composed of a filament core protein, fibroin, and a glue-like coating, sericin. Silk proteins have robust mechanical properties and good cellular compatibility and therefore have been used as medical sutures and scaffolds for tissue engineering (Altman et al., 2003). Silk fibroins are natural block copolymers composed of hydrophilic blocks with ordered hydrophobic blocks that tend to form β-sheets or crystals through hydrogen bonding and hydrophobic interactions, forming the basis for their mechanical strength. However, silk fibroins do not have native cell-binding regions, and so cell-binding domains have to be synthetically incorporated into silk to improve cell adhesion (Bini et al., 2006). Many researchers have focused on the development of fibroin, because some studies suggest that the sericin glue-like proteins are the cause of adverse problems with biocompatibility and hypersensitivity to silk (Altman et al., 2003). However, more recent research has demonstrated that sericin has antioxidative properties (Dash et al., 2008) and can promote cell adhesion and survival of a variety of cells including fibroblasts (Aramwit et al., 2010), epithelial cells (Nagai et al., 2009) and osteoblasts (Motta et al., 2011), although the mechanism remains to be elucidated.

9.2.2 Mammalian-based natural hydrogel materials

Natural hydrogels have also been designed based on mammalian polymers, which can be broken down into several broad classifications, such as proteins, glycosaminoglycans (GAGs) and DNA (see Table 9.2). Each of these broad types of polymers has its own benefits and drawbacks, as outlined below.

9.2.2.1 Proteins

There is a large variety of proteins in the body. Despite the large variety of proteins, the cost and expertise needed to purify proteins and ensure that they are stable means that only a few proteins have been extensively utilised in the biomaterials literature for hydrogel design. Below are some of the most commonly used proteins for hydrogel formulation.

Collagen

Collagen is the main protein of the ECM, comprising 25% of protein in most mammals (Lee et al., 2001a). Collagen hydrogels have found widespread use for cell encapsulation because collagen molecules can self-aggregate via hydrogen and covalent bonds to form stable fibres in the presence of cells. Furthermore, collagen has native binding motifs, which provides for cell attachment and integrin signalling (Levental et al., 2009) and degradation by enzymes, such as metalloproteases and serine proteases. Because of the bioactive capabilities of collagen gels, they have been utilised for tissue engineering a variety of organs such as liver (Kaufmann et al., 1997), skin (Auger et al., 1998) and blood vessels (Seliktar et al., 2000). However, collagen gels are often soft, comparable to fat tissue (i.e. elastic moduli <5 kPa) (Lau et al., 2006). Therefore to enhance the mechanical properties and retard hydrogel degradation, the density of collagen must be increased or the collagen needs to be chemically modified. Collagens have been crosslinked by methods such as chemical crosslinking (e.g. glutaraldehyde, formaldehyde, carbodiimide), UV crosslinking or thermal gelation (Lee et al., 2001b).

Table 9.2 Examples of common mammalian-based natural polymers used for cell encapsulation and their method of crosslinking with a variety of cell types

Polymer	Crosslinking groups	Cell type	References
Collagen	Protein self-assembly	Smooth muscle cell	Seliktar et al. (2000)
	Protein self-assembly	Keratinocyte	Auger et al. (1998)
	Protein self-assembly	Hepatocyte	Kaufmann et al. (1997)
Fibrin	Protein self-assembly	Mesenchymal stem cell	Neumann et al. (2013)
	Protein self-assembly	Chondrocyte	Scotti et al. (2010)
	Protein self-assembly	Infrapatellar fat pad-derived stem cell	Ahearne et al. (2011)
	Protein self-assembly	Vascular smooth muscle cell	Rowe et al. (2007)
Chondroitin sulphate	Methacrylate	Mesenchymal stem cell	Steinmetz and Bryant (2012)
	Methacrylate	Chondrocyte	Bryant et al. (2004)
	Thiol, acrylate	Fibroblast	Shu et al. (2006)
Heparin	No modification	Fibroblast	Wieduwild et al. (2013)
	Methacrylamide	Osteoblast, mesenchymal stem cell	Seto et al. (2012)
	Thiol, acrylate	Hepatocyte	Kim et al. (2010)
	Methacrylate	Mesenchymal stem cell	Benoit et al. (2007)
Hyaluronan	Thiol	Mesenchymal stem cell, endothelial progenitor cell, neural progenitor cell	Burdick and Prestwich (2011)
	Methacrylate	Chondrocyte, valvular interstitial cells	Burdick and Prestwich (2011)
DNA	Protein self-assembly	Chinese hamster ovary cell	Um et al. (2006)

Researchers will also form hydrogels out of the collagen derivative, gelatin. Gelatin is a single-stranded protein formed by hydrolysing the triple-helix structure of collagen. Gelatin retains cell-binding regions and thus can promote cell adhesion, migration, differentiation and proliferation. However, the weakness of gelatin hydrogels is problematic, and chemical modifications have been investigated to improve their mechanical properties (Lee and Mooney, 2001).

Fibrin

Fibrin is a protein that natively forms fibrous matrices (i.e. clots) at wound sites when fibrinogen found in plasma is cleaved by thrombin (Mosesson, 2005). Fibrin has found extensive use in the design of hydrogels for cell encapsulation because fibrin hydrogels are cytocompatible and promote cell migration, proliferation and adhesion (Ahmed et al., 2008; Geer and Andreadis, 2003). Additionally, fibrin gels have multiple domains that can bind with heparin, fibronectin and integrins (Hogg and Jackson, 1989). Fibrin-based hydrogels have been widely used for controlled drug delivery (Ahearne et al., 2011), wound healing (Hall, 2007) and tissue engineering (Neumann et al., 2013; Scotti et al., 2010). For example, Neumann et al. found that encapsulating stem cells in 3D within fibrin hydrogels led to more effective gene transduction than traditional 2D transduction methods (Neumann et al., 2013), although the use of purely fibrin hydrogels is limited by their fast gelation time and their low mechanical properties (1−30 kPa) (DeVolder and Kong, 2012). Moreover, fibrin gels can be enzymatically degraded by molecules such as plasmin, and will undergo uncontrolled loss of mechanical integrity (Rowe et al., 2007).

9.2.2.2 Glycosaminoglycans

Glycosaminoglycans are ubiquitous linear polysacchraides found in mammalian tissue. GAGs are a major class of natural compounds found in the ECM and are often conjugated to a protein backbone and expressed as proteoglycans. GAGs are highly polar, attracting water, which is ideal for the development of hydrogels. Glycosaminoglycan polymers are involved in cell signalling, proliferation, adhesion and motility (Theocharis et al., 2010) making them attractive bioactive polymers for cell encapsulation. However, GAGs do not natively self-assemble, and therefore must be covalently modified to form hydrogels, which may affect their bioactivity (Nilasaroya et al., 2008). There are a variety of sulphated (i.e. heparin sulphate, chondroitin sulphate, keratin sulphate and dermatan sulphate) and nonsulphated (i.e. hyaluronan) GAGs that differ based on the type of sugar in their disaccharide repeating unit. The cell-signalling properties of GAGs are dictated by their structure, with the negatively charged sulpho and carboxyl groups believed to be critical to interaction (Weyers and Linhardt, 2013). Three GAGs commonly employed for cell encapsulation are outlined below.

Chondroitin sulphate

Chondroitin sulphate (CS) is a linear polysaccharide with a structure based on (1−3)-β-*N*-acetyl-D-galactosamine and (1−4)-β-glucuronic acid. CS is found attached to proteoglycans, such as aggrecan, or as a receptor on cells or basement membranes. CS can be degraded by the native enzyme, chondroitinase. To allow for polymerisation into a hydrogel, CS has been modified with a variety of functional groups including methacrylates (Steinmetz and Bryant, 2012) and thiols (Shu et al., 2006). A main use of functionalised CS has been as a component of hydrogels for cartilage tissue engineering (Bryant et al., 2004; Steinmetz and Bryant, 2012).

Heparin

Heparin is a linear polysaccharide with the highest charge density of any biological molecule. Its heterogeneous structure is made up of α-L-iduronic acid, β-D-glucuronic acid and a-D-glucosamine repeat units. The high charge density of heparin makes it attractive for cell encapsulation in applications using growth factors and cytokines, because heparin helps to localise and stabilise these proteins (Bhatia, 2012). Physically and chemically crosslinked heparin hydrogels have been used for a variety of biomedical applications including the encapsulation of fibroblasts (Wieduwild et al., 2013), differentiation of stem cells (Seto et al., 2012) and liver tissue-engineering applications (Kim et al., 2010). In spite of these advantages, heparin is degraded in vivo by heparanase, and as such, caution must be taken when using heparin for biomaterials, as it is a potent anticoagulant and can cause bleeding (Lever et al., 2012; Melloni et al., 2008).

Hyaluronan

Hyaluronan (HA) hydrogels are one of the most prominent materials for cell encapsulation (Burdick and Prestwich, 2011). Hyaluronan is found in nearly all animal tissues, but is particularly prevalent in joints and the wound healing cascade because of its role in tissue hydration, nutrient diffusion and proteoglycan organisation (Peppas et al., 2006; Alberts, 1994). A variety of cell-surface proteins, including intercellular adhesion molecules (ICAM-1), cluster of differentiation (CD 44) and the receptor for hyaluronan-mediated motility, are known to enable binding to HA and promote cell adhesion and proliferation (Toole, 2004). The repeating dissacharide of HA is comprised of 1,4-linked β-D-glucuronic acid and *N*-acetyl-β-D-glucosamine units, of which the primary and secondary hydroxyl groups, glucuronic acid carboxylic acid, and the *N*-acetyl group (following deamidation) have been targeted for modification. Common modifications include carbodiimide-mediated reactions, esterification, amidation, etherification, addition of thiols, hydrazide derivation, divinylsulphone crosslinking and methacrylate crosslinking (Burdick and Prestwich, 2011). Native enzymes (i.e. hyaluronidase) can degrade hyaluronan hydrogels, allowing the cells in the body to locally regulate clearance of the hyaluronan. However, for HA hydrogels there is a fine balance between forming gels with weak mechanical properties and rapid, uncontrollable degradation versus forming mechanically robust hydrogels that have reduced capability for enzymatic degradation because of too much modification. Additionally, enzymatically degraded HA fragments from hydrogels can regulate ECM production (Nuttelman et al., 2008), and low-molecular-weight hyaluronan oligomers can be pro-inflammatory (Noble, 2002).

9.2.2.3 Deoxyribonucleic acid

Deoxyribonucleic acid (DNA) is composed of two polynucleotide chains held together by weak intermolecular forces. DNA has been probed for its ability to form hydrogels (Um et al., 2006). Hydrogels made from DNA can efficiently self-assemble into predictable networks under physiological conditions and can be biodegraded by nucleases. The mechanical properties of DNA hydrogels can be tuned by adjusting the concentration and type of DNA monomers. Their unique properties make DNA hydrogel networks ideal for specific biomedical applications, such as 3D cell culture, cell transplant therapy, controlled drug delivery and cell-free protein production (Zhu and Marchant, 2011). However, limited supply and purification cost are challenges that will need to be overcome for scale-up of DNA hydrogels.

9.2.3 Summary of natural polymers

Natural polymers are commonly proteins and polysaccharide chains derived from non-mammalian and mammalian sources. Depending on the source, natural polymers can recapitulate many aspects of the native ECM, such as fibrous 3D hierarchy, adhesive ligands and cell-mediated enzymatic degradation. However, natural polymer hydrogels can be limited by their low mechanical properties, batch-to-batch variation and uncontrolled loss of integrity due to enzymatic degradation, suggesting a need for the design of biosynthetic hydrogels.

9.3 Synthetic polymers

Synthetic polymers overcome many of the limitations of biological polymers by minimising batch-to-batch variations and having tunable mechanical and degradation properties. Synthetic polymers can be easily purchased or prepared from commercially available monomers. These polymers can have much tighter control over the molecular weights and have a broad working range for pH, ionic strength and chemical conditions for macromer (i.e. macromolecular monomer) and hydrogel synthesis. Purely synthetic systems can provide a blank slate environment, with controllable and reproducible chemistries and properties. This allows the effects of mechanics to be better isolated than in biological polymer hydrogels because cell-adhesive ligands can be presented in a controlled manner (Mann and West, 2002). For example, poly(ethylene glycol) hydrogels with tunable mechanics have been designed, providing for the study of stiffness on cells in 3D (Burdick and Anseth, 2002). However, a convolution in this 3D system is that molecular diffusion properties through the hydrogel network change as crosslinking density changes.

Synthetic polymers can be designed with specific molecular weights, block structures, crosslinking modes and degradable linkages. These factors dictate key hydrogel properties such as gelation kinetics, swelling, crosslinking density, molecule transport, mechanical strength and degradation rates. The selection of the molecular weight of the nondegradable segments of synthetic polymers is critical because small molecules may be cytotoxic and large molecules cannot pass renal clearance thresholds. There are a variety of mild gelation conditions for synthetic hydrogels that provide for cell encapsulation, utilising both physical (e.g., ionic interaction, hydrogen bonding, hydrophobic interaction) and covalent crosslinking (Abdel-Mottaleb et al., 2009; Hunt et al., 2011; Griffin and Kasko, 2012; Kharkar et al., 2013). Covalent crosslinking has been evaluated using a variety of chemistries that are cytocompatible (Kharkar et al., 2013). Radical photopolymerisation using acrylates (Roberts and Bryant, 2013; Fairbanks et al., 2009a), methacrylates (Roberts et al., 2011a) or thiol-norbornenes (Roberts and Bryant, 2013; Fairbanks et al., 2009b) are commonly used because photopolymerisation affords spatial and temporal control over in situ hydrogel gelation and can be performed using light sources with cytocompatible wavelengths, intensities and concentrations of photoinitators (e.g. LAP and Irgacure 2959) (Fairbanks et al., 2009a; Bryant et al., 2000). Other common covalent crosslinking techniques include Micheal Addition (Phelps et al., 2012; McGann et al., 2013), radical polymerisation (Temenoff et al., 2003), hydrazine (Alves et al., 2012; McKinnon et al., 2014), oxime (Grover et al., 2012) and Schiff-base crosslinking (Kharkar et al., 2013; Zhao et al., 2011). Depending on the polymer backbone selected and the crosslinking functionality used to create the macromer, this chemistry will dictate hydrogel degradability. The ability to design nondegradable synthetic hydrogels provides studies of encapsulated cells without the convolution of evolving mechanical properties. Additionally, nondegradable synthetic hydrogels can be utilised to isolate cells (Young et al., 2012), which may be important for cells such as pancreatic β-cells that need to be immunoisolated to treat diabetes (Hume et al., 2011). However, when cells are encapsulated for tissue engineering applications it is critical that hydrogels degrade in parallel with tissue deposition (Roberts et al., 2011b).

Despite the numerous advantages of synthetic materials, many were originally not designed for use in biology and medicine, but instead were off-the-shelf materials that clinicians found useful to solve a problem (Peppas et al., 2006). As such they have inferior biocompatibility and cell-mediated biodegradability to natural polymers. This is exacerbated by the hydrophilic nature of hydrogels, which do not absorb ECM proteins. Additionally, the mesh size, or crosslinking density, of many commonly used synthetic hydrogels (e.g. poly(ethylene glycol) and poly (vinyl alcohol)) is on the order of nanometers, which is several orders of magnitude smaller than cells (microns) (Roberts et al., 2011b; Bryant and Anseth, 2002). This will alter the transport of large solute molecules and limit cellular migration and cell–cell interactions. Mesh size has to be considered when designing synthetic materials and may require alterations in crosslink density or controlled degradation. Although there are design challenges to overcome before placing synthetic polymer materials in the body, the high degree of control and repeatability of synthetic materials accounts for their widespread use in cell encapsulation (see Table 9.3).

9.3.1 Poly(ethylene glycol)

Poly(ethylene glycol) (PEG), which at high molecular weight is also known as poly(ethylene oxide) (PEO), is one of the most commonly applied synthetic polymers for tissue-engineering applications. PEG is widely used for hydrogels because it is soluble in both water and organic solvents, nontoxic, nonimmunogenic, has low protein adhesion and is approved by the U.S. Food and Drug Administration (FDA) for several medical applications (Merrill et al., 1982; Peppas et al., 2006). The end hydroxyl groups of linear

Table 9.3 Examples of common synthetic polymers used for cell encapsulation and their method of crosslinking with a variety of cell types

Polymer	Crosslinking groups	Cell type	Reference
PEG	Acrylate	Myoblast	Linnenberger et al. (2013)
	Norbornene, thiol	Mesenchymal stem cells	Fairbanks et al. (2009b)
	Vinylsulphone, thiol	Fibroblasts	Lutolf et al. (2003b)
PEG-poly(lactic acid)	Methacrylate	Chondrocyte	Roberts et al. (2011b)
PEG-poly(propylene fumarate)	Methacrylate	Marrow stromal cells	Qiu et al. (2011)
PEG-poly(caprolactone)	Methacrylate	Chondrocyte	Rice and Anseth (2007)
PVA	Tyramine	Fibroblasts	Lim et al. (2013)
	Methacrylate	Fibroblasts	Young et al. (2012)
	Hydrazide, aldehyde	Fibroblasts	Alves et al. (2012)
PHEMA	Methacrylate	Corneal epithelial cells	Paterson et al. (2012)
	Methacrylate	Fibroblasts	Uludag and Sefton (1993)
PNIPAAm	Hydrophobic interactions	Fibroblasts	Mortisen et al. (2010)
	Hydrophobic interactions	Mesenchymal stem cells	Peroglio et al. (2013)

and multi-armed PEG allow for easy modification with a variety of functional groups, including thiols, acrylates and methacrylates (Fairbanks et al., 2009a; Roberts et al., 2011b; Roberts and Bryant, 2013; Gould and Anseth, 2013).

PEG macromers have been used alone to create hydrophilic, nondegradable networks for encapsulation of cells (Roberts et al., 2011b; Bryant and Anseth, 2002), but PEG has also been synthesised into triblock copolymers using polyester functional groups to incorporate degradability (Roberts et al., 2011b; Rice and Anseth, 2007;

Qiu et al., 2011). Polyesters, such as lactic acid, glycolic acid and caprolactone, are hydrophobic polymers that are FDA approved for medical applications. Polyesters were originally developed into porous, rigid constructs that were seeded with cells but later found application in the PEG-based hydrogels (Vunjak-Novakovic et al., 1998). These copolymers can degrade via hydrolysis of their ester bonds, and the degradation rate can be controlled by changing the ratio of the hydrophilic/hydrophobic component and via the addition of esterase enzymes (Rice and Anseth, 2007). Methacrylated, triblock copolymers of caprolactone-PEG-caprolactone were found to support cell-secreted collagen deposition, and the rate of degradation of these hydrogels could be controlled via the exogenous addition of lysozyme (Rice and Anseth, 2007). An alternative triblock copolymer based on PEG and the polyester poly(propylene fumarate) has been evaluated as an injectable carrier for tendon and blood vessel engineering and supported the encapsulation of viable cells that secreted ECM during hydrogel degradation (Qiu et al., 2011; Suggs and Mikos, 1999).

9.3.2 Poly(vinyl alcohol)

Poly(vinyl alcohol) (PVA) is prepared by a partial or complete hydrolysis of poly(vinyl acetate). The physical characteristics of PVA depend on both the degree of polymerisation and the degree of hydrolysis of the acetate groups. The solubility of PVA is highest at 87–89% acetate hydrolysis (Chaouat et al., 2008), and at higher degrees of hydrolysis PVA forms strong intra- and intermolecular hydrogen bonds based on its many repeating hydroxyl groups. PVA is widely used in areas such as pharmaceuticals, medicine and biotechnology, and PVA biomaterials have been approved by the FDA and other regulatory organisations (Chaouat et al., 2008). PVA hydrogels are nontoxic, cytocompatible, gas permeable and hydrophilic. Depending on the processing parameters, such as concentration, molecular weight and degree of functional group substitution, PVA hydrogels can have excellent mechanical properties for tissue engineering applications (i.e. soft tissue imitation, flexibility). Moreover, cells and proteins do not adhere to PVA, making it an attractive blank-slate material for cell encapsulation (Dini et al., 2005). Unmodified PVA has been formed into rigid constructs, by freeze thawing, that can be seeded with cells (Cascone et al., 1995). However, in order to ensure homogeneous cell encapsulation, PVA must be modified and formed into covalently bound hydrogels. PVA has been modified with a variety of groups such as tyramines (Lim et al., 2013), meth(acrylates) (Nilasaroya et al., 2008; Martens et al., 2003), hydrazides and aldehydes (Alves et al., 2012; Ossipov et al., 2007) that allow for in situ gelation. Every repeat of vinyl alcohol has accessible hydroxyl groups that can be modified (as compared to linear PEG, which only has two end groups), and it is therefore possible to have a large range of number and type of modifications on the PVA backbone. This means that a variety of crosslinking functional groups could be attached, and one could postulate that these could be used for multimodal crosslinking and degradation. The pendant hydroxyls could also be used for the addition of bioactive molecules, such as peptides, to signal cell attachment, proliferation, differentiation or migration (Schmedlen et al., 2002). This flexibility in design makes PVA a versatile polymer and results in a broad range of applications.

9.3.3 Poly(hydroxyethyl) methacrylate

Poly(hydroxyethyl) methacrylate (PHEMA) is a stable, optically transparent hydrophilic polymer that is one of the most widely applied hydrogel biomaterials. PHEMA-based hydrogels can be engineered to possess similar water content and mechanical properties as tissue, and exhibit excellent cytocompatibility. It has been applied to a variety of medical applications including contact lenses, dressings and drug delivery (Peppas et al., 2006). PHEMA hydrogels are generally synthesised via the free radical polymerisation of meth(acrylates). Because PHEMA hydrogels are nondegradable in vivo, its application in tissue engineering has been restricted. Many studies aim to modify the properties of PHEMA to improve the degree of hydration, degradation, mechanical properties and transport properties. To introduce controlled degradation into PHEMA hydrogels, hydrolytically (Atzet et al., 2008) and enzymatically (Paterson et al., 2012) cleavable sequences have been incorporated. By copolymerising PHEMA with functional groups, the swelling and mechanical properties can be tuned to allow for the encapsulation of cells, such as fibroblasts (Uludag and Sefton, 1993).

9.3.4 Poly(N-isopropylacrylamide)

Poly(*N*-isopropylacrylamide) (PNIPAAm) is an environmentally sensitive "smart" hydrogel that gels due to changes in temperature. PNIPAAm undergoes a reversible phase transition because it has a lower critical solution temperature (LCST) of approximately 31 °C in aqueous solution. Below the LCST, the hydrophilic moieties (-CONH-) in PNIPAAm interact with water molecules through hydrogen bonding, but above the LCST the hydrogen bonding becomes weakened and hydrophobic interactions (-$CH(CH_3)_2$) become strong and the polymer chains entangle to form a hydrogel. This is ideal for the design of an injectable materials, because at room temperature PNIPAAm is a liquid, but at body temperature it becomes a hydrogel solid when dissolved in aqueous medium (Zhang et al., 2008). To adjust the phase transition temperature of PNIPAAm hydrogels, NIPAAm can be copolymerised with more hydrophilic or hydrophobic monomers. The addition of a hydrophilic monomer generally increases the LCST, while a more hydrophobic monomer will generally lower the LCST. PNIPAAm-based hydrogels have been extensively studied for drug delivery, as well as for tissue engineering applications (Zhang et al., 2008; Santos et al., 2010; Mortisen et al., 2010; Peroglio et al., 2013). For example, Peroglio et al. demonstrated that stem cells encapsulated in thermoreversible, PNIPAAm-based hydrogels can be differentiated toward the intervertebral disc phenotype without the need for growth factor supplementation in vitro (Peroglio et al., 2013).

9.3.5 Summary of synthetic polymers

By providing a relatively bioinert platform for cell delivery and cell localisation, synthetic polymeric hydrogels can be used to engineer tissues in a 3D, highly hydrated environment. The chemistry of the synthetic polymer is easily adapted to contain hydrolytically or enzymatically degradable polymers, as well as a large variety of crosslinking functional groups that provide spatial and temporal control over hydrogel gelation. Adaptations in the polymer molecular weight, number of crosslinking molecules and polymer density can be used to create hydrogels that range from Pa to MPa in strength with highly varied mass-transport properties. However, the lack of bioactivity of purely synthetic hydrogels limits their ability to support cell survival and growth and suggests the need for biosynthetic hydrogel development.

9.4 Biosynthetic polymers

It has been shown by many researchers that using purely biological or synthetic materials has limitations in creating cell encapsulation systems. Therefore, there has been an evolution towards the development of biosynthetic gels that combine the strengths of biological and synthetic polymers for cellular encapsulation. By using hybrid, biosynthetic materials we can synergistically combine the bulk properties of synthetic polymers, while exploiting biological polymer attributes, such as high affinity and specificity of binding. Tailoring the molecular design of biosynthetic hydrogels allows for their biological (e.g. cell viability, adhesion, migration and differentiation), degradation (e.g. enzymatic, hydrolytic) and physical properties (e.g. diffusion, molecular architecture, mechanical properties) to be controlled to deliver desired signals. The design of these new materials requires a variety of new considerations, such as the selection of the specific biological and synthetic polymers and the method to combine the polymers for the specific cell encapsulation application of interest.

9.4.1 Design considerations

Combining multiple polymers into a hydrogel material poses new challenges to researchers. There are a variety of standard considerations to encapsulating cells within biosynthetic materials and subsequently placing those materials in vivo (see Figure 9.2). The materials need to retain their biological activity as well as biocompatibility, that is not elicit any local or systemic effects when placed in vivo. Additionally, the new materials have to be capable of sterilisation, without any material degradation or functional changes. It is important when selecting and designing materials that they meet the regulatory guidelines of the governing body (e.g. the FDA). It may be quicker and easier to get market approval of biomaterials that combine already commercially available medical materials. Many materials, such as PEG, PVA, heparin, hyaluronan, alginate, collagen and fibrin, have already been approved for specific clinical applications by the FDA. However, care needs to be taken when using particular biological polymers, as often undesirable and unintended biological properties are also maintained in the hydrogel. One example of this is the use of heparin in hydrogels. Heparin has been used due to its ability to sequester growth factors and signal cells (Nilasaroya et al., 2008); however, heparin is most commonly used in the hospital as a blood thinner and anticoagulant.

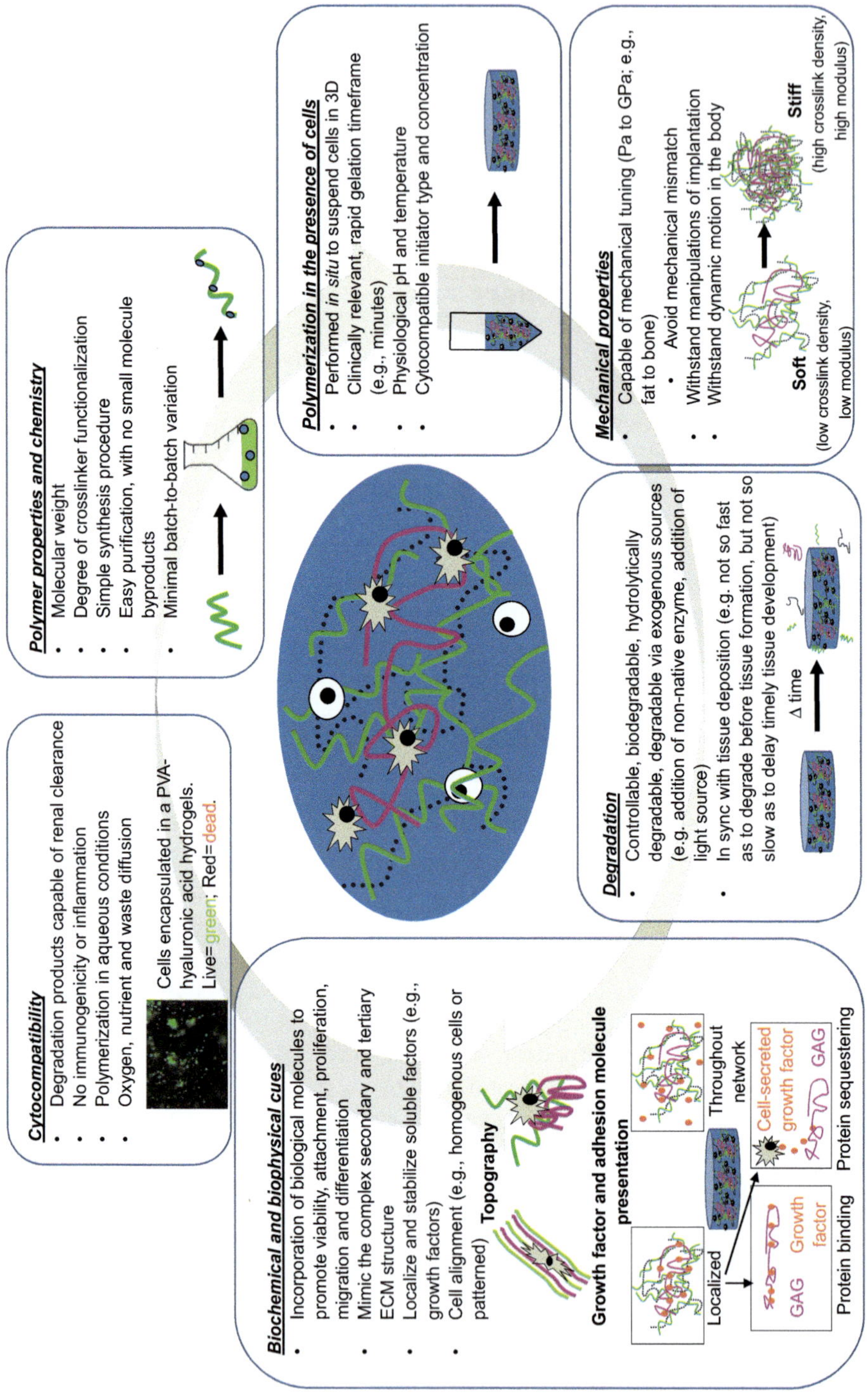

Figure 9.2 Design criteria for a biosynthetic encapsulation system.

Care has to be taken when designing new synthesis and formulation techniques to combine biological and synthetic materials. Small molecules (e.g. unreacted monomers or crosslinkers) must be removed before placing cells with macromers, as they can be cytotoxic. To obtain a 3D hydrogel with homogenous cell suspension, the cells must be mixed with macromers and initiating agents before polymerisation, and this may require extra consideration during formulation because of the relative charges and solubility of the biological and synthetic components, which could lead to phase separation. The chemical transformation from a liquid hydrogel precursor to a solid may involve changes in temperature, pH or radical concentration, which all have the potential to damage cells. Depending on the type of cell and the type of crosslinking functionality, macromers have been shown to affect cell viability (Bryant et al., 2000) and phenotype (Roberts and Bryant, 2013). Careful selection of gelation mechanism will allow for the creation of biosynthetic hydrogels that do not damage the biological polymer and do not alter cellular viability, genotype or phenotype.

In addition to basic material considerations, the target microenvironment needs to be considered. The target microenvironment may be a disease state, an organ or a tissue type of interest. The ECM of different tissues is made up of a variety of complex biological molecules that have different spatial and temporal regulations by the resident cells, and which may change during disease or injury. When selecting biological polymers for hydrogels, the specific cell type to be encapsulated and the concentration and type of biomolecules present within a tissue need to be considered to recapitulate that environment. Materials that mimic the mechanical and biochemical environment will help researchers better guide cell behaviour. For example, tailoring hydrogel mechanical properties to be similar to native tissue has been shown to guide stem cells down specific lineages (Trappmann and Chen, 2013). Also, overcoming mechanical mismatch between device mechanical properties and the tissue may reduce fibrotic encapsulation (Baek et al., 2014). Because the crosslinked polymer mesh is dense in many hydrogels, degradation is required for normal cell processes such as migration, matrix synthesis and matrix remodelling. Degradation will allow us to better mimic the dynamic, native ECM, understand in vivo cell behaviour, and for tissue engineering applications allows for the timely infiltration of cells and blood vessels (Novosel et al., 2011). By combining biological and synthetic polymers, there is potential for improved hydrogel mechanics and unique, bimodal degradation due to cell-secreted enzyme degradation and synthetic polymer hydrolysis.

9.4.2 Selecting fragments or entire biological molecules

The first choice that researchers face in designing biosynthetic gels is whether to utilise fragments or whole biological molecules. The answer to this choice is often dependent on the intended application. The use of peptide sequences to functionalise synthetic hydrogels has widespread appeal because short peptide sequences are relatively easily synthesised and modified and are stable (Zhu and Marchant, 2011). A big advantage of peptide sequences is their ease of incorporation. For example, DeForest and Anseth were able to spatially and temporally control the presentation of RGD in PEG hydrogels using thiolene and strain-promoted azide–alkyne cycloaddition click chemistries (DeForest and Anseth, 2011). Peptides can also be designed to mimic the complex, nanofibrous structure of natural ECM. For instance, collagen mimetic peptides that undergo triple helical assembly have been incorporated into PEG hydrogels and utilised to differentiate stem cells down a chondrogenic lineage (Yu et al., 2011). Additionally, peptides can be used to probe how cells sense stiffness without the convolution of other signals provided by whole proteins. Huebsch et al. varied the concentration of peptide in alginate, agarose and PEG hydrogels laden with mesenchymal stem cells. They found that varying the polymer concentration, and as a result the crosslink density, allowed them to direct differentiation to specific lineages (i.e. adipogenic at 2.5–5 kPa and osteogenic at 11–30 kPa) depending on the stiffness of the hydrogel (Huebsch et al., 2010). However, the use of peptides assumes that they retain their biological specificity and function when isolated from the tertiary protein structure. This is especially unlikely if the sequence is located within the β-sheets or α-helixes that make up the secondary structure of proteins. For example, RGD retains its integrin-binding ability, although not with as high of an affinity as the full fibronectin protein (Zhu and Marchant, 2011). Therefore, the use of full proteins has also been evaluated to impart attachment, as well as other inherent signalling from the biological polymers of interest. For example, collagen proteins coated on polyacrylamide materials have shown stem cell differentiation towards adipogenic (0.5–2 kPa) or osteogenic (20–115 kPa) lineages (Trappmann et al., 2012).

9.4.3 Methods to combine biologicals and synthetic polymers

To create biosynthetic hydrogels, the biological and synthetic components can be combined via techniques such as physical entrapment (Roberts et al., 2014; Unterman et al., 2012), interpenetrating networks (Rennerfeldt et al., 2013; Daniele et al., 2014) or covalent crosslinking (Nilasaroya et al., 2008; Lim et al., 2013). When utilising any of these techniques the biological molecule must be evaluated after any modification and after encapsulation, to ensure that processing does not change or destroy bioactivity.

9.4.3.1 Physical entrapment

Physical entanglement has generally been applied with a synthetic or biosynthetic network that has entrapped biological molecules and cells. The biological polymers can be physically entangled in the network, or be incorporated via ionic interactions, hydrogen bonding or hydrophobic interactions. This system allows for the cells to be entrapped within a mechanically robust network and have localised bioactive cues. Care needs to be taken when selecting the crosslinking strategy so as to not damage or denature encapsulated proteins. For example, photopolymerisation of acrylate PEG hydrogels led to a loss of 50% bioactivity of lysozyme, whereas lysozyme retained nearly 100% of its pre-reaction activity in thiolene PEG networks (McCall and Anseth, 2012). Additionally, physical entrapment of biological polymers does have the risk of the biomolecules diffusing out, depending on the relative size of the biomolecule compared to the hydrogel network (Roberts et al., 2011a). To minimise diffusion of entrapped molecules, researchers have covalently tethered ECM-binding peptides to synthetic hydrogel networks to localise encapsulated ECM molecules for stem cell differentiation (Unterman et al., 2012).

9.4.3.2 Interpenetrating networks

Hydrogel interpenetrating newtorks (IPNs) consist of two or more physically interlocked polymers. These native ECM-mimetics can have a heterogeneous and hierarchical network architecture that surrounds cells, providing mechanical support and a biologically interactive environment. The different interlocked networks may have different degradation rates and methods (e.g. enzymatic, hydrolytic), and thus there may be bimodal changes in network swelling and mechanical properties. IPNs of PEG and gelatin have been shown to support endothelial cell growth adhesion, viability and proliferation (Daniele et al., 2014). By combining two biocompatible hydrogel materials, agarose and PEG, an IPN was designed with greatly enhanced mechanical performance (DeKosky et al., 2010). The PEG-agarose IPNs had over four-fold higher modulus than agarose or PEG alone, and supported the encapsulation of viable chondrocytes that secreted chondrocyte-specific tissue molecules (DeKosky et al., 2010).

9.4.3.3 Covalent crosslinking

Covalent crosslinking of biological polymers into a synthetic network localises the biological signal of interest (McCall et al., 2012). Covalently attaching biological polymers into hydrogels typically requires chemical modification of the biological molecules. For example, grafting polymers (e.g. PEGylation) or chemical modification using crosslinkable functional groups, such as acrylates or thiols, are popular techniques for functionalising glycosaminoglycans (Nilasaroya et al., 2008; Steinmetz and Bryant, 2012; Choh et al., 2011) and proteins (McCall et al., 2012; Gonen-Wadmany et al., 2011). For example, thiol-modified hyaluronan has been copolymerised with PEG-dithiol, and the resulting networks have shown high viability of fibroblasts, endothelial cells, and mesenchymal stem cells up to 7 days after encapsulation (Choh et al., 2011). However, chemical modification of proteins can cause degradation, denaturation or loss of biological activity. Therefore, recent studies have explored integrating biological polymers by exploiting the observation that proteins can be crosslinked without prior modification via their tyrosine residues (Lim et al., 2013). Lim et al. demonstrated that PVA-tyramine hydrogels could be used to crosslink unmodified gelatin, which was released in a controlled manner as the hydrogels hydrolytically degraded and that these hydrogels supported the growth of fibroblasts (Lim et al., 2013). Although these techniques may not result in identical biopolymer activity as prior to crosslinking, it is important to recognise the physiochemical benefits of covalently crosslinking biopolymers into hydrogels (i.e. localisation for cell-mediated degradation, adhesion, etc.) (Gonen-Wadmany et al., 2011).

9.4.4 Biosynthetic hydrogels for specific applications

Biosynthetic hydrogels for cell encapsulation are used to deliver signals to cells and act as support for cell growth and function. It is well known that cell genotype and phenotype are guided by the extracellular microenvironment. Soluble factors, cell—cell communication (e.g. via gap junctions) and ECM mechanical properties are only a few of the multitude of factors directing cells down specific lineages. Therefore, tissue engineers are exploring methods to exploit the extracellular environment to modulate cell behaviour and guide cells to regenerate tissues. For certain cell types, adhesion is critical to viability, or growth factors aid in differentiation and accelerate tissue formation and angiogensis, or hydrogel degradation is required for migration and tissue production. Biological polymers can be combined with synthetic polymers to design hydrogels aimed at accomplishing these specific applications (i.e. increased cell adhesion, cell-mediated enzymatic degradation and growth factor delivery).

9.4.4.1 Cell adhesive hydrogels

Cell attachment to the ECM is necessary for cell migration, and for many cell types it is critical for their viability and proliferation (Scott, 1995). Cell binding to ECM molecules plays key roles in tissue development, organisation, maintenance and repair by providing anchorage and signals that direct cell function. To mimic these cell—matrix interactions, a variety of ECM-derived peptides and ECM proteins have been used to modify and design biosynthetic hydrogels (Figure 9.3).

Peptides designed to promote cell adhesion are generally derived from ECM proteins, such as fibronectin, laminin, collagen and elastin. Commonly used peptides include the amino acid sequences RGD (derived from proteins such as collagen, fibronectin or laminin), YIGSR and IKVAV (both derived from laminin) (Liu et al., 2010; Mann and West, 2002; Fittkau et al., 2005; Weber and Anseth, 2008; Weiss et al., 2012; Gould and Anseth, 2013). Vascular smooth muscle cells have been shown to have minimal attachment to PEG-diacrylate hydrogels, whereas the incorporation of the adhesion peptides RGDS, KQAGDV and VAPG led to increased cell attachment on and within the scaffolds (Zhu and Marchant, 2011). A variety of whole-cell adhesion proteins, such as laminin, fibronectin and collagen, have also been incorporated into hydrogels to create

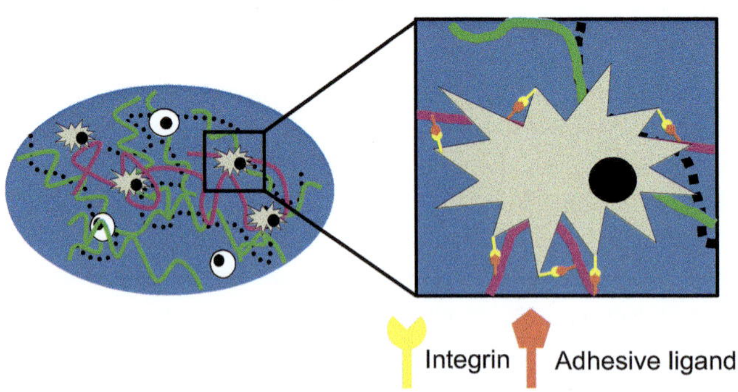

Figure 9.3 Cells encapsulated within biosynthetic hydrogels can interact with adhesive ligands on biological polymers via cell-surface integrands.

biosynthetics. The proteins are commonly PEGylated using acrylate-PEG-*N*-hydroxyl succinimidyl ester, Micheal addition, and other techniques (DeVolder and Kong, 2012; Zhu, 2010). For example, PEGylated fibrinogen has been shown to facilitate the adhesion of smooth muscle cells (Peyton et al., 2008). PVA-based hydrogels have been made adhesive through modification with the complete fibronectin protein (Nuttelman et al., 2001). Another protein that has recently been used for its cell-adhesion properties, despite not being mammalian, is the glue-like silk protein sericin. For example, Lim et al. covalently crosslinked methacrylated sericin within PVA hydrogels and observed a significant increase in the attachment of fibroblasts (Lim et al., 2012).

9.4.4.2 Growth factor presenting hydrogels

Native ECM has a variety of signalling molecules, including growth factors, that guide cell responses and resultant tissue development. Controlling growth factor presentation in hydrogels can modulate cellular function, such as differentiation (e.g. gene expression), migration (e.g. cell homing for recruitment of endogenous cells) and proliferation (Chen and Mooney, 2003). Growth factors have been loaded into pre-formed hydrogels, encapsulated during gelation, covalently bound, and indirectly bound using GAGs (Figure 9.4) (Benoit et al., 2007; Mann et al., 2001b; Ehrbar et al., 2007; Park et al., 2007; Tae et al., 2007; McCall et al., 2012). McCall et al. covalently tethered the

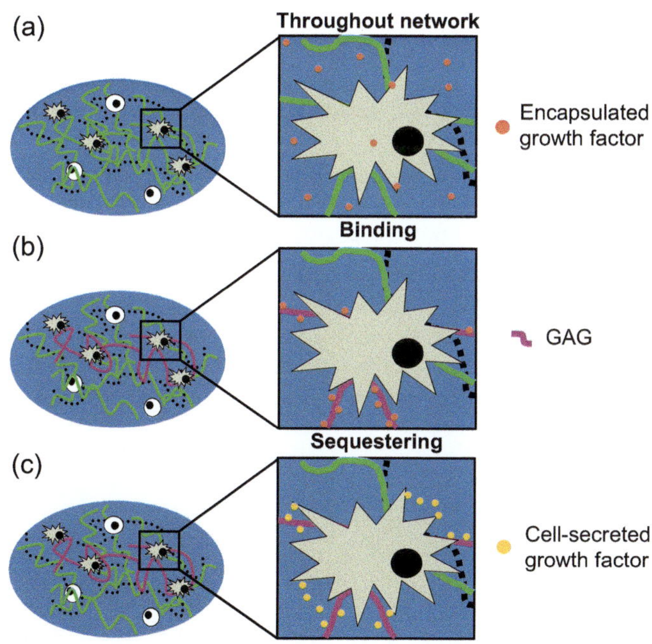

Figure 9.4 There are a variety of approaches to deliver growth factors to encapsulated cells. (a) Growth factors can be encapsulated within the hydrogel network allowing for diffusion throughout the hydrogel and gradual growth factor release. (b) Biological polymers, such as GAGs, can be used to localise encapsulated growth factors within the hydrogel. (c) Biological polymers can be used to sequester and localise cell-secreted growth factors.

cytokine transforming growth factor β (TGFβ) into PEG hydrogels, and observed that after 21 days tethered TGFβ promoted chondrogenesis of encapsulated mesenchymal stem cells (McCall et al., 2012). The encapsulation of multiple growth factors (i.e. TGFβ and insulin-like growth factor-I) within PEG hydrogels resulted in increased GAG production by encapsulated chondrocytes, enhancing the ECM content of the engineered neocartilage (Elisseeff et al., 2001). Alternatively, GAGs, such as heparin sulphate, have been used to sequester or localise growth factors within hydrogels (Tae et al., 2007; Benoit et al., 2007). These GAGs can act to stabilise the growth factors' active conformation and localise it so that it does not have immediate clearance. For example, heparin-PEG biosynthetic hydrogels were used to sequester bone morphogenic protein-2 to promote mesenchymal stem cell osteogenesis (Benoit et al., 2007). By localising growth factors near encapsulated cells, tissue engineers can guide cell behaviour and the resulting type and quantity of tissue production.

9.4.4.3 Enzymatically degradable hydrogels

The native ECM is a dynamic environment, constantly allowing for cell proliferation, migration and differentiation in order to develop, maintain and regenerate the local tissue. During migration and signalling, cells produce proteolytic enzymes, such as matrix metalloproteinases (MMPs), which are a component of the matrix remodelling and assembly process. Enzymatically degradable hydrogels (Figure 9.5) have been used to study angiogenesis (Lutolf et al., 2003b), valve disease (Gould and Anseth, 2013) and wound healing (Raeber et al., 2007) amongst other applications. The commonly used enzymatically degradable sequence include GPQGIAGQ, GPQGIWGQ and GPQGILGQ (degraded by collagenase and various MMPs such as -1, -2, -3, -7, -8 and -9) (Fairbanks et al., 2009b; Lutolf et al., 2003a), GGLGPAGGK (degraded by collagenase) (Mann et al., 2001a) and AAAAAAAAK (Mann et al., 2001a), AAPVR and AAP(Nva) (Aimetti et al., 2009) (degraded by elastase). Varying the amount of MMP-cleavable crosslinker within hydrogels allows for modulation of the migration rate of fibroblasts (Lutolf et al., 2003a). The incorporation of enzymatic degradation into synthetic hydrogels has been shown to allow cells to migrate and produce more collagen than in nondegradable hydrogels (Mann et al., 2001a). HA-PNIPAAm hydrogels have been demonstrated to undergo enzyme degradation using hyaluronidase (Mortisen et al., 2010), and have been employed towards

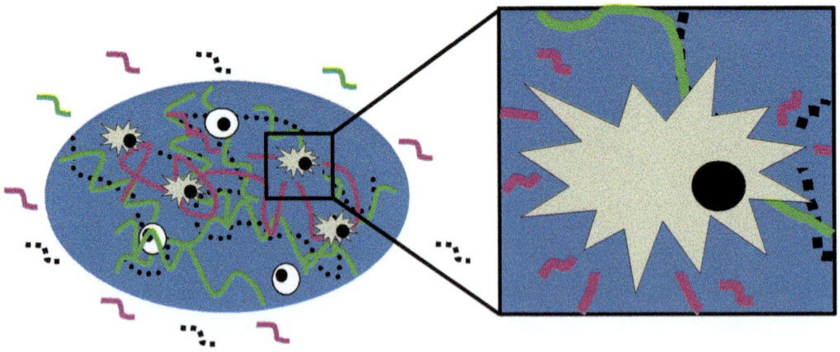

Figure 9.5 Depending on the selected biological polymer, cell-secreted or exogenously added enzymes can be used to degrade biological polymers in sync with cellular activity.

regenerating the nucleus pulposus in intervertebral discs (Peroglio et al., 2013). Additionally, bimodal degradation, where hydrogels degrade both enzymatically and hydrolytically, has been investigated for cell encapsulation. Although the inclusion of cell-mediated degradable enzymes is attractive, further control over hydrogel degradation may be desirable if the enzyme degradation is slow, or the enzymes are not present. HA macromers that are both hydrolytically (via ester hydrolysis of lactic acid or caprolactone) and enzymatically degradable offer control over the kinetics of degradation through the crosslinking density, type of degradable unit and copolymerisation with the enzymatically degradable macromers (Sahoo et al., 2008). These hydrogels supported the encapsulation of mesenchymal stem cells and controlled the distribution of the ECM molecules that they produced via changes in the copolymer concentration.

9.5 Future trends

There are numerous challenges that remain in the field of biosynthetic hydrogels for cell encapsulation. Some long-standing questions include whether it is better to select protein fragments (i.e. peptides) or whole proteins, and if nondegradable or degradable hydrogels are better for cell encapsulation. A more recent question is if the material needs to be "smart." Smart hydrogels can take on many connotations; however, smart hydrogels are generally those that are capable of responding to their environment, and there are numerous excellent reviews that cover these topics in detail. Some examples of environmental response include hydrogel changes due to alterations in pH (Qiu and Park, 2001), temperature (Ruel-Gariepy and Leroux, 2004), electrical stimuli or chemical stimuli (Kulkarni and Biswanath, 2007; Soppimath et al., 2002). In the design of all smart hydrogels, the timing and control of the response is crucial and remains an ongoing area of research. Another area to be probed in the development of biosynthetic hydrogels is the exact effect of the chemical modification and the fabrication process on the cells being encapsulated. Most studies demonstrate that the designed hydrogel material is capable of keeping encapsulated cells viable and metabolically active for short periods of time. However, the long-term effects of hydrogel chemistries and fabrication processes on the genotype and phenotype of cells remain to be systematically evaluated. Thus, while the use of biosynthetic hydrogels for cell encapsulation is growing in popularity, there are still many new avenues of research to explore and improve upon the current designs.

References

Abdel-Mottaleb, M.M., Mortada, N.D., El-Shamy, A.A., Awad, G.A., 2009. Physically cross-linked polyvinyl alcohol for the topical delivery of fluconazole. Drug Dev. Ind. Pharm. 35, 311–320.

Ahearne, M., Buckley, C.T., Kelly, D.J., 2011. A growth factor delivery system for chondrogenic induction of infrapatellar fat pad-derived stem cells in fibrin hydrogels. Biotechnol. Appl. Biochem. 58, 345–352.

Ahmed, T.A., Dare, E.V., Hincke, M., 2008. Fibrin: a versatile scaffold for tissue engineering applications. Tissue Eng. Part B Rev. 14, 199–215.

Aimetti, A.A., Tibbitt, M.W., Anseth, K.S., 2009. Human neutrophil elastase responsive delivery from poly(ethylene glycol) hydrogels. Biomacromolecules 10, 1484–1489.

Alberts, B., 1994. Molecular Biology of the Cell. Garland Publication, New York.

Alshamkhani, A., Duncan, R., 1995. Radioiodination of alginate via covalently-bound tyrosinamide allows monitoring of its fate in-vivo. J. Bioact. Compat. Polym. 10, 4–13.

Altman, G.H., Diaz, F., Jakuba, C., Calabro, T., Horan, R.L., Chen, J., Lu, H., Richmond, J., Kaplan, D.L., 2003. Silk-based biomaterials. Biomaterials 24, 401–416.

Alves, M.H., Young, C.J., Bozzetto, K., Poole-Warren, L.A., Martens, P.J., 2012. Degradable, click poly(vinyl alcohol) hydrogels: characterization of degradation and cellular compatibility. Biomed. Mater. 7, 024106.

Aramwit, P., Kanokpanont, S., Nakpheng, T., Srichana, T., 2010. The effect of sericin from various extraction methods on cell viability and collagen production. Int. J. Mol. Sci. 11, 2200–2211.

Atzet, S., Curtin, S., Trinh, P., Bryant, S., Ratner, B., 2008. Degradable poly(2-hydroxyethyl methacrylate)-co-polycaprolactone hydrogels for tissue engineering scaffolds. Biomacromolecules 9, 3370–3377.

Auger, F.A., Rouabhia, M., Goulet, F., Berthod, F., Moulin, V., Germain, L., 1998. Tissue-engineered human skin substitutes developed from collagen-populated hydrated gels: clinical and fundamental applications. Med. Biol. Eng. Comput. 36, 801–812.

Baek, S., Green, R.A., Poole-Warren, L.A., 2014. Effects of dopants on the biomechanical properties of conducting polymer films on platinum electrodes. J. Biomed. Mater. Res. A 102 (8), 2743–2754.

Baldwin, A.D., Kiick, K.L., 2010. Polysaccharide-modified synthetic polymeric biomaterials. Biopolymers 94, 128–140.

Benoit, D.S., Durney, A.R., Anseth, K.S., 2007. The effect of heparin-functionalized PEG hydrogels on three-dimensional human mesenchymal stem cell osteogenic differentiation. Biomaterials 28, 66–77.

Bhatia, S.K., 2012. Engineering Biomaterials for Regenerative Medicine: Novel Technologies for Clinical Applications. Springer, New York, NY.

Bini, E., Foo, C.W., Huang, J., Karageorgiou, V., Kitchel, B., Kaplan, D.L., 2006. RGD-functionalized bioengineered spider dragline silk biomaterial. Biomacromolecules 7, 3139–3145.

Bryant, S.J., Anseth, K.S., 2002. Hydrogel properties influence ECM production by chondrocytes photoencapsulated in poly(ethylene glycol) hydrogels. J. Biomed. Mater. Res. 59, 63–72.

Bryant, S.J., Davis-Arehart, K.A., Luo, N., Shoemaker, R.K., Arthur, J.A., Anseth, K.S., 2004. Synthesis and characterization of photopolymerized multifunctional hydrogels: water-soluble poly(vinyl alcohol) and chondroitin sulfate macromers for chondrocyte encapsulation. Macromolecules 37, 6726–6733.

Bryant, S.J., Nuttelman, C.R., Anseth, K.S., 2000. Cytocompatibility of UV and visible light photoinitiating systems on cultured NIH/3T3 fibroblasts in vitro. J. Biomater. Sci. Polym. Ed. 11, 439–457.

Burdick, J.A., Anseth, K.S., 2002. Photoencapsulation of osteoblasts in injectable RGD-modified PEG hydrogels for bone tissue engineering. Biomaterials 23, 4315–4323.

Burdick, J.A., Prestwich, G.D., 2011. Hyaluronic acid hydrogels for biomedical applications. Adv. Mater. 23, H41–H56.

Buschmann, M.D., Gluzband, Y.A., Grodzinsky, A.J., Kimura, J.H., Hunziker, E.B., 1992. Chondrocytes in agarose culture synthesize a mechanically functional extracellular matrix. J. Orthop. Res. 10, 745–758.

Cascone, M.G., Laus, M., Ricci, D., Delguerra, R.S., 1995. Evaluation of poly(vinyl alcohol) hydrogels as a component of hybrid artificial tissues. J. Mater. Sci. Mater. Med. 6, 71–75.
Chaouat, M., Le Visage, C., Baille, W.E., Escoubet, B., Chaubet, F., Mateescu, M.A., Letourneur, D., 2008. A novel cross-linked poly(vinyl alcohol) (PVA) for vascular grafts. Adv. Funct. Mater. 18, 2855–2861.
Chen, R.R., Mooney, D.J., 2003. Polymeric growth factor delivery strategies for tissue engineering. Pharm. Res. 20, 1103–1112.
Chenite, A., Chaput, C., Wang, D., Combes, C., Buschmann, M.D., Hoemann, C.D., Leroux, J.C., Atkinson, B.L., Binette, F., Selmani, A., 2000. Novel injectable neutral solutions of chitosan form biodegradable gels in situ. Biomaterials 21, 2155–2161.
Choh, S.Y., Cross, D., Wang, C., 2011. Facile synthesis and characterization of disulfide-cross-linked hyaluronic acid hydrogels for protein delivery and cell encapsulation. Biomacromolecules 12, 1126–1136.
Daniele, M.A., Adams, A.A., Naciri, J., North, S.H., Ligler, F.S., 2014. Interpenetrating networks based on gelatin methacrylamide and PEG formed using concurrent thiol click chemistries for hydrogel tissue engineering scaffolds. Biomaterials 35, 1845–1856.
Dash, R., Acharya, C., Bindu, P.C., Kundu, S.C., 2008. Antioxidant potential of silk protein sericin against hydrogen peroxide-induced oxidative stress in skin fibroblasts. Bmb Rep. 41, 236–241.
DeForest, C.A., Anseth, K.S., 2011. Cytocompatible click-based hydrogels with dynamically tunable properties through orthogonal photoconjugation and photocleavage reactions. Nat. Chem. 3, 925–931.
DeKosky, B.J., Dormer, N.H., Ingavle, G.C., Roatch, C.H., Lomakin, J., Detamore, M.S., Gehrke, S.H., 2010. Hierarchically designed agarose and poly(ethylene glycol) interpenetrating network hydrogels for cartilage tissue engineering. Tissue Eng. Part C Methods 16, 1533–1542.
DeVolder, R., Kong, H.J., 2012. Hydrogels for in vivo-like three-dimensional cellular studies. Wiley Interdiscip. Rev. Syst. Biol. Med. 4, 351–365.
Dini, L., Panzarini, E., Miccoli, M.A., Miceli, V., Protopapa, C., Ramires, P.A., 2005. In vitro study of the interaction of polyalkilimide and polyvinyl alcohol hydrogels with cells. Tissue Cell 37, 479–487.
Drury, J.L., Mooney, D.J., 2003. Hydrogels for tissue engineering: scaffold design variables and applications. Biomaterials 24, 4337–4351.
Ehrbar, M., Rizzi, S.C., Hlushchuk, R., Djonov, V., Zisch, A.H., Hubbell, J.A., Weber, F.E., Lutolf, M.P., 2007. Enzymatic formation of modular cell-instructive fibrin analogs for tissue engineering. Biomaterials 28, 3856–3866.
Elisseeff, J., Mcintosh, W., Fu, K., Blunk, B.T., Langer, R., 2001. Controlled-release of IGF-I and TGF-beta1 in a photopolymerizing hydrogel for cartilage tissue engineering. J. Orthop. Res. 19, 1098–1104.
Emerich, D.F., Winn, S.R., Hantraye, P.M., Peschanski, M., Chen, E.Y., Chu, Y., Mcdermott, P., Baetge, E.E., Kordower, J.H., 1997. Protective effect of encapsulated cells producing neurotrophic factor CNTF in a monkey model of Huntington's disease. Nature 386, 395–399.
Fairbanks, B.D., Schwartz, M.P., Bowman, C.N., Anseth, K.S., 2009a. Photoinitiated polymerization of PEG-diacrylate with lithium phenyl-2,4,6-trimethylbenzoylphosphinate: polymerization rate and cytocompatibility. Biomaterials 30, 6702–6707.
Fairbanks, B.D., Schwartz, M.P., Halevi, A.E., Nuttelman, C.R., Bowman, C.N., Anseth, K.S., 2009b. A versatile synthetic extracellular matrix mimic via thiol-norbornene photopolymerization. Adv. Mater. 21, 5005–5010.

Ferreira, L.S., Gerecht, S., Fuller, J., Shieh, H.F., Vunjak-Novakovic, G., Langer, R., 2007. Bioactive hydrogel scaffolds for controllable vascular differentiation of human embryonic stem cells. Biomaterials 28, 2706–2717.

Fittkau, M.H., Zilla, P., Bezuidenhout, D., Lutolf, M., Human, P., Hubbell, J.A., Davies, N., 2005. The selective modulation of endothelial cell mobility on RGD peptide containing surfaces by YIGSR peptides. Biomaterials 26, 167–174.

Geer, D.J., Andreadis, S.T., 2003. A novel role of fibrin in epidermal healing: plasminogen-mediated migration and selective detachment of differentiated keratinocytes. J. Invest. Dermatol. 121, 1210–1216.

Gonen-Wadmany, M., Goldshmid, R., Seliktar, D., 2011. Biological and mechanical implications of PEGylating proteins into hydrogel biomaterials. Biomaterials 32, 6025–6033.

Gould, S.T., Anseth, K.S., 2013. Role of cell-matrix interactions on VIC phenotype and tissue deposition in 3D PEG hydrogels. J. Tissue Eng. Regen. Med. http://dx.doi.org/10.1002/term.1836.

Griffin, D.R., Kasko, A.M., 2012. Photodegradable macromers and hydrogels for live cell encapsulation and release. J. Am. Chem. Soc. 134, 13103–13107.

Grover, G.N., Lam, J., Nguyen, T.H., Segura, T., Maynard, H.D., 2012. Biocompatible hydrogels by oxime click chemistry. Biomacromolecules 13, 3013–3017.

Hall, H., 2007. Modified fibrin hydrogel matrices: both, 3D-scaffolds and local and controlled release systems to stimulate angiogenesis. Curr. Pharm. Des. 13, 3597–3607.

Hao, S.G., Su, L.P., Gu, X.L., Moyana, T., Xiang, J., 2005. A novel approach to tumor suppression using microencapsulated engineered J558/TNF-alpha cells. Exp. Oncol. 27, 56–60.

Hiemstra, C., Van Der Aa, L.J., Zhong, Z.Y., Dijkstra, P.J., Feijen, J., 2007. Rapidly in situ-forming degradable hydrogels from dextran thiols through michael addition. Biomacromolecules 8, 1548–1556.

Hogg, P.J., Jackson, C.M., 1989. Fibrin monomer protects thrombin from inactivation by heparin-antithrombin III: implications for heparin efficacy. Proc. Natl. Acad. Sci. U.S.A. 86, 3619–3623.

Hoshiba, T., Lu, H., Kawazoe, N., Chen, G., 2010. Decellularized matrices for tissue engineering. Expert Opin. Biol. Ther. 10, 1717–1728.

Huebsch, N., Arany, P.R., Mao, A.S., Shvartsman, D., Ali, O.A., Bencherif, S.A., Rivera-Feliciano, J., Mooney, D.J., 2010. Harnessing traction-mediated manipulation of the cell/matrix interface to control stem-cell fate. Nat. Mater. 9, 518–526.

Hume, P.S., Bowman, C.N., Anseth, K.S., 2011. Functionalized PEG hydrogels through reactive dip-coating for the formation of immunoactive barriers. Biomaterials 32, 6204–6212.

Hunt, J.N., Feldman, K.E., Lynd, N.A., Deek, J., Campos, L.M., Spruell, J.M., Hernandez, B.M., Kramer, E.J., Hawker, C.J., 2011. Tunable, high modulus hydrogels driven by ionic coacervation. Adv. Mater. 23, 2327–2331.

Ingber, D.E., 1990. Fibronectin controls capillary endothelial cell growth by modulating cell shape. Proc. Natl. Acad. Sci. U.S.A. 87, 3579–3583.

Ishihara, M., Nakanishi, K., Ono, K., Sato, M., Kikuchi, M., Saito, Y., Yura, H., Matsui, T., Hattori, H., Uenoyama, M., Kurita, A., 2002. Photocrosslinkable chitosan as a dressing for wound occlusion and accelerator in healing process. Biomaterials 23, 833–840.

Iwata, H., Takagi, T., Amemiya, H., Shimizu, H., Yamashita, K., Kobayashi, K., Akutsu, T., 1992. Agarose for a bioartificial pancreas. J. Biomed. Mater. Res. 26, 967–977.

Jin, R., Teixeira, L.S., Dijkstra, P.J., Van Blitterswijk, C.A., Karperien, M., Feijen, J., 2010. Enzymatically-crosslinked injectable hydrogels based on biomimetic dextran-hyaluronic acid conjugates for cartilage tissue engineering. Biomaterials 31, 3103–3113.

Kaufmann, P.M., Heimrath, S., Kim, B.S., Mooney, D.J., 1997. Highly porous polymer matrices as a three-dimensional culture system for hepatocytes. Cell Transplant. 6, 463–468.
Kharkar, P.M., Kiick, K.L., Kloxin, A.M., 2013. Designing degradable hydrogels for orthogonal control of cell microenvironments. Chem. Soc. Rev. 42, 7335–7372.
Kim, M., Lee, J.Y., Jones, C.N., Revzin, A., Tae, G., 2010. Heparin-based hydrogel as a matrix for encapsulation and cultivation of primary hepatocytes. Biomaterials 31, 3596–3603.
Kim, S., Bell, K., Mousa, S.A., Varner, J.A., 2000. Regulation of angiogenesis in vivo by ligation of integrin alpha5beta1 with the central cell-binding domain of fibronectin. Am. J. Pathol. 156, 1345–1362.
Kim, Y.T., Hitchcock, R., Broadhead, K.W., Messina, D.J., Tresco, P.A., 2005. A cell encapsulation device for studying soluble factor release from cells transplanted in the rat brain. J. Control. Release 102, 101–111.
Kulkarni, R.V., Biswanath, S., 2007. Electrically responsive smart hydrogels in drug delivery: a review. J. Appl. Biomater. Biomech. 5, 125–139.
Langer, R., Peppas, N.A., 2003. Advances in biomaterials, drug delivery, and bionanotechnology. Aiche J. 49, 2990–3006.
Langer, R., Tirrell, D.A., 2004. Designing materials for biology and medicine. Nature 428, 487–492.
Lau, Y.K., Gobin, A.M., West, J.L., 2006. Overexpression of lysyl oxidase to increase matrix crosslinking and improve tissue strength in dermal wound healing. Ann. Biomed. Eng. 34, 1239–1246.
Lee, C.H., Singla, A., Lee, Y., 2001a. Biomedical applications of collagen. Int. J. Pharm. 221, 1–22.
Lee, C.R., Grodzinsky, A.J., Spector, M., 2001b. The effects of cross-linking of collagen-glycosaminoglycan scaffolds on compressive stiffness, chondrocyte-mediated contraction, proliferation and biosynthesis. Biomaterials 22, 3145–3154.
Lee, K.Y., Ha, W.S., Park, W.H., 1995. Blood compatibility and biodegradability of partially N-acylated chitosan derivatives. Biomaterials 16, 1211–1216.
Lee, K.Y., Mooney, D.J., 2001. Hydrogels for tissue engineering. Chem. Rev. 101, 1869–1879.
LeRoux, M.A., Guilak, F., Setton, L.A., 1999. Compressive and shear properties of alginate gel: effects of sodium ions and alginate concentration. J. Biomed. Mater. Res. 47, 46–53.
Levental, K.R., Yu, H., Kass, L., Lakins, J.N., Egeblad, M., Erler, J.T., Fong, S.F., Csiszar, K., Giaccia, A., Weninger, W., Yamauchi, M., Gasser, D.L., Weaver, V.M., 2009. Matrix crosslinking forces tumor progression by enhancing integrin signaling. Cell 139, 891–906.
Lever, R., Mulloy, B., Page, C.P., 2012. Heparin – A Century of Progress. Springer, New York.
Lim, F., Sun, A.M., 1980. Microencapsulated islets as bioartificial endocrine pancreas. Science 210, 908–910.
Lim, K.S., Alves, M.H., Poole-Warren, L.A., Martens, P.J., 2013. Covalent incorporation of non-chemically modified gelatin into degradable PVA-tyramine hydrogels. Biomaterials 34, 7097–7105.
Lim, K.S., Kundu, J., Reeves, A., Poole-Warren, L.A., Kundu, S.C., Martens, P.J., 2012. The influence of silkworm species on cellular interactions with novel PVA/silk sericin hydrogels. Macromol. Biosci. 12, 322–332.
Lima, E.G., Bian, L., Ng, K.W., Mauck, R.L., Byers, B.A., Tuan, R.S., Ateshian, G.A., Hung, C.T., 2007. The beneficial effect of delayed compressive loading on tissue-engineered cartilage constructs cultured with TGF-beta3. Osteoarthritis Cartilage 15, 1025–1033.

Linnenberger, A., Bodine, M.I., Fiedler, C., Roberts, J.J., Skaalure, S.C., Quinn, J.P., Bryant, S.J., Cole, M., Mcleod, R.R., 2013. Three dimensional live cell lithography. Opt. Express 21, 10269–10277.

Liu, S.Q., Tian, Q.A., Wang, L., Hedrick, J.L., Hui, J.H.P., Yang, Y.Y., Ee, P.L.R., 2010. Injectable biodegradable poly(ethylene glycol)/RGD peptide hybrid hydrogels for in vitro chondrogenesis of human mesenchymal stem cells. Macromol. Rapid Commun. 31, 1148–1154.

Lokeshwar, V.B., Selzer, M.G., 2000. Differences in hyaluronic acid-mediated functions and signaling in arterial, microvessel, and vein-derived human endothelial cells. J. Biol. Chem. 275, 27641–27649.

Lutolf, M.P., Lauer-Fields, J.L., Schmoekel, H.G., Metters, A.T., Weber, F.E., Fields, G.B., Hubbell, J.A., 2003a. Synthetic matrix metalloproteinase-sensitive hydrogels for the conduction of tissue regeneration: engineering cell-invasion characteristics. Proc. Natl. Acad. Sci. U.S.A. 100, 5413–5418.

Lutolf, M.P., Raeber, G.P., Zisch, A.H., Tirelli, N., Hubbell, J.A., 2003b. Cell-responsive synthetic hydrogels. Adv. Mater. 15, 888–892.

Maguire, T., Novik, E., Schloss, R., Yarmush, M., 2006. Alginate-PLL microencapsulation: effect on the differentiation of embryonic stem cells into hepatocytes. Biotechnol. Bioeng. 93, 581–591.

Mann, B.K., Gobin, A.S., Tsai, A.T., Schmedlen, R.H., West, J.L., 2001a. Smooth muscle cell growth in photopolymerized hydrogels with cell adhesive and proteolytically degradable domains: synthetic ECM analogs for tissue engineering. Biomaterials 22, 3045–3051.

Mann, B.K., Schmedlen, R.H., West, J.L., 2001b. Tethered-TGF-beta increases extracellular matrix production of vascular smooth muscle cells. Biomaterials 22, 439–444.

Mann, B.K., West, J.L., 2002. Cell adhesion peptides alter smooth muscle cell adhesion, proliferation, migration, and matrix protein synthesis on modified surfaces and in polymer scaffolds. J. Biomed. Mater. Res. 60, 86–93.

Martens, P.J., Bryant, S.J., Anseth, K.S., 2003. Tailoring the degradation of hydrogels formed from multivinyl poly(ethylene glycol) and poly(vinyl alcohol) macromers for cartilage tissue engineering. Biomacromolecules 4, 283–292.

Mason, B.N., Starchenko, A., Williams, R.M., Bonassar, L.J., Reinhart-King, C.A., 2013. Tuning three-dimensional collagen matrix stiffness independently of collagen concentration modulates endothelial cell behavior. Acta Biomater. 9, 4635–4644.

McCall, J.D., Anseth, K.S., 2012. Thiol-ene photopolymerizations provide a facile method to encapsulate proteins and maintain their bioactivity. Biomacromolecules 13, 2410–2417.

McCall, J.D., Luoma, J.E., Anseth, K.S., 2012. Covalently tethered transforming growth factor beta in PEG hydrogels promotes chondrogenic differentiation of encapsulated human mesenchymal stem cells. Drug Deliv. Transl. Res. 2, 305–312.

McGann, C.L., Levenson, E.A., Kiick, K.L., 2013. Resilin-based hybrid hydrogels for cardiovascular tissue engineering. Macromolecules 214, 203–213.

McKinnon, D.D., Domaille, D.W., Cha, J.N., Anseth, K.S., 2014. Biophysically defined and cytocompatible covalently adaptable networks as viscoelastic 3D cell culture systems. Adv. Mater. 26, 865–872.

Melloni, C., Alexander, K.P., Chen, A.Y., Newby, L.K., Roe, M.T., Allen Lapointe, N.M., Pollack Jr., C.V., Gibler, W.B., Ohman, E.M., Peterson, E.D., Investigators, C., 2008. Unfractionated heparin dosing and risk of major bleeding in non-ST-segment elevation acute coronary syndromes. Am. Heart J. 156, 209–215.

Merrill, E.W., Salzman, E.W., Wan, S., Mahmud, N., Kushner, L., Lindon, J.N., Curme, J., 1982. Platelet-compatible hydrophilic segmented polyurethanes from polyethylene glycols and cyclohexane diisocyanate. Trans. Am. Soc. Artif. Intern. Organs 28, 482–487.

Mi, F.L., Kuan, C.Y., Shyu, S.S., Lee, S.T., Chang, S.F., 2000. The study of gelation kinetics and chain-relaxation properties of glutaraldehyde-cross-linked chitosan gel and their effects on microspheres preparation and drug release. Carbohydr. Polym. 41, 389–396.

Mortisen, D., Peroglio, M., Alini, M., Eglin, D., 2010. Tailoring thermoreversible hyaluronan hydrogels by "click" chemistry and RAFT polymerization for cell and drug therapy. Biomacromolecules 11, 1261–1272.

Mosesson, M.W., 2005. Fibrinogen and fibrin structure and functions. J. Thromb. Haemost. 3, 1894–1904.

Motta, A., Barbato, B., Foss, C., Torricelli, P., Migliaresi, C., 2011. Stabilization of *Bombyx mori* silk fibroin/sericin films by crosslinking with PEG-DE 600 and genipin. J. Bioact. Compat. Polym. 26, 130–143.

Nagai, N., Murao, T., Ito, Y., Okamoto, N., Sasaki, M., 2009. Enhancing effects of sericin on corneal wound healing in rat debrided corneal epithelium. Biol. Pharm. Bull. 32, 933–936.

Neumann, A.J., Schroeder, J., Alini, M., Archer, C.W., Stoddart, M.J., 2013. Enhanced adenovirus transduction of hMSCs using 3D hydrogel cell carriers. Mol. Biotechnol. 53, 207–216.

Nilasaroya, A., Poole-Warren, L.A., Whitelock, J.M., Martens, P.J., 2008. Structural and functional characterisation of poly(vinyl alcohol) and heparin hydrogels. Biomaterials 29, 4658–4664.

Noble, P.W., 2002. Hyaluronan and its catabolic products in tissue injury and repair. Matrix Biol. 21, 25–29.

Normand, V., Lootens, D.L., Amici, E., Plucknett, K.P., Aymard, P., 2000. New insight into agarose gel mechanical properties. Biomacromolecules 1, 730–738.

Novosel, E.C., Kleinhans, C., Kluger, P.J., 2011. Vascularization is the key challenge in tissue engineering. Adv. Drug Deliv. Rev. 63, 300–311.

Nuttelman, C.R., Mortisen, D.J., Henry, S.M., Anseth, K.S., 2001. Attachment of fibronectin to poly(vinyl alcohol) hydrogels promotes NIH3T3 cell adhesion, proliferation, and migration. J. Biomed. Mater. Res. 57, 217–223.

Nuttelman, C.R., Rice, M.A., Rydholm, A.E., Salinas, C.N., Shah, D.N., Anseth, K.S., 2008. Macromolecular monomers for the synthesis of hydrogel niches and their application in cell encapsulation and tissue engineering. Prog. Polym. Sci. 33, 167–179.

Ossipov, D.A., Brannvall, K., Forsberg-Nilsson, K., Hilborn, J., 2007. Formation of the first injectable poly(vinyl alcohol) hydrogel by mixing of functional PVA precursors. J. Appl. Polym. Sci. 106, 60–70.

Park, H., Temenoff, J.S., Tabata, Y., Caplan, A.I., Mikos, A.G., 2007. Injectable biodegradable hydrogel composites for rabbit marrow mesenchymal stem cell and growth factor delivery for cartilage tissue engineering. Biomaterials 28, 3217–3227.

Pashuck, E.T., Cui, H.G., Stupp, S.I., 2010. Tuning supramolecular rigidity of peptide fibers through molecular structure. J. Am. Chem. Soc. 132, 6041–6046.

Paterson, S.M., Shadforth, A.M.A., Brown, D.H., Madden, P.W., Chirila, T.V., Baker, M.V., 2012. The synthesis and degradation of collagenase-degradable poly(2-hydroxyethyl methacrylate)-based hydrogels and sponges for potential applications as scaffolds in tissue engineering. Mater. Sci. Eng. C Mater. Biol. Appl. 32, 2536–2544.

Peppas, N.A., Hilt, J.Z., Khademhosseini, A., Langer, R., 2006. Hydrogels in biology and medicine: from molecular principles to bionanotechnology. Adv. Mater. 18, 1345–1360.

Peroglio, M., Eglin, D., Benneker, L.M., Alini, M., Grad, S., 2013. Thermoreversible hyaluronan-based hydrogel supports in vitro and ex vivo disc-like differentiation of human mesenchymal stem cells. Spine J. 13, 1627–1639.

Peyton, S.R., Kim, P.D., Ghajar, C.M., Seliktar, D., Putnam, A.J., 2008. The effects of matrix stiffness and RhoA on the phenotypic plasticity of smooth muscle cells in a 3-D biosynthetic hydrogel system. Biomaterials 29, 2597–2607.

Phelps, E.A., Enemchukwu, N.O., Fiore, V.F., Sy, J.C., Murthy, N., Sulchek, T.A., Barker, T.H., Garcia, A.J., 2012. Maleimide cross-linked bioactive PEG hydrogel exhibits improved reaction kinetics and cross-linking for cell encapsulation and in situ delivery. Adv. Mater. 24, 64–70, 2.

Qiu, Y., Lim, J.J., Scott Jr., L., Adams, R.C., Bui, H.T., Temenoff, J.S., 2011. PEG-based hydrogels with tunable degradation characteristics to control delivery of marrow stromal cells for tendon overuse injuries. Acta Biomater. 7, 959–966.

Qiu, Y., Park, K., 2001. Environment-sensitive hydrogels for drug delivery. Adv. Drug Deliv. Rev. 53, 321–339.

Raeber, G.P., Lutolf, M.P., Hubbell, J.A., 2007. Mechanisms of 3-D migration and matrix remodeling of fibroblasts within artificial ECMs. Acta Biomater. 3, 615–629.

Rault, I., Frei, V., Herbage, D., Abdulmalak, N., Huc, A., 1996. Evaluation of different chemical methods for cross-linking collagen gel, films and sponges. J. Mater. Sci. Mater. Med. 7, 215–221.

Read, T.A., Sorensen, D.R., Mahesparan, R., Enger, P.O., Timpl, R., Olsen, B.R., Hjelstuen, M.H., Haraldseth, O., Bjerkvig, R., 2001. Local endostatin treatment of gliomas administered by microencapsulated producer cells. Nat. Biotechnol. 19, 29–34.

Rennerfeldt, D.A., Renth, A.N., Talata, Z., Gehrke, S.H., Detamore, M.S., 2013. Tuning mechanical performance of poly(ethylene glycol) and agarose interpenetrating network hydrogels for cartilage tissue engineering. Biomaterials 34, 8241–8257.

Rice, M.A., Anseth, K.S., 2007. Controlling cartilaginous matrix evolution in hydrogels with degradation triggered by exogenous addition of an enzyme. Tissue Eng. 13, 683–691.

Roberts, J.J., Bryant, S.J., 2013. Comparison of photopolymerizable thiol-ene PEG and acrylate-based PEG hydrogels for cartilage development. Biomaterials 34, 9969–9979.

Roberts, J.J., Elder, R.M., Neumann, A.J., Jayaraman, A., Bryant, S.J., 2014. Interaction of hyaluronan binding peptides with glycosaminoglycans in poly(ethylene glycol) hydrogels. Biomacromolecules 15, 1132–1141.

Roberts, J.J., Nicodemus, G.D., Giunta, S., Bryant, S.J., 2011a. Incorporation of biomimetic matrix molecules in PEG hydrogels enhances matrix deposition and reduces load-induced loss of chondrocyte-secreted matrix. J. Biomed. Mater. Res. A 97, 281–291.

Roberts, J.J., Nicodemus, G.D., Greenwald, E.C., Bryant, S.J., 2011b. Degradation improves tissue formation in (un)loaded chondrocyte-laden hydrogels. Clin. Orthop. Relat. Res. 469, 2725–2734.

Rowe, S.L., Lee, S., Stegemann, J.P., 2007. Influence of thrombin concentration on the mechanical and morphological properties of cell-seeded fibrin hydrogels. Acta Biomater. 3, 59–67.

Ruel-Gariepy, E., Leroux, J.C., 2004. In situ-forming hydrogels - review of temperature-sensitive systems. Eur. J. Pharm. Biopharm. 58, 409–426.

Sahoo, S., Chung, C., Khetan, S., Burdick, J.A., 2008. Hydrolytically degradable hyaluronic acid hydrogels with controlled temporal structures. Biomacromolecules 9, 1088–1092.

Salasznyk, R.M., Williams, W.A., Boskey, A., Batorsky, A., Plopper, G.E., 2004. Adhesion to vitronectin and collagen I promotes osteogenic differentiation of human mesenchymal stem cells. J. Biomed. Biotechnol. 2004, 24–34.

Santos, J.R., Alves, N.M., Mano, J.F., 2010. New thermo-responsive hydrogels based on poly (*N*-isopropylacrylamide)/hyaluronic acid semi-interpenetrated polymer networks: swelling properties and drug release studies. J. Bioact. Compat. Polym. 25, 169–184.
Schmedlen, R.H., Masters, K.S., West, J.L., 2002. Photocrosslinkable polyvinyl alcohol hydrogels that can be modified with cell adhesion peptides for use in tissue engineering. Biomaterials 23, 4325–4332.
Scott, J.E., 1995. Extracellular matrix, supramolecular organisation and shape. J. Anat. 187 (Pt 2), 259–269.
Scotti, C., Mangiavini, L., Boschetti, F., Vitari, F., Domeneghini, C., Fraschini, G., Peretti, G.M., 2010. Effect of in vitro culture on a chondrocyte-fibrin glue hydrogel for cartilage repair. Knee Surg. Sports Traumatol. Arthrosc. 18, 1400–1406.
Seliktar, D., Black, R.A., Vito, R.P., Nerem, R.M., 2000. Dynamic mechanical conditioning of collagen-gel blood vessel constructs induces remodeling in vitro. Ann. Biomed. Eng. 28, 351–362.
Seto, S.P., Casas, M.E., Temenoff, J.S., 2012. Differentiation of mesenchymal stem cells in heparin-containing hydrogels via coculture with osteoblasts. Cell Tissue Res. 347, 589–601.
Sharma, N.S., Nagrath, D., Yarmush, M.L., 2010. Adipocyte-derived basement membrane extract with biological activity: applications in hepatocyte functional augmentation in vitro. FASEB J. 24, 2364–2374.
Shu, X.Z., Ahmad, S., Liu, Y., Prestwich, G.D., 2006. Synthesis and evaluation of injectable, in situ crosslinkable synthetic extracellular matrices for tissue engineering. J. Biomed. Mater. Res. A 79, 902–912.
Smidsrod, O., Skjak-Braek, G., 1990. Alginate as immobilization matrix for cells. Trends Biotechnol. 8, 71–78.
Soppimath, K.S., Aminabhavi, T.M., Dave, A.M., Kumbar, S.G., Rudzinski, W.E., 2002. Stimulus-responsive "smart" hydrogels as novel drug delivery systems. Drug Dev. Ind. Pharm. 28, 957–974.
Steinmetz, N.J., Bryant, S.J., 2012. Chondroitin sulfate and dynamic loading alter chondrogenesis of human MSCs in PEG hydrogels. Biotechnol. Bioeng. 109, 2671–2682.
Suggs, L.J., Mikos, A.G., 1999. Development of poly(propylene fumarate-co-ethylene glycol) as an injectable carrier for endothelial cells. Cell Transplant. 8, 345–350.
Suh, J.K., Matthew, H.W., 2000. Application of chitosan-based polysaccharide biomaterials in cartilage tissue engineering: a review. Biomaterials 21, 2589–2598.
Sun, G., Mao, J.J., 2012. Engineering dextran-based scaffolds for drug delivery and tissue repair. Nanomed. (Lond.) 7, 1771–1784.
Sun, G., Zhang, X., Shen, Y.I., Sebastian, R., Dickinson, L.E., Fox-Talbot, K., Reinblatt, M., Steenbergen, C., Harmon, J.W., Gerecht, S., 2011. Dextran hydrogel scaffolds enhance angiogenic responses and promote complete skin regeneration during burn wound healing. Proc. Natl. Acad. Sci. U.S.A. 108, 20976–20981.
Tae, G., Kim, Y.J., Choi, W.I., Kim, M., Stayton, P.S., Hoffman, A.S., 2007. Formation of a novel heparin-based hydrogel in the presence of heparin-binding biomolecules. Biomacromolecules 8, 1979–1986.
Temenoff, J.S., Shin, H., Conway, D.E., Engel, P.S., Mikos, A.G., 2003. In vitro cytotoxicity of redox radical initiators for cross-linking of oligo(poly(ethylene glycol) fumarate) macromers. Biomacromolecules 4, 1605–1613.
Theocharis, A.D., Skandalis, S.S., Tzanakakis, G.N., Karamanos, N.K., 2010. Proteoglycans in health and disease: novel roles for proteoglycans in malignancy and their pharmacological targeting. FEBS J. 277, 3904–3923.

Toole, B.P., 2004. Hyaluronan: from extracellular glue to pericellular cue. Nat. Rev. Cancer 4, 528–539.

Trappmann, B., Chen, C.S., 2013. How cells sense extracellular matrix stiffness: a material's perspective. Curr. Opin. Biotechnol. 24, 948–953.

Trappmann, B., Gautrot, J.E., Connelly, J.T., Strange, D.G., Li, Y., Oyen, M.L., Cohen Stuart, M.A., Boehm, H., Li, B., Vogel, V., Spatz, J.P., Watt, F.M., Huck, W.T., 2012. Extracellular-matrix tethering regulates stem-cell fate. Nat. Mater. 11, 642–649.

Uludag, H., Sefton, M.V., 1993. Metabolic activity and proliferation of CHO cells in hydroxyethyl methacrylate-methyl methacrylate (HEMA-MMA) microcapsules. Cell Transplant. 2, 175–182.

Um, S.H., Lee, J.B., Park, N., Kwon, S.Y., Umbach, C.C., Luo, D., 2006. Enzyme-catalysed assembly of DNA hydrogel. Nat. Mater. 5, 797–801.

Unterman, S.A., Gibson, M., Lee, J.H., Crist, J., Chansakul, T., Yang, E.C., Elisseeff, J.H., 2012. Hyaluronic acid-binding scaffold for articular cartilage repair. Tissue Eng. Part A 18, 2497–2506.

VanWinkle, W.B., Snuggs, M.B., Buja, L.M., 1996. Cardiogel: a biosynthetic extracellular matrix for cardiomyocyte culture. In Vitro Cell Dev. Biol. Anim. 32, 478–485.

Vunjak-Novakovic, G., Obradovic, B., Martin, I., Bursac, P.M., Langer, R., Freed, L.E., 1998. Dynamic cell seeding of polymer scaffolds for cartilage tissue engineering. Biotechnol. Prog. 14, 193–202.

Weber, L.M., Anseth, K.S., 2008. Hydrogel encapsulation environments functionalized with extracellular matrix interactions increase islet insulin secretion. Matrix Biol. 27, 667–673.

Weiss, M.S., Bernabe, B.P., Shikanov, A., Bluver, D.A., Mui, M.D., Shin, S.J., Broadbelt, L.J., Shea, L.D., 2012. The impact of adhesion peptides within hydrogels on the phenotype and signaling of normal and cancerous mammary epithelial cells. Biomaterials 33, 3548–3559.

Weyers, A., Linhardt, R.J., 2013. Neoproteoglycans in tissue engineering. FEBS J. 280, 2511–2522.

Wieduwild, R., Tsurkan, M., Chwalek, K., Murawala, P., Nowak, M., Freudenberg, U., Neinhuis, C., Werner, C., Zhang, Y., 2013. Minimal peptide motif for non-covalent peptide-heparin hydrogels. J. Am. Chem. Soc. 135, 2919–2922.

Xiong, J.Y., Narayanan, J., Liu, X.Y., Chong, T.K., Chen, S.B., Chung, T.S., 2005. Topology evolution and gelation mechanism of agarose gel. J. Phys. Chem. B 109, 5638–5643.

Yannas, I.V., Burke, J.F., 1980. Design of an artificial skin. I. Basic design principles. J. Biomed. Mater. Res. 14, 65–81.

Young, C.J., Poole-Warren, L.A., Martens, P.J., 2012. Combining submerged electrospray and UV photopolymerization for production of synthetic hydrogel microspheres for cell encapsulation. Biotechnol. Bioeng. 109, 1561–1570.

Yu, J., Du, K.T., Fang, Q., Gu, Y., Mihardja, S.S., Sievers, R.E., Wu, J.C., Lee, R.J., 2010. The use of human mesenchymal stem cells encapsulated in RGD modified alginate microspheres in the repair of myocardial infarction in the rat. Biomaterials 31, 7012–7020.

Yu, S.M., Li, Y., Kim, D., 2011. Collagen mimetic peptides: progress towards functional applications. Soft Matter 7, 7927–7938.

Zhang, W.J., Laue, C., Hyder, A., Schrezenmeir, J., 2001. Purity of alginate affects the viability and fibrotic overgrowth of encapsulated porcine islet xenografts. Transplant. Proc. 33, 3517–3519.

Zhang, X.Z., Xu, X.D., Cheng, S.X., Zhuo, R.X., 2008. Strategies to improve the response rate of thermosensitive PNIPAAm hydrogels. Soft Matter 4, 385–391.

Zhang, Y., Zhang, M.Q., 2001. Synthesis and characterization of macroporous chitosan/calcium phosphate composite scaffolds for tissue engineering. J. Biomed. Mater. Res. 55, 304−312.

Zhao, L., Zhu, L., Liu, F., Liu, C., Shan, D., Wang, Q., Zhang, C., Li, J., Liu, J., Qu, X., Yang, Z., 2011. pH triggered injectable amphiphilic hydrogel containing doxorubicin and paclitaxel. Int. J. Pharm. 410, 83−91.

Zhu, J., 2010. Bioactive modification of poly(ethylene glycol) hydrogels for tissue engineering. Biomaterials 31, 4639−4656.

Zhu, J., Marchant, R.E., 2011. Design properties of hydrogel tissue-engineering scaffolds. Expert Rev. Med. Devices 8, 607−626.

Part Four

Conjugated conducting polymers

Conducting polymers and their biomedical applications

10

N. Yi[1], M.R. Abidian[2]
[1]Pennsylvania State University, PA, USA; [2]Biomedical Engineering Department, University of Houston, Houston, TX, USA

10.1 Introduction

10.1.1 History

Polymers are typically used as insulators. Wires are coated with plastics, and switches are made of plastics for insulation purpose. But in fact, not all polymers are insulators. They can be conductive just like metals. The first conducting polymer, poly(sulphur nitride), was discovered by Greene and Street in 1975 [1]. They found that poly(sulphur nitride) was electronically conductive at a low temperature and that a super conduction transition occurs at a temperature of 0.26 K [2]. In latter studies, chemist Alan MacDiarmid and physicist Alan Heeger collaborated to examine the electrical properties of poly(sulphur nitride). At this time, Hideki Shirikawa was focusing on the Ziegler-Natta-catalyzed polymerisation of acetylene and found that when the concentration of catalyst was near to molar, shiny film would appear on the surface of the reaction vessel [1]. This type of 'metallic' polymer attracted MacDiarmid Heeger and Shirikawa to collaborate on poly(acetylene). Acceptors and donors were doped on poly(acetylene) and the conductivity and structure of this polymer were examined [1]. After their discoveries on the doping of poly(acetylene) in 1977, more researchers have been interested in conducting polymers. In less than one decade, most of the monomers that researchers currently use to produce conducting polymers were found. In 2000, the Nobel Prize was awarded to Heeger, MacDiarmid and Shirakawa for their contribution in the discovery and development of conducting polymers.

10.1.2 Why conducting polymers attract researchers

Polymers, either natural or synthetic, are widely applied in daily life due to their good processability, thermal stability, various optical and mechanical properties, and relative low cost fabrication [3]. Polymers can be shaped into more complicated structures than other materials such as metals and ceramics. However, most of these applications were non-electronic prior to the discovery of conducting polymers. Since then, scientists from different disciplines have rushed into this field and boosted the development of conducting polymers. What attracts researchers to this polymer is that conducting polymers have a wide range of electrical conductivity like metals while they maintain their polymeric mechanical properties at the same time. Investigators can control the

Biosynthetic Polymers for Medical Applications. http://dx.doi.org/10.1016/B978-1-78242-105-4.00010-9

doping level of conducting polymer and use different counter-ions (dopants) to modify the conductivity [4]. In addition, conductivity of conducting polymers is not only determined by the type of monomers and dopants but also determined by the conditions under which the polymers are fabricated [5].

10.2 Conducting mechanism

The alternating single- and double-bond structure (conjugated backbone) can be electronically conductive because the carbon atoms on the polymer backbone are sp^2 hybridised. The *p* orbitals of carbon atoms in the *z* direction are parallel to each other and therefore can form a continuous π bond, which can be a pathway for the charge carriers to move along the polymer chain [6]. A conducting polymer is not conductive if there are no charge carriers within the polymer structure. Most organic conjugated polymers do not have intrinsic charge carriers. Therefore, external charge carriers should be introduced to the polymers to make them conductive. Conducting polymers can be either partially oxidised by electron acceptors or partially reduced by electron donors [6]. The process by which charge carriers are introduced into a conducting polymer is called the doping process. Band theory is applied for conducting polymers to explain the change of electronic structure during the doping process. Usually band theory is used to describe the electronic structure of inorganic semiconductors. The lowest empty band is called the conduction band, the highest occupied band is called the valence band and the energy difference between them is called the band gap. Insulators have a large band gap and semiconductors have a relatively small band gap. As for metals, partially filled bands exist, and there is no band gap between the conduction band and valence band; thus metals are more conductive. When a conducting polymer is doped with a dopant, either the conduction band or valence band is partially filled or polarons are created during this process [7].

Molecular orbital theory can be applied to support the band theory. One *p* orbital from one carbon atom and another *p* orbital from another carbon atom can form two new molecular orbitals. One of the newly formed orbitals has a lower energy than the original *p* orbital and the other has a higher energy than the original *p* orbital. The lower-energy orbital is called the bonding molecular orbital. The orbital that has a higher energy is called the anti-bonding molecular orbital. Since electrons in the bonding molecular orbital are more stable, two electrons from two carbon atoms fill the bonding molecular orbital. These two electrons share the same orbital and form the π bond. (The π bond is part of the carbon–carbon double bond. The double bond contains one σ bond and one π bond.) In this case, the bonding molecular orbital has the highest occupied molecular orbital (HOMO), and the anti-bonding molecular orbital has the lowest unoccupied molecular orbital (LUMO). The energy band of HOMO is called the valence band, and the energy band of LUMO is called the conduction band. The energy difference between HOMO and LUMO is the band gap energy, which is the energy for the activation of electrons [8]. A conducting polymer with an infinitely long polymer chain has infinite *p* orbitals and the countless molecular orbitals finally form a band between the valence band and conduction band. While the band gap disappears, electrons are able to transit from one state in that band to another state with less activation energy, and eventually the polymer becomes metallic.

10.3 Electrochemical polymerisation of conducting polymers

Chemical methods can be used to produce conducting polymers. However, conducting polymers are synthesised in chemical routes only when a large amount of product is needed rather than a thin layer of conducting polymer film [9]. Electrochemical polymerisation can produce a thin layer of polymer, and the thickness of the film can be precisely controlled by adjusting electrochemical polymerisation parameters such as current density and time of electropolymerisation [10,11]. The polymerisation reaction is often an oxidative reaction [10,12,13], but reduction reactions may also be used [14] for electrochemical polymerisation, several factors should be considered (e.g. the choice of electrolyte and applied current versus applied voltage). These factors have a significant influence on electrical and physical properties of conducting polymers [10,11].

10.3.1 Polyaniline

Polyaniline (PANI) is a common conducting polymer. PANI has some advantages over other type of conducting polymers, such as its ease of synthesis, cheap monomers, tunable properties, high capacitance values and better chemical stability [15]. Thermal degradation of PANI doped with different counter-ions always occurs when the temperature is higher than 200 °C [16]. PANI is less noble than silver but more noble than copper, which makes it broadly used in printed circuit board manufacturing and corrosion protection [17]. Electrical conductivity of PANI ranges from 10 to 100 S/cm [18]. This conductivity is controlled by molecular weight, oxidation level, percentage of crystallinity and degree of doping. As shown in Figure 10.1, there are two different monomers of PANI. The monomer unit on the left side is a result of oxidation of the monomer unit on the right hand side. PANI can either be oxidised and transfer all its monomers to the deprotonated form, or be reduced to the protonated form [8]. Figure 10.2 demonstrates the different oxidisation states of PANI. Several

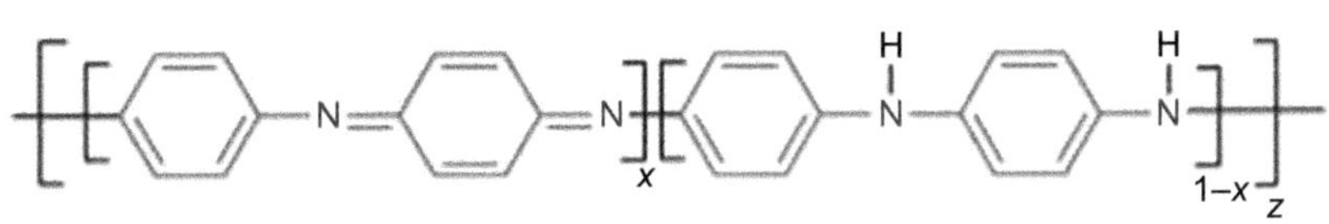

Figure 10.1 Chemical formula of PANI.
Reproduced with permission from Ref. [87].

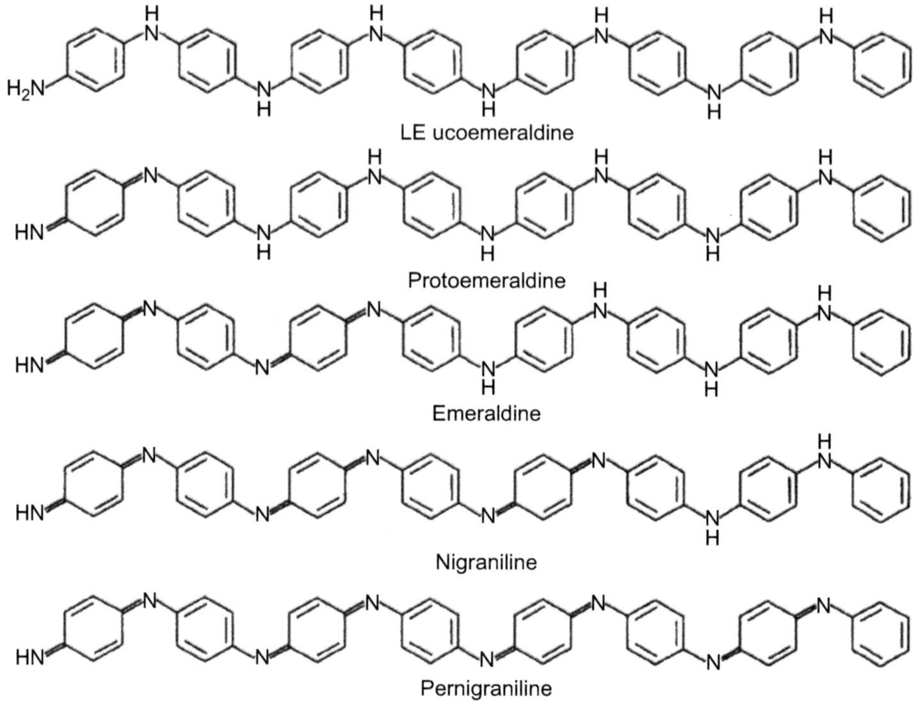

Figure 10.2 Different oxidation states of PANI.
Reproduced with permission from Ref. [19].

methods have been proposed by researchers for synthesising PANI [13]. Different polymerisation mechanisms have been proposed due to different synthesis conditions.

10.3.1.1 Electrochemical polymerisation mechanism

There are several proposed methods for synthesising PANI [13]. Here the synthesising mechanism proposed by Genies, Boyle and Lapkowski is described. In their electrochemical polymerisation process, a low oxidation potential is applied (0.7 V) and a copper electrode is used [13]. The first step of the polymerisation is the formation of a cation radical, which is a consensus among different mechanisms. Figure 10.3(a) shows the formation of a cation radical by oxidation.

Then the cation radical alters its structure. Figure 10.3(b) demonstrates the different structure of the cation radicals. The unpaired electrons can be localised at either the nitrogen atom or other carbon atoms in the benzene ring. At this time, cation radicals are concentrated near the surface of the electrode. The diffusion rate of the radical is smaller than the diffusion rate of new radicals that are created. Therefore, the radicals are more likely to react with each other rather than react with a neutral monomer. Figure 10.3(c) shows the formation of a precursor of a dimer. This new structure can undergo a deprotonation process and forms an intermediate product of the

(a) (b) (c) (d) (e) (f) (g)

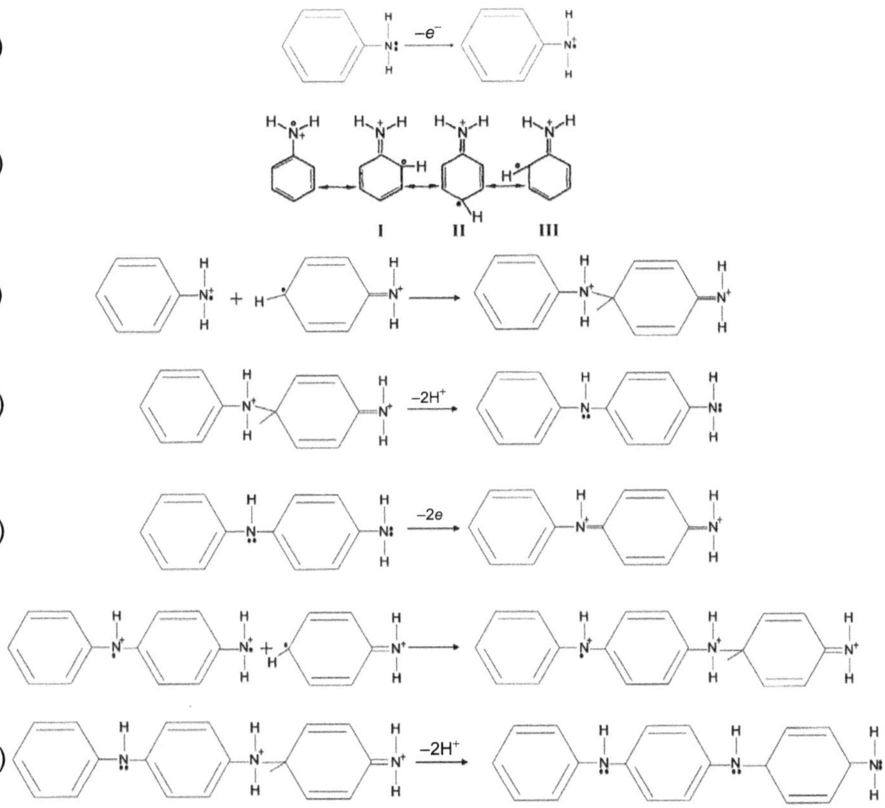

Figure 10.3 (a) Formation of cation radical. (b) Different form of aniline cation radical. (c) Dimerisation of aniline. (d) Formation of PADPA. (e) Oxidation of PADPA. (f) Formation of a protonated trimer. (g) Deprotonation of a trimer.
Reproduced with permission from Ref. [13].

polymerisation of PANI called *p*-aminodiphenylamine (PADPA). Since the oxidation potential for PADPA is lower than that for an aniline monomer, it is easier to oxidise the dimer and continue the cation radical reaction. Thus, the oxidation of the aniline monomer is the key reaction and affects the total reaction rate of polymerisation [13]. Figure 10.3(d) demonstrates the formation of PADPA by deprotonation. Then the PADPA can be oxidised and become another cation radical (Figure 10.3(e)). The oxidised PADPA should continue reacting with an aniline monomer cation radical to extend the polymer chain (Figure 10.3(f)). By deprotonation, a trimer is formed (Figure 10.3(g)). By repeating this oxidation-addition-deprotonation cycle, the aniline monomers are added to the chain and finally the PANI is produced. This is one of the possible electrochemical polymerisation mechanisms. When the polymerisation conditions are changed, some other reactions may occur. For example, if the formed cation radicals diffuse more quickly, the radicals may find several neutral aniline monomers. Then the radicals react with the neutral monomers. In some other conditions, neutral aniline monomers can react with the radical on the chain by nucleophilic addition. Sometimes the monomer radicals can react with the neutral polymer chain through electrophilic addition [13].

PANI is always prepared in an acidic environment because side products are generated during the electrochemical polymerisation if the pH value is too high. The final product has a lower electrical conductivity if the PANI is polymerised in a basic, neutral or weak acidic environment [12]. Galvanostatic, potentiostatic and potential scanning methods are used to electrochemically polymerise PANI [19]. It has been reported that passing a constant current with a density of 1 mA/cm^2 leads to deposition of PANI on a platinum electrode. However, applying a constant potential, powders of PANI can be formed, which will poorly adhere to the electrode surface. When the potential is swept between predetermined potentials, a PANI film is deposited, which strongly adheres to electrodes [19]. Several dopants (i.e. counter-ions) have been used for polymerisation of PANI, including F^- [20], Cl^- [21], ClO_4^- [22], SO_4^{2-} [23] and BF_4^- [24].

10.3.2 Polypyrrole

Polypyrrole (PPy) is of particular interest due to its high conductivity and stability in oxidised states. PPy has some advantages over other conducting polymers, such as easier oxidation reaction, more water solubility and low-cost process. However, compared to PANI, the cost of pyrrole monomers is greater than aniline, which makes it less attractive for some potential applications [25]. PPy's colour is a result of the degree of oxidation, changing from yellow to blue and finally to black as the oxidation degree increases [26]. The chemical stability of oxidised PPy is very good at room temperature. PPy degradation only happens when the temperature is greater than 150–300 °C [26]. Electrical conductivity of PPy ranges from 10 to 1000 S/cm [18] depending on the counter-ions. Electropolymerised PPy can be well adhered to the electrode when the thickness of PPy film is less than 10 μm [26]. However, when the thickness is larger than 10 μm, the PPy film can be easily peeled off [27].

10.3.2.1 Electrochemical polymerisation mechanism

Researchers have investigated the polymerisation mechanism of PPy. Since the polymerisation process happens quickly, it is difficult to investigate this process stage by stage. Different models have been proposed to explain the mechanism of PPy polymerisation [10]. However, there is no consensus on which mechanism is correct. The Diaz mechanism is the most frequently used mechanism by researchers [28]. Similar to the polymerisation mechanism of PANI, the first step is the oxidation of the pyrrole monomers. When the polymerisation begins, the monomers near the electrode are oxidised. Figure 10.4 shows the oxidation reaction of pyrrole monomers. After the pyrrole monomer is oxidised, the cation radical form several different structures because the unpaired electrons are not localised at the nitrogen atom but localised at the carbon atoms in the ring. Figure 10.4(b)

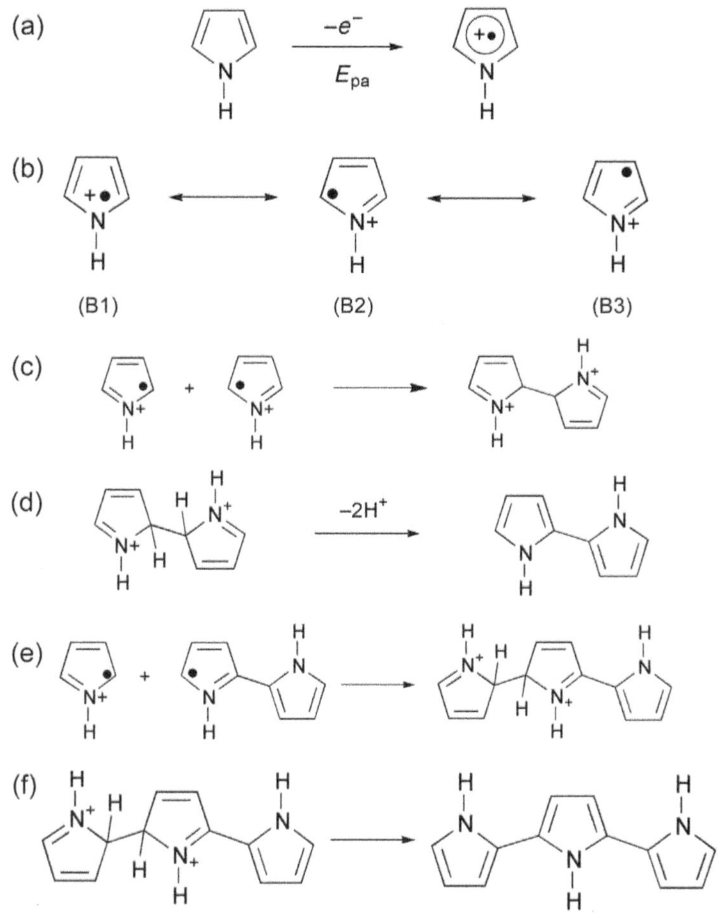

Figure 10.4 (a) Oxidation of pyrrole monomer. (b) Pyrrole cation radicals. (c) The combination of two pyrrole cation radicals. (d) Deprotonation of the dimer. (e) Formation of a pyrrole trimer. (f) Deprotonation of pyrrole trimer.
Reproduced with permission from Ref. [10].

shows the different forms of the pyrrole cation radical. The pyrrole cation radicals in the form B2 have the unpaired electrons in the α-position, which has the lowest total energy. Thus, the pyrrole cation radicals in form B2 are more commonly observed. Then according to the Diaz mechanism, two cation radicals bond with each other by the combination of the two unpaired electron in the α-position (Figure 10.4(c)). This is called α-position coupling. There are two hydrogen atoms bonded to the α-position carbons. The hydrogen atoms can be removed by the deprotonation process (Figure 10.4(d)).

The deprotonated dimer can be further oxidised and forms another cation radical. Again, the oxidised dimer has a unique structure due to the different position that the unpaired electron can occupy. Most of the dimers usually have the electrons localised at the α-position. The oxidised dimer should react with the monomer cation to form a trimer (Figure 10.4(e)). Deprotonation happens after the trimer is formed (Figure 10.4(f)). By repeating the oxidation, addition and the deprotonation process, the polymer chain is extended. However, as the polymer chain gets longer, α-position coupling is not the only way that the monomer can be added to the polymer chain because most of the α-position carbon atoms are used to form a single bond, leaving lots of β-position unused. The probability of the unpaired electrons to localise at the β-position carbon is increased when the polymer chain become longer. As a result, the structure of the PPy chain is more irregular [10]. There are other proposed mechanisms for polymerisation of PPy that are not discussed in this chapter [29–31].

Electrochemical polymerisation of PPy can be performed either in aqueous media or non-aqueous media such as acetonitrile [32], propylene carbonate [33] and dichloromethane [26]. However, film growth is inhibited when the nucleophilicity of solvent increases due to the reaction between the solvent and the oxidation product of pyrrole monomers [26]. Potentiostatic, galvanostatic and potential scanning methods can be applied to perform electrochemical polymerisation of PPy. Corrosion-resistant materials such as Pt, Au, Pd, Rh, Ir, etc. [30,34] are used as the working electrodes. Three-electrode cells always yield PPy film with higher quality [26].

10.3.3 Polythiophene

Polythiophene (PT) has a similar structure to pyrrole, with the NH group in pyrrole substituted by S in PT. It has been reported that the electrical conductivity of PT particles prepared by chemical polymerisation is poor (2×10^{-2} S/cm) [35]. However, the electrical conductivity of electrochemical polymerised PT is comparable with PPy with a value of more than 100 S/cm [36]. Both chemical and electrochemical reduction reaction can reduce oxidised PT to neutral [36]. The electrochemical synthesis mechanism of polythiophene is demonstrated by Schopf and Koβmehl [37]. At the first step, the monomer is oxidised. The structure of thiophene is similar to the pyrrole and the synthesis mechanism is also similar to PPy. Figure 10.5 shows the polymerisation of a thiophene monomer. The unpaired electron is more likely localised at the α-position. However, as the polymer chain grows, the unpaired electrons have a higher possibility to localise at the β-position. After the cation radicals are formed during oxidation, these radicals react with each other to form a dimer (Figure 10.5(a)). Figure 10.5(b) shows the dimerisation of thiophene. By deprotonation (Figure 10.5(c)), the dimer becomes neutral. Then by repeating the process of oxidation, addition and deprotonation, the thiophene chain extends. Polythiophenes are electrochemical polymerised in non-aqueous solution. Acetonitrile [38,39], propylene carbonate [40] and benzonitrile [41] are the most-used electrolytes for polymerisation. Indium tin oxide (ITO), conducting glass [40] and platinum [38,40] are commonly used working electrodes for electrochemical polymerisation where the PT forms. Reported counter-ions for PT are BF_4^- [42], ClO_4^- [39] and $CF_3SO_3^-$ [42].

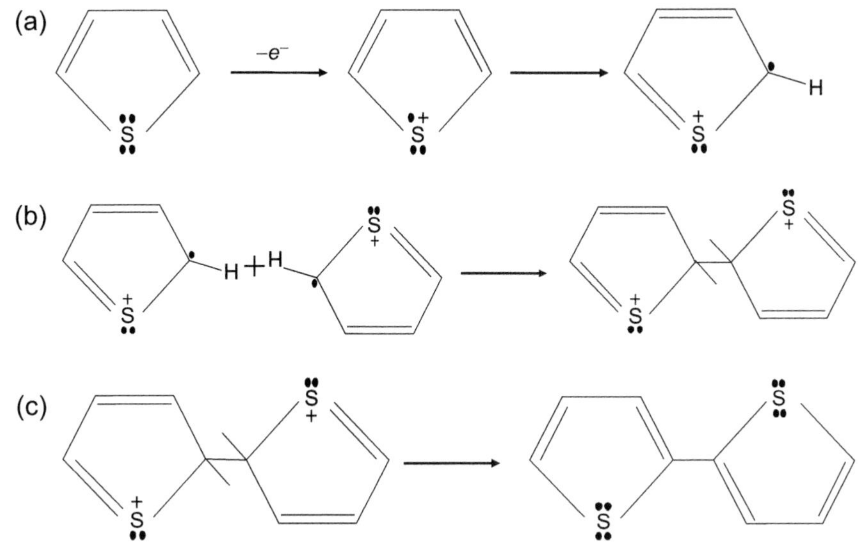

Figure 10.5 (a) Oxidation of thiophene monomer. (b) Dimerisation of thiophene. (c) Deprotonation of thiophene dimer.

10.4 Applications of conducting polymers in biomedical fields

Conducting polymers have similar electrical and optical properties as metals and semiconductors and at the same time have mechanical properties of the polymers. Conducting polymers are easy to synthesise and process. This makes conducting polymers attractive for many applications such as batteries [43], light-emitting diodes [44], antistatic coatings [45] and chemical sensors [46−50]. Conducting polymers also have several applications in biomedical fields due to their unique properties: (1) their organic nature, (2) responsiveness to electrical stimuli, (3) easy functionalisation with biomolecules and (4) ionic and electronic conductivity. Conducting polymers can be used in biosensors, neural prosthetic devices, drug delivery and actuators.

Conventional conducting polymers are stiff and friable, with typical elastic moduli on the order of 1−8 GPa [51,52]; therefore, the application of conducting polymers in biomedical fields is limited as stand-alone materials. This issue has driven the development and design of new hybrid or composite conducting polymer-based materials with softer, more robust mechanics. These include composites of conducting polymers and hydrogels [53−57], elastomers [58] and CP nanotubes with gel-like cores [47,48].

10.4.1 Biosensors

Biosensors are analytical devices used to detect specific analytes. Typically, a biosensor is composed of a biological sensing element and a transducer [11]. The biological sensing element can be enzymes, antibodies, cell receptors and DNA probes [11], which interact with a specific analyte. The transducer can be a piezoelectric, optical or physicochemical material [11] that translates the biological signals to electrical and optical signals. Biosensors can be divided into different categories depending on how the signals are translated by the transducers [11]: (1) amperometric biosensors (measure the electrical current); (2) potentiometric biosensors (measure electrical voltage); (3) conductometric biosensors (measure electrical conductance); (4) optical biosensors (measure the absorbed or emitted light) (5) calorimetric biosensors (measure the change of enthalpy) and (6) piezoelectric biosensors (detect stress). Figure 10.6 is a schematic of a biosensor.

By incorporating different biological sensing elements within the conducting polymers, the produced biosensors can detect various types of biological material. Gao et al. employed a composite of carbon nanotubes (CNTs) and PPy to fabricate biosensors for detection of glucose [59]. They used aligned CNTs as substrate materials to provide a large surface area (Figure 10.7(a)). Then, PPy was electropolymerised to coat CNTs (Figure 10.7(b)). During the polymerisation, an enzyme of glucose oxidase (biological sensing element for glucose) was mixed with the monomers and electrolyte solution. Therefore, the glucose oxidase was entrapped into the PPy. Since the glucose oxidase had good contact with the PPy film, signals could be transduced. An amperometric method was used to detect the electrical current produced during the oxidation of hydrogen peroxide, a by-product of the electrochemical reaction [59].

Abidian and co-workers recently reported another type of glucose biosensor by using different conducting polymers [60]. Poly(3,4-ethylenedioxythiophene) (PEDOT) was used in this new type of glucose biosensor due to its high chemical stability and superior conductivity [61]. PEDOT film and PEDOT nanofibre biosensors were electrochemically fabricated on platinum (Pt) neural microelectrodes. PEDOT film was directly deposited on the surface of Pt microelectrode arrays. PEDOT

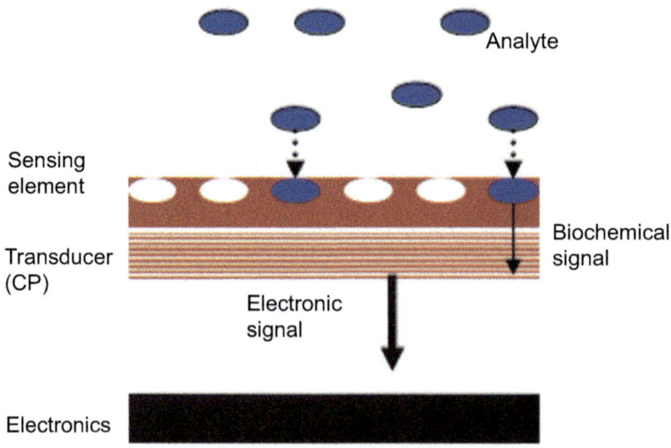

Figure 10.6 Schematic of a biosensor.
Reproduced with permission from Ref. [11].

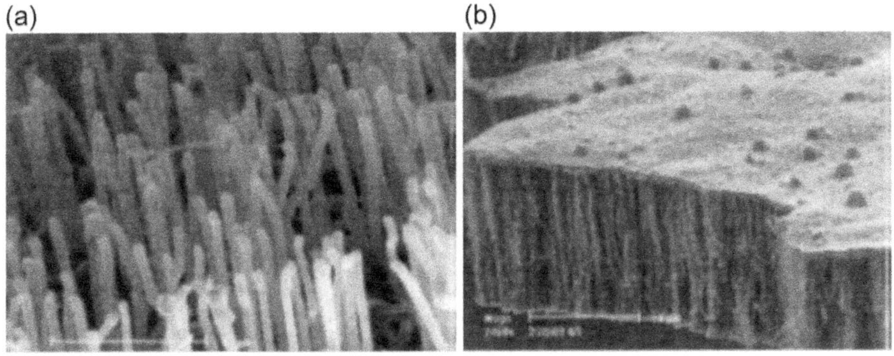

Figure 10.7 (a) Carbon nanotube array before coating. (b) Carbon nanotubes array after coating. Reproduced with permission from Ref. [59].

nanofibre biosensors were produced by electrodeposition of PEDOT on Pt microelectrodes and around electrospun nanofibres (Figure 10.8(b) and (c)) [60]. During electropolymerisation processes, glucose oxidase was immobilised into the PEDOT films and PEDOT nanofibres. The difference between the two biosensors on the amount of glucose oxidase incorporated was determined by electrochemical quartz crystal microbalance (EQCM). The sensitivity of two biosensors was determined by amperometric change in the current when an increase of glucose concentration was added to the electrolyte solution. As a result, they found that PEDOT nanofibre biosensors had more glucose oxidase incorporated within the nanofibres and had higher sensitivity in comparison with PEDOT film biosensors [60]. Figure 10.8(a) shows the current response to an injection of glucose in solution by the two different PEDOT glucose biosensors.

Gu et al. investigated polyaniline/polyacrylate modified boron-doped diamond (BDD) DNA biosensors. The polyaniline/polyacrylate thin film was coated on the surface of diamond electrodes using the electrochemical polymerisation method (Figure 10.9(a)). Carboxylic groups in polyaniline/polyacrylate were employed to immobilise the DNA-sensing probes [62]. The DNA probes could detect DNA with complementary nucleotide sequences to the probe.

Hybridisation happens when the DNA probe pairs with the target DNA sequence. Since double-strand DNA has a higher conductivity than single-strand DNA, the hybridisation of the DNA probe and target DNA could decrease the impedance of the whole diamond-conducting polymer–DNA system [62]. Therefore, they were able to detect specific DNA by measuring the change of the impedance [62]. Bode and Nyquist plots of impedance plots are shown in Figure 10.9(a) and (b).

Conducting polymer-based biosensors can also be modified by CNTs. For example, Luo et al. used CNTs to modify a PANI-based biosensor [63]. The CNTs could enhance the mechanical strength and conductivity of the PANI biosensor [64]. In this study, they demonstrated CNTs could improve the efficiency of enzyme absorption and immobilisation. Horseradish peroxidase (HRP) was incorporated into the PANI layer during electrochemical polymerisation on glassy carbon electrodes.

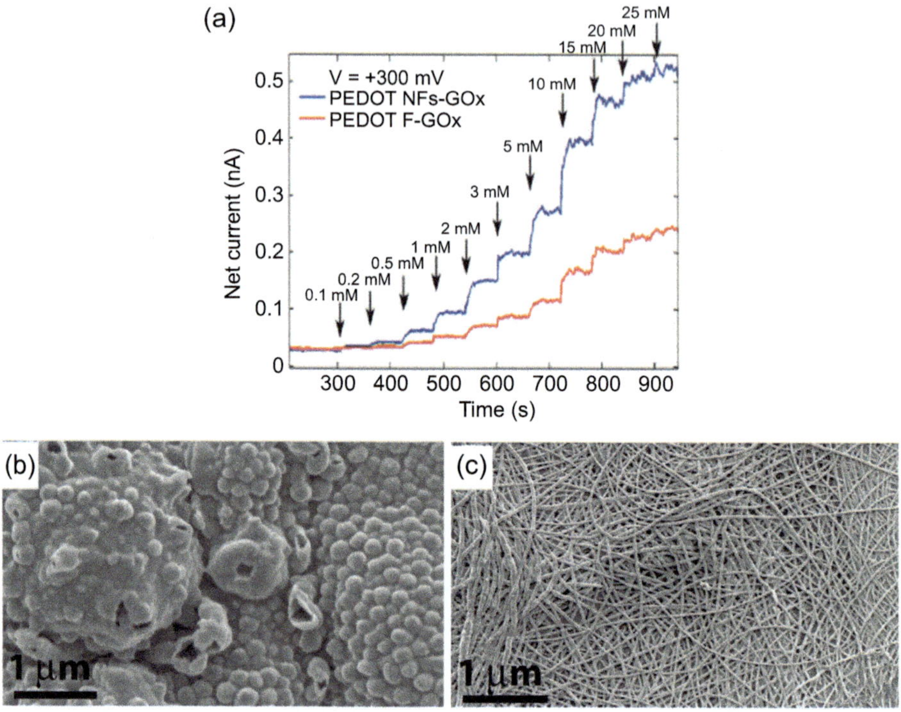

Figure 10.8 (a) Glucose biosensor response to increased glucose concentration. PEDOT nanofibre-glucose oxidase (PEDOT NFs-GOx) was the biosensor, with nanofibres electrospun on the surface of electrode. PEDOT film glucose oxidase (PEDOT F-GOx) is the glucose biosensor with PEDOT film on the surface of electrode. (b) Scanning micrograph (SEM) of PEDOT F-GOx. (c) SEM of PEDOT NFs-GOx.
Reproduced with permission from Ref. [60].

Then CNTs were added to the surface by dropping demethyl formamide with CNTs dispersed at one of the electrodes. By incorporating CNTs into the PANI electrodes, they found that CNTs increased the amount of incorporated HRP in the biosensors [63]. Then the performance of the PANI/CNTs biosensor and the PANI biosensor was compared. They found that the biosensor with CNTs had a stronger signal, presumably due to more stable attachment of HRP when CNTs were mixed with PANI [63]. Figure 10.10 shows the current-detection time relationship for PANI electrodes with and without CNTs.

10.4.2 Neural electrodes

Conducting polymers have been used for neural recording and stimulation [65] of neural prostheses such as cochlear implants and deep brain stimulators. These implantable electrodes are designed to evoke specific responses in neurons by applying electrical stimulation or alternately record neuronal electrical activity from the brain to

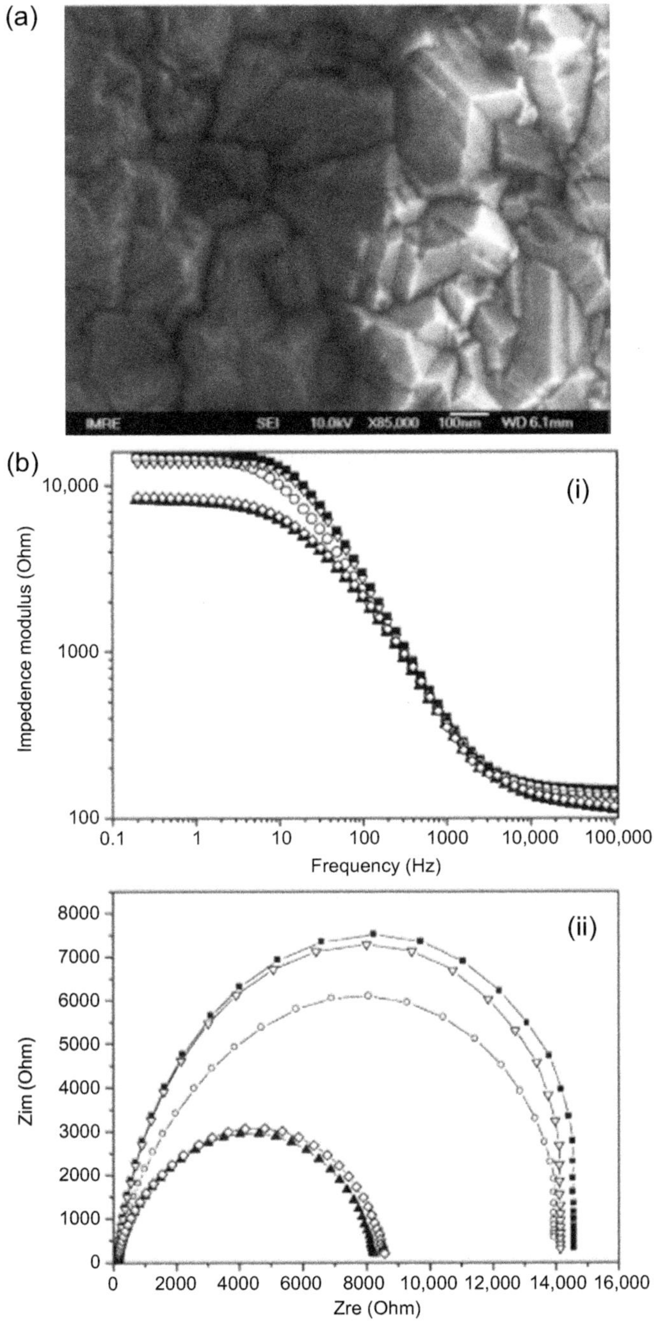

Figure 10.9 (a) Polyaniline/polyacrylate modified boron-doped diamond DNA sensor under SEM. (b) Impedance (i) Bode plot and (ii) Nyquist plot of DNA probe-immobilised, PANI/PAA-modified BDD before (■) and after hybridisation to fully complementary target (▲) or one base mismatch target (○), and after denature (∇) and renature (◇) with the fully complementary target, measured at −1.0 V open circuit potential versus Ag/AgCl. Reproduced with permission from Ref. [54].

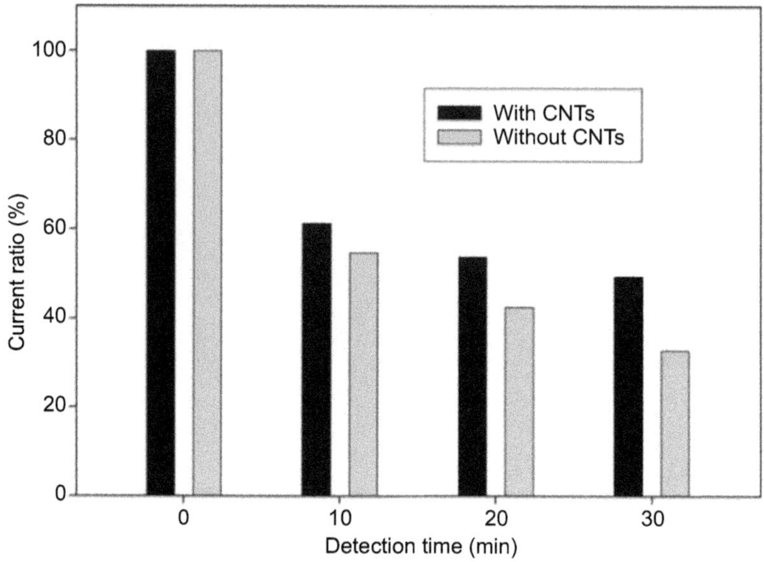

Figure 10.10 Signal of PANI HRP-based biosensors with CNTs and without CNTs. Reproduced with permission from Ref. [63].

provide diagnostics or drive external robotics. Traditional metal electrode implants have a poor long-term performance for neural stimulation and recording, presumably due to high mechanical mismatch between brain tissue and metal electrodes [65]. This results in a large amount of fibrous tissue formation at the electrode–tissue interface and reducing the signal intensity [65]. By applying conducting polymers at the electrode–tissue interface, the thickness of the fibrous tissue can be reduced. In addition, the conducting polymers can increase the effective surface, which further reduces the impedance and therefore improves the signal intensity [65].

Martin and co-workers investigated the surface-modification neural recording electrodes using PPy coatings [66]. In this research, they electrochemically deposited PPy along with silk-like polymer with fibronectin (SLPF) fragments and nanopeptides CDPGYIGSR onto gold-electrode sites of a neural probe [66]. Then rat glial cells and human neuroblastoma cells were grown separately on the neural electrode under appropriate conditions (Figure 10.11(a)). A decrease of electrode impedance and increase of charge capacity were measured after electrochemical deposition of PPy (Figure 10.11(b)). Finally, they found that glial cells could attach better on the PPy/SLPF-coated electrodes than the bare-gold electrode, and the human neuroblastoma cells could grow better on the PPy/CDPGYIGSR-coated electrode [66]. Figure 10.11(a) shows the impedance spectroscopy gold electrode coated with different PPy/SLFP and PPy/PSS. Figure 10.11(b) demonstrates the attachment of human neuroblastoma cells on different electrodes. As shown in this figure, neuroblastoma cells grow better on PPy/CDPGYIGSR-coated electrode.

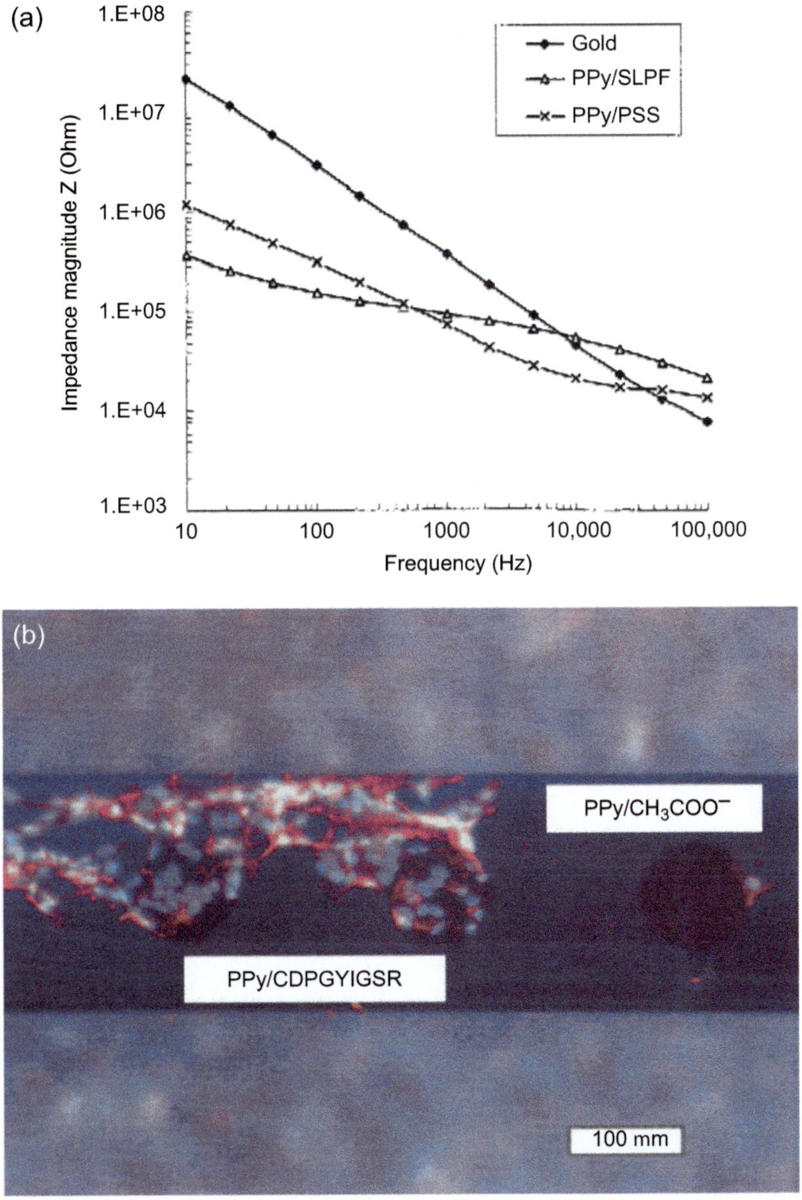

Figure 10.11 (a) Impedance of pure gold and coated electrodes. (b) Attachment of human neuroblastoma cells on electrodes coated with polypyrrole/CDPGYIGSR and polypyrrole/ CH_3COO^-.
Reproduced with permission from Ref. [66].

More recently, Green et al. examined the performance of PEDOT coatings in neuroprosthetic applications. In this research, they employed electrochemical deposition to coat paratoluene sulphonate (pTS) doped PEDOT on the surface of Pt electrode arrays and tested the physical and electrical stability of the PEDOT coating under biologically relevant environment [67]. Figure 10.12 shows the scanning electron micrographs (SEM) of different electrodes. The voltage excursion over the electrode decreased less for the coated electrode than the bare Pt electrode since the conducting polymer provided a large surface area [67] (Figure 10.13(b)). They also demonstrated that the charge injection limit of PEDOT-coated electrodes was improved (Figure 10.13(a)). The charge injection limit is the maximum amount of charge that moves out form the electrode without an irreversible chemical reaction [68]. Thus, by coating PEDOT on the Pt electrode, more charges were allowed to transfer to neural tissues without damage to the electrode. In addition, the stability of the PEDOT was better in comparison with Pt electrodes after three billion cycles of electrical stimulation [67].

Studies have shown that electrodes are more compatible with biological system when the electrical, bioactivity, softness and topography of the electrodes are similar to human tissue [69]. Martin and co-workers studied the polymerisation of conducting polymer around living neural cells (Figure 10.14) [69]. They fabricated a composite of conducting polymer and neural cells and tested the property of this composite electrode (Figure 10.15). Figure 10.15 shows the PEDOT and neural cells. The blue area is the neural cells and the dark area is the PEDOT [69]. As shown in Figure 10.15, the PEDOT was not only polymerised around the cells but also had direct contact with the cells. As a result, they found that the PEDOT electrodes with neurons had higher impedance than PEDOT electrode without neurons [69]. Cyclic voltammetry (CV) was used to compare the charge capacity of PEDOT-coated electrodes, bare-metal electrodes, bare-metal electrodes with neurons, electrodes with PEDOT coated around neurons and neuron-template PEDOT-coated electrodes (Figure 10.16). The result showed that the charge capacity of PEDOT neurons was lower than PEDOT coated electrodes, and the shapes of the CV curve were different (Figure 10.16). During the polymerisation process, 80% of the neural cells could keep viable in EDOT monomer solution for nearly 72 h. After the neurons were embedded in PEDOT, they could

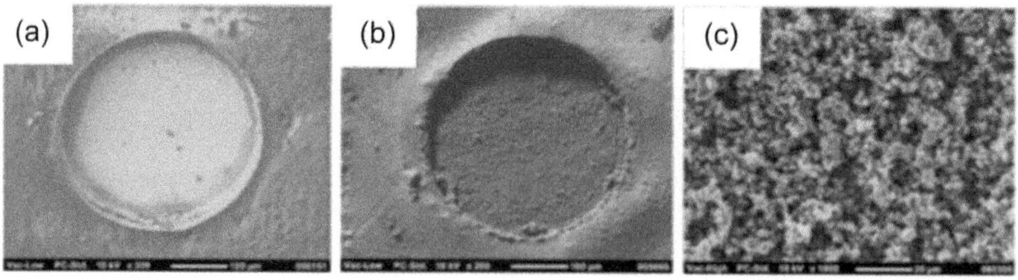

Figure 10.12 SEM images of electrodes. (a) Bare Pt electrode. (b) Pt electrode coated with PEDOT/pTS at 200× magnification. (c) Pt electrode coated with PEDOT/pTS at 1000× magnification.
Reproduced with permission from [67].

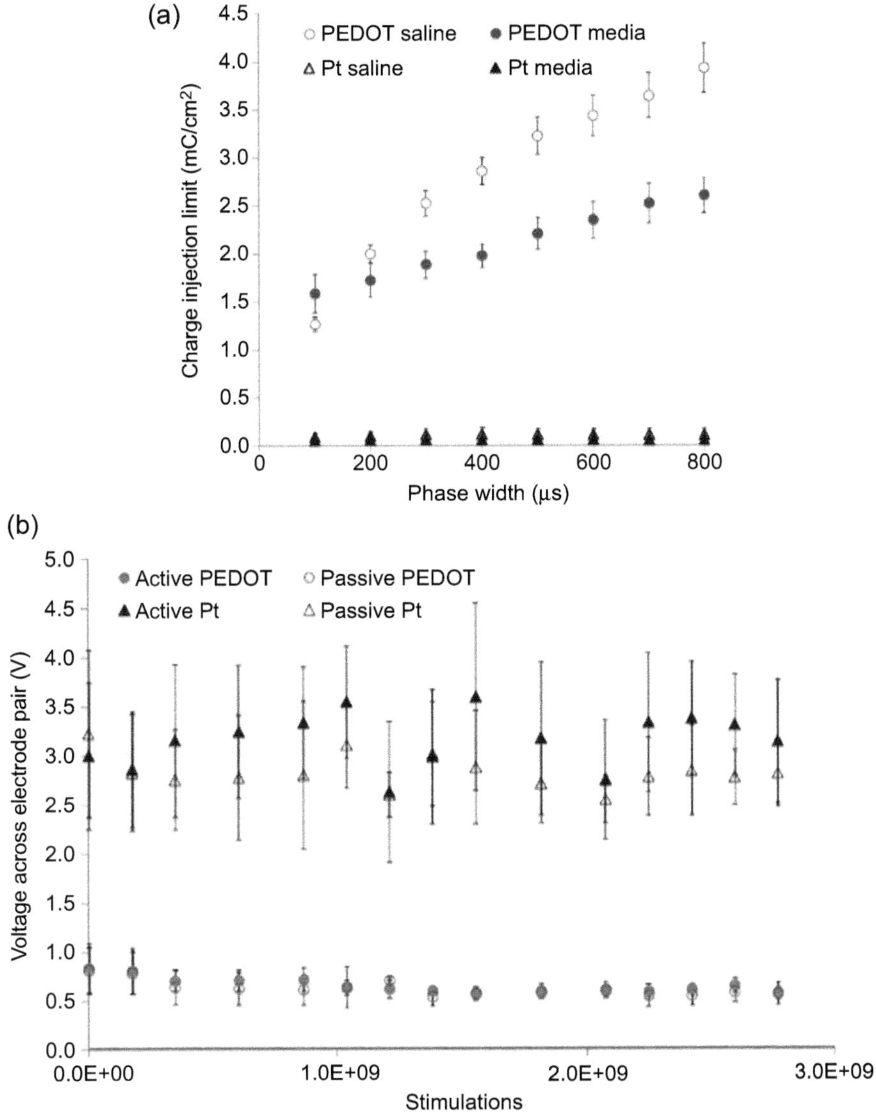

Figure 10.13 (a) Charge injection limit of PEDOT-coated and uncoated electrodes. (b) Voltage drop for different electrodes.
Reproduced with permission from Ref. [67].

still live for a week. This implied that the PEDOT coating did not affect the nutrition transportation greatly [69]. The experimental result showed that it was possible to establish a long-term communication between electrical device and neural cells. Also, polymerisation of conducting polymer on living cells demonstrated a new method to immobilise cells on electrodes.

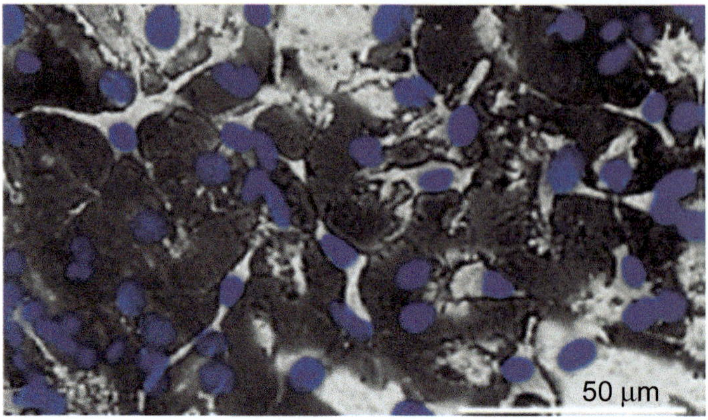

Figure 10.14 PEDOT polymerised around neural cells.
Reproduced with permission from Ref. [69].

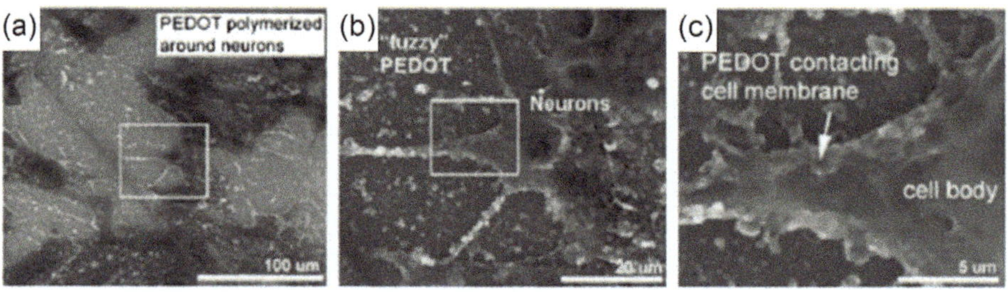

Figure 10.15 SEM images of PEDOT polymerised near neurons.
Reproduced with permission from Ref. [69].

Abidian et al. examined the improvement of the signal recording of neural electrodes in vivo after coating the microelectrodes with PEDOT nanotubes (PEDOT NTs). PEDOT NTs were fabricated by electrochemical polymerisation of PEDOT on a gold site and around electrospun poly(L-lactide) (PLLA) nanofibres followed by dissolving PLLA nanofibres (Figure 10.17(a)). Chronic neural microelectrodes modified by PEDOT NTS were inserted in the barrel cortex of rats [70].

Microelectrodes without PEDOT NTs were considered control groups. Electrochemical impedance spectroscopy was used to examine the impedance of neural electrodes before and after implantation for both coated and uncoated sites. PEDOT NTs sites had significantly lower impedance, especially at 1 kHz, than control sites (uncoated sites) over 7 weeks of implantation (Figure 10.17(b)), which may help improve the quality of signal recording. The change of impedance could be explained by protein absorption and biological response at the neural–electrode interface [70]. Chronic neural recording from animal brain revealed that PEDOT NTs recorded brain activity with a higher signal-to-noise ratio (SNR); in particular, the percentage of sites for quality unites (SNR > 4) in the case of PEDOT NTs was 35% higher than uncoated sites over the course of implantation. The percentage of sites with SNR larger

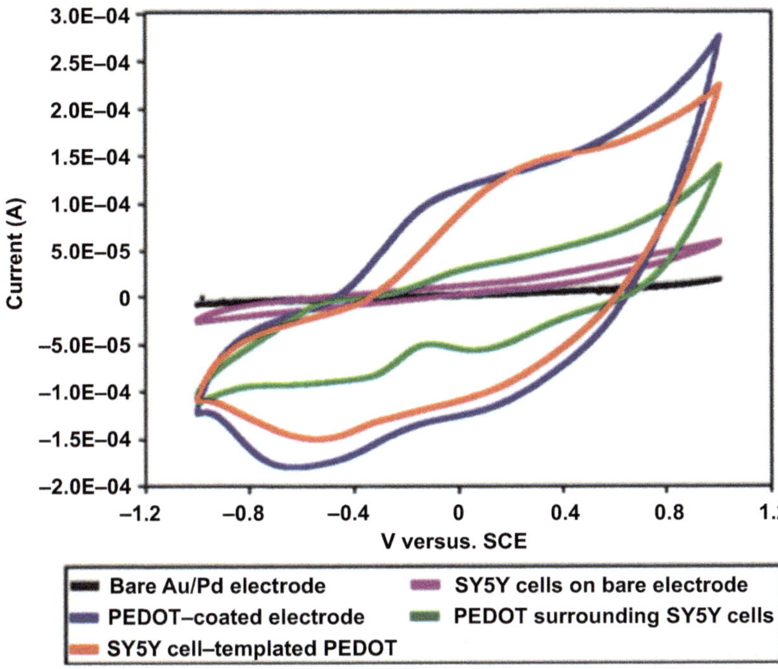

Figure 10.16 Cyclic voltammetry for bare Au/Pd electrode, PEDOT-coated electrode, SY5Y cell-templated PEDOT-coated electrode, bare electrode with SY5Y cells and electrode with PEDOT around SY5Y cells.
Reproduced with permission from Ref. [69].

than 4 of PEDOT-coated electrodes was always higher than uncoated electrodes (Figure 10.17(c)). As a result, the conducting polymers, PEDOT NTs, could effectively decreased the impedance of microelectrodes and lower the noise level.

10.4.3 Drug-delivery systems

Drug delivery has a great impact on the efficiency of therapy. Traditional drug-delivery systems always release the drug immediately after entering the human circulatory system. At the beginning, the drug concentration always exceeds the therapeutic range, and then the drug concentration immediately falls below the therapeutic range. Thus, the total effective time for the drug is short [71]. Researchers have focused on designing controlled drug-delivery systems. For example, Langer and co-workers have designed a polymeric microchip device that could release drugs at different times (Figure 10.18(a)). The mechanism for the multiple release of drug was based on the different degradation rates of the reservoir membrane. The reservoir membrane was made of poly(lactic-co-glycolic acid) (PLGA). By controlling the molecular weight, chemical composition and thickness of PLGA, the degradation of the membrane was controlled. Figure 10.18(b) shows the release of dextran as a drug model over

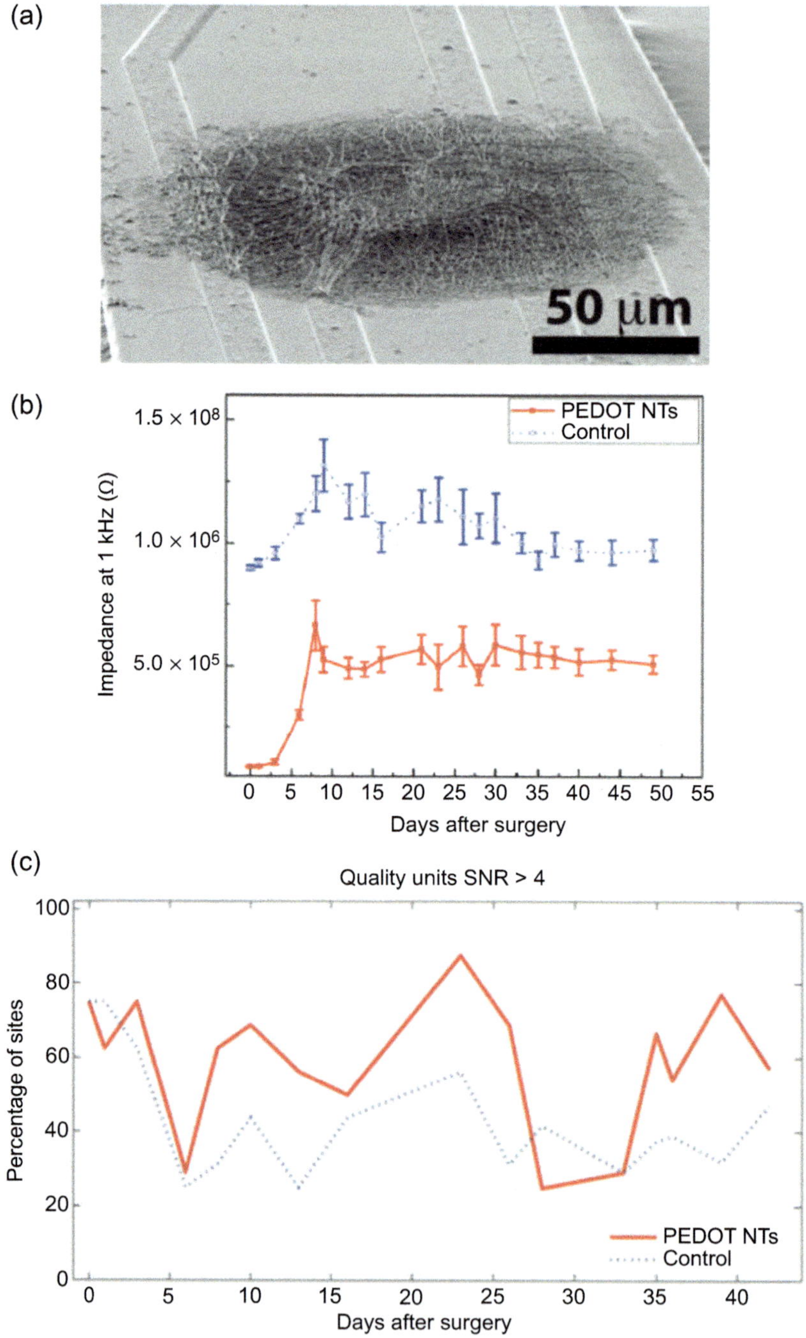

Figure 10.17 (a) PEDOT nanotube-coated electrode site. (b) Impedance change of PEDOT-coated electrodes and uncoated electrodes over 7 weeks after implantation. (c) Percentage of electrode sites with SNR > 4.
Reproduced with permission from Ref. [70].

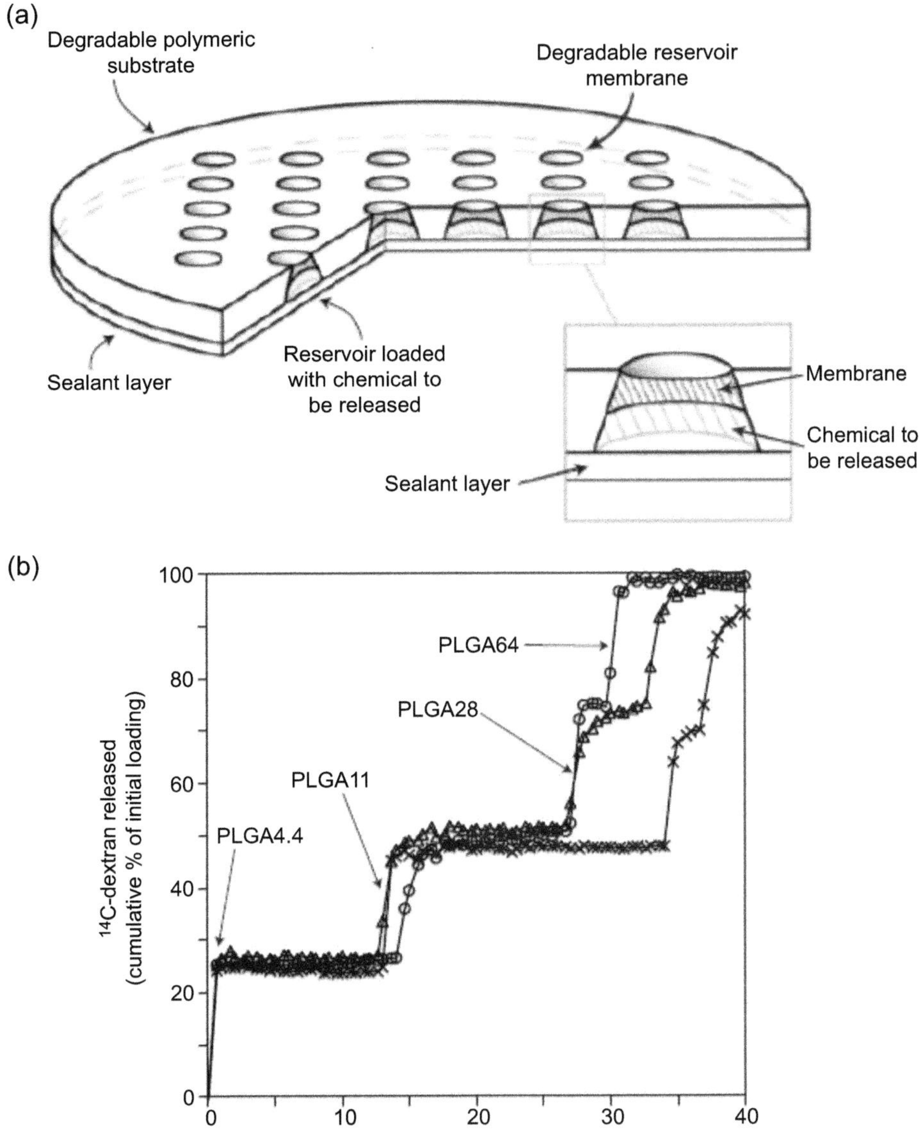

Figure 10.18 (a) Diagram of polymeric microchip device. (b) Percentage of released dextran from microchip devices in vitro.
Reproduced with permission from Ref. [72].

time by PLGA microchip. However, this microchip device can release drug without external stimulation to provide on-demand and a more triggered release system [72].

Conducting polymer can be used to precisely release drugs and biomolecules by applying electrical stimulation. Wadhwa et al. investigated the controlled drug release of dexamethasone from a PPy-coated electrode. The electrode was made of plastic coverslips coated with 40-nm thick gold. Electrochemical deposition was carried out to deposit PPy and dexamethasone (as dopant) on the gold electrodes. In this study, CV scan was performed to study the drug-release behaviour in a phosphate-buffered saline (PBS). The voltage ranged from −0.8 to 1.4 V, with a scanning rate of 100 mV/s for 30 cycles. They found that the dexamethasone was not released at first several cycles. However, after about two to three cycles the incorporated dexamethasone was released linearly in respect to the numbers of CV cycles. Figure 10.19 shows the dexamethasone release for both stimulated and unstimulated electrodes [73]. As shown in this figure, the drug was released at a higher rate with an external electrical stimulation.

Abidian et al. developed a method for fabrication of drug-loaded conducting polymer nanotubes [74]. Dexamethasone was incorporated within the PLGA electrospun nanofibres (Figure 10.20(a)) and PEDOT was electropolymerised on the electrode sites (Figure 10.20(b)) and around the PLGA nanofibres to create dexamethasone-loaded PEDOT nanotubes. PLGA is an ideal biodegradable material for making electrospun microfibres and nanofibres. In this research, PLGA incorporated with dexamethasone was electrospun on gold-coated silicon wafer electrodes. Electrochemical polymerisation was carried out in a solution containing PEDOT monomer and PBS.

After that, the response of the drug-release system to electrical stimulation as low as 1 V was tested in PBS. The drug-loaded PEDOT nanotubes were stimulated by applying a positive voltage of 1 V with a scan rate of 0.1 V/s for 10 s (charge density 0.8 C/cm^2) at five specific time points (blue line in Figure 10.20(c)). A control experiment was done to demonstrate that dexamethasone did diffuse through the PEDOT nanotube walls. In this experiment, the expansion and contraction of the PEDOT nanotube provided an additional means for controlling the kinetics of drug release. They predicted that the amount of released drug would be directly corresponded to the contraction force and the duration of the contraction [74].

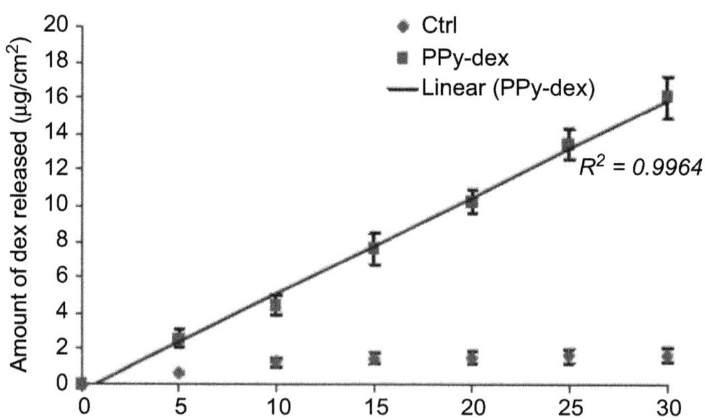

Figure 10.19 Release of dexamethasone over CV cycles.
Reproduced with permission from Ref. [73].

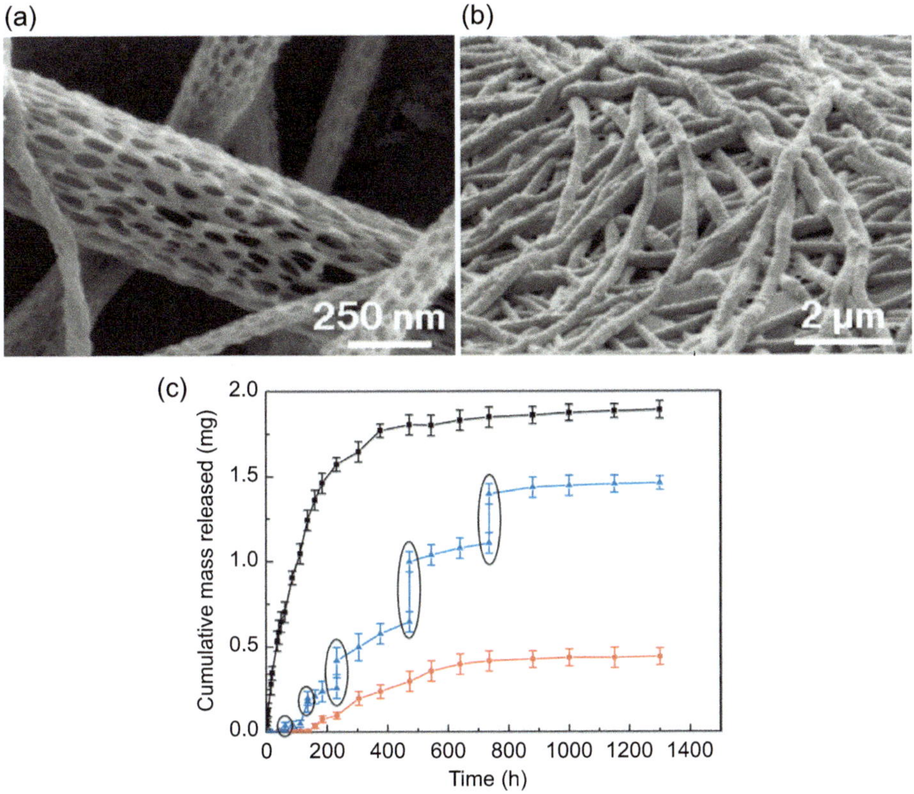

Figure 10.20 (a) SEM of PLGA fibres. (b) SEM of electropolymerised PEDOT nanotubes on the electrode. (c) Dexamethasone released from PEDOT nanotubes as a function of time. (Black line, PLGA fibres; blue line, PEDOT-coated PLGA fibres with 1 V electrical stimulation applied at five specific times; red line, PEDOT-coated PLGA fibres without electrical stimulation.)
Reproduced with permission from Ref. [74].

Conducting polymer-based drug-delivery systems has some restrictions on the choice of dopant and drug molecular weight [75]. The molecular weight of drugs should be small, for expelling of drugs out from the conducting polymer film. To overcome this restriction, George et al. attached drug molecules on the surface of the conducting polymer rather than incorporating them into conducting polymer structure [75]. They employed PPy as the conducting polymer substrate and biotin as the dopant during the electrochemical polymerisation. Biotin is negatively charged in solution, and therefore can be considered a counter-ion for PPy. The electrical attraction between negatively charged biotin and positively charged PPy ensured the attachment of biotin to the PPy film. They carried out several experiments to examine the stability of the attachment of biotin to the PPy surface. They found that biotin attachment to the PPy surface was very stable when no activation occurred. Then streptavidine was used to bind the biotins. The streptavidine has four binding sites, which can not

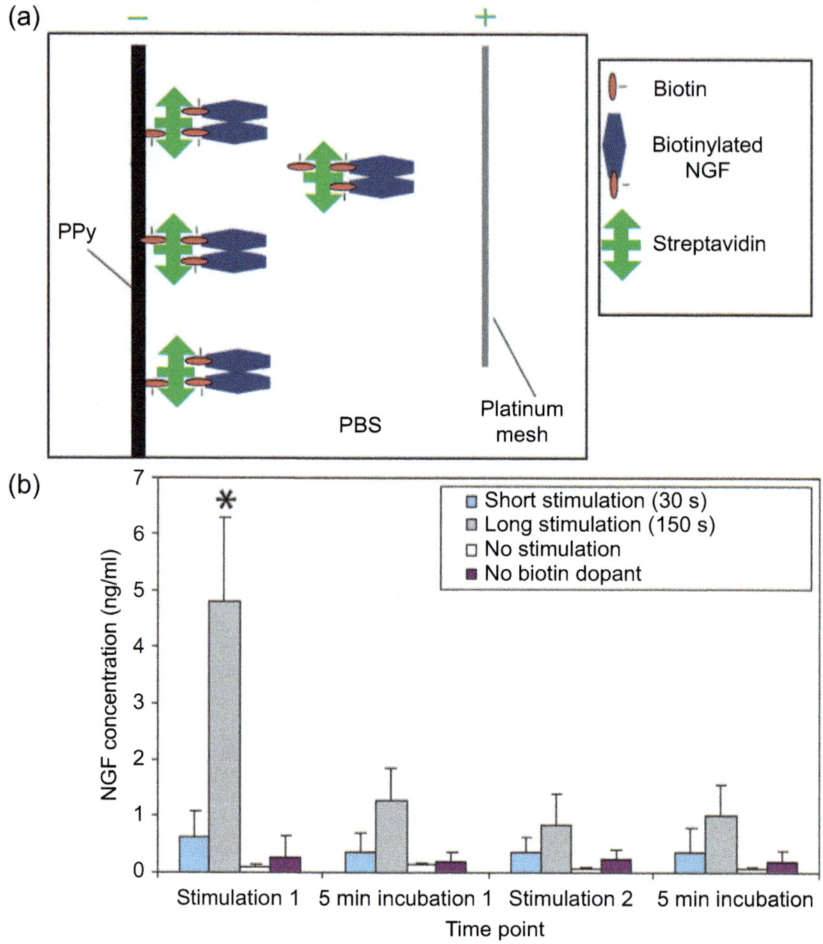

Figure 10.21 (a) Schematic of biotin-doped conducting polymer drug-delivery system for incorporation of NGF [75]. (b) Amount of NGF released at different conditions [75].

only bind to biotin but also to biotinylated drugs such as nerve growth factor (NGF). Figure 10.21(a) shows the schematic of this type of drug-delivery system. When an external stimulation of 3 V was applied to the PPy, a reduction reaction occurred and PPy became electrically neutral [75]. As a result, the PPy no longer attracted biotins and NGF was released from the PPy surface. Figure 10.21(b) shows the result of NGF-releasing experiment using electrical stimulation of PPy film.

Cho et al. fabricated a mesoporous silica nanosphere-based drug-delivery system [76]. Mesoporous silica nanospheres (MSNs) were employed due to their biocompatibility, chemical stability and nontoxic property [76]. NGF was loaded into the pores of MSNs (Figure 10.22(a)) and then the MSN−NGF composites were immobilised by electrochemical polymerisation of PPy at the surface of the electrode [76]. The amount

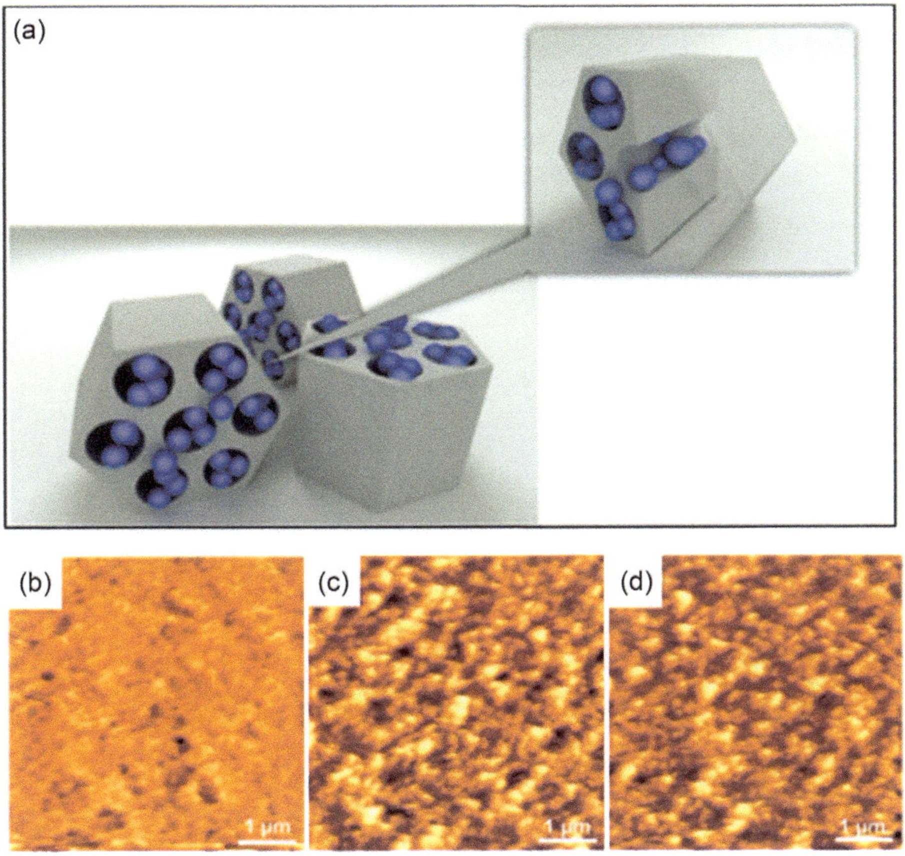

Figure 10.22 (a) Schematic of NGF-filled MSNs. (b) AFM image of polypyrrole-coated electrode. (c) AFM image of polypyrrole-MSN coated electrode. (d) AFM image of polypyrrole–MSN–NGF-coated electrode.
Reproduced with permission from Ref. [76].

of NGF incorporated into MSNs was examined. The drug-release profile and the attachment and neurite outgrowth of PC12 cells were evaluated. Figure 10.22(a) shows the schematic of the MSNs with NGF filled into the pores. The NGF was filled into the pores of MSNs due to electrostatic interactions because the signs of charges of the MSNs walls and NGFs are opposite [76]. Then the MSN–NGF composite acted as a dopant together with poly(styrene sulphonate) (PSS) during the electropolymerisation of PPy. The MSNs have a large surface-to-volume ratio, which makes them more efficient in drug loading [77]. The MSNs can also protect the drugs during the implantation [76]. They found that the surface roughness of porous MSNs improved the PC12 attachment [78]. Figure 10.22(b), (c) and (d) shows the atomic force microscopy (AFM) images of the electrode surfaces. The surface of PPy–MSN–NGF composite was compared with the surface of PPy and the surface of PPy–MSN composite.

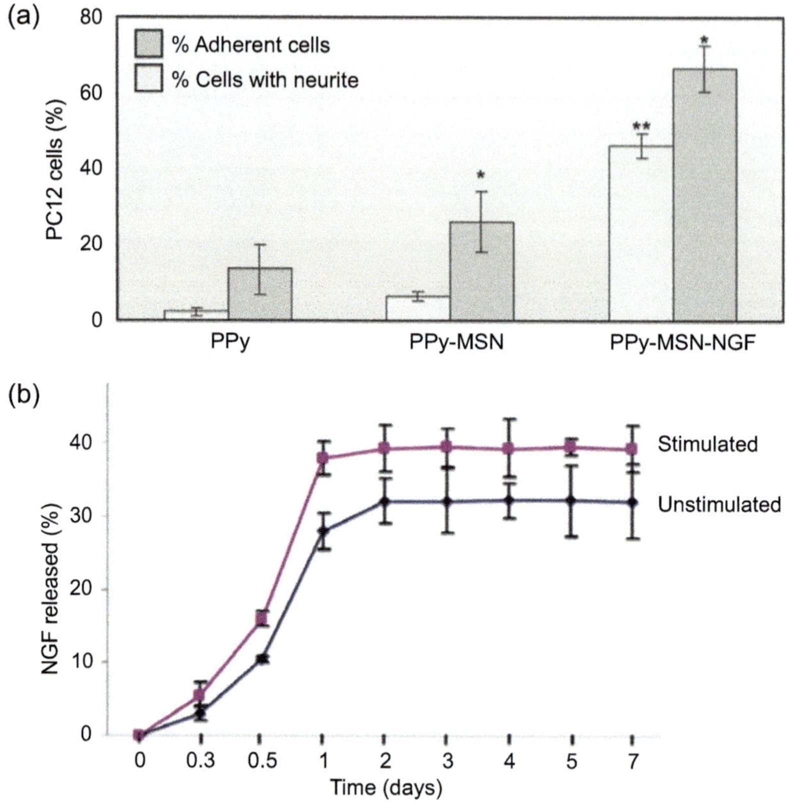

Figure 10.23 (a) Characterisation of adherent cells percentage and cells with neurite percentage on PPy, Ppy−MSN and Ppy−MSN−NGF surfaces. (b) NGF released over time. Reproduced with permission from Ref. [76].

The PC12 cell attachment and neurite outgrowth on different surfaces were characterised (Figure 10.23(a)). They concluded that the cell attachment on PPy−MSN films was significantly facilitated and the NGF promoted the growth of neurite. Cho et al. also compared the NGF release profile for stimulated and unstimulated PPy. Stimulation of a 0.6-m/Acm^2 constant current density was applied to stimulate the conducting polymer for NGF release. Figure 10.23(b) shows the obvious increase of the amount of released NGF under electrical stimulation.

10.4.4 Bioactuators

Conducting polymer can also be used as biomedical actuators due to the volume change during reduction or oxidation reactions [79]. Conducting polymer-based actuators have been employed as artificial muscles [80] and biomedical devices [81]. Shape-memory alloys [82], piezoelectric polymers [79] and electrostrictive polymers [83] have been investigated as potential actuator materials. When an electrical current passes through the alloy, the current heats the alloy and the shape-memory alloy undergoes a phase transformation, and then the alloy bends [79]. As for electrostrictive and piezoelectric polymers, the external electric field should force them to change their shapes. After discovery of conducting polymers, researchers have investigated conducting polymers as materials for mechanical actuators.

Conducting polymer has several advantages over other actuator materials. For example, the strain of a conducting polymer actuator can be as high as 30% [80], which is much larger than piezoelectric polymers and shape-memory alloys. Conducting polymers have a high Young's modulus and tensile strength, which makes them suitable for exertion of large forces. In addition, the required voltage for the conducting polymers to exert a considerable force is lower than other materials [79]. Lastly, conducting polymers can operate in an aqueous environment without any protection due to their high resistance to the corrosive environment, such as blood. However, conducting polymers have a low efficiency to convert electrical energy to mechanical energy. It has been reported that the mechanical work transferred from electrical work was less than 1% for conducting polymer actuators [84]. Even so, conducting polymers are more attractive than other actuator materials due to their unique properties for biomedical applications.

The mechanism of actuation of conducting polymers is simple. When conducting polymer is doped with counter-ions, the carbon–carbon bond length of the polymer backbone is changed during the actuation. This contributes to the volume change of conducting polymer. However, the most primary mechanism for the volume change is the movement of counter-ions and solvent inside and outside the conducting polymer. When conducting polymer is oxidised by a positive voltage, negatively charged counter ions enter the polymer to maintain the electrical neutrality of the polymer structure, and then polymer expands. When a conducting polymer undergoes a reduction reaction, if the counter ions are small enough to be expelled from the polymer, then the conducting polymer contracts. If the counter-ions are large, small cations enter the polymers to compensate the charge balance [79]. Figure 10.24 shows the schematic of the expansion of conducting polymer under redox process. The strain of the polymer is determined by how many ions are attracted into the polymers. PANI and PPy are the most investigated conducting polymers for actuator applications.

Otero and co-workers fabricated bilayer conducting polymer actuators as a potential device for artificial muscle [80]. One layer of conducting polymer (PPy) and a nonconductive plastic layer were used to create the bilayer structure. The PPy was electrochemically polymerised on a square stainless-steel electrode. Then a plastic tape was pasted to the PPy layer and the bilayer polymer was removed from the stainless-steel electrode. By adding a 1 V external voltage, the PPy was oxidised and a dimensional change occurred. Since there was no volume change in the nonconductive plastic tape, the bilayer would bend [80]. Different currents (5–25 mA) were used to examine the speed of actuator's response at different stimulation intensity. Later, they successfully fabricated a PPy-based triple-layer artificial muscle, which could push an obstacle with a mass of 6000 mg immersed in the electrolyte solution [85].

Mazzoldi et al. developed steerable catheters that might be used as an optical endoscope for minimally invasive surgery. A steerable catheter is able to pass around a

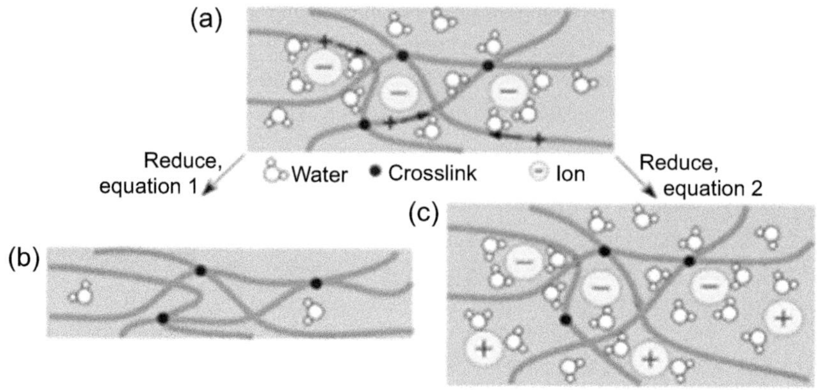

Figure 10.24 Schematic of conducting polymer expansion. (a) Oxidised state of conducting polymer. (b) Reduced state of conducting polymer. (c) Reduced state of conducting polymer with large anions.
Reproduced with permission from Ref. [79].

divergence or through a sharp turn in human vessels. They employed a composite structure made of PANI fibres and solid polymer electrolyte elastomeric matrix. When two opposite electrical stimulations were applied at different region of the same end of the catheter, one side of the catheter would expand and the other side would contract, which caused the catheter to bend. Figure 10.25 shows the structure of the conducting polymer-based steerable catheter. They found that the maximum bending angle could be adjusted by controlling the catheter diameter, the conducting polymer fibre elastic modulus and matrix elastic modulus [81].

Conducting polymer actuators can also be used in some microfabricated systems. For example, Jager et al. fabricated a stretchable microvial for single-cell manipulation. Traditionally, cells are studied by monitoring a group of cells in a Petri dish. By applying this microvial, researchers could study cell biology by investigating a single cell. The microvial had a very small dimension ($100 \times 100 \times 20$ μm), which could only contain one or few cells [86]. Figure 10.26 shows the design of this microvial.

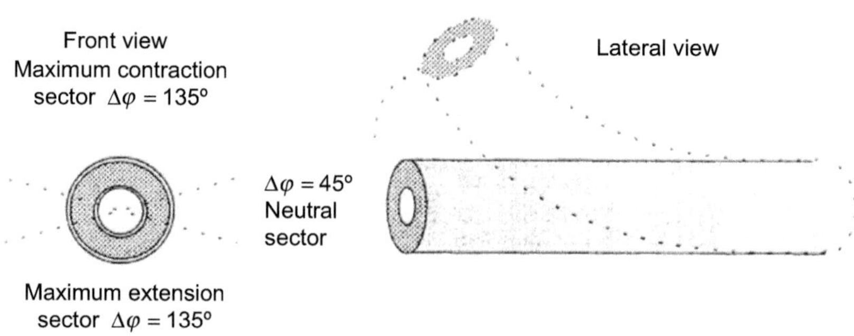

Figure 10.25 Schematic of a conducting polymer-based steerable catheter.
Reproduced with permission from Ref. [81].

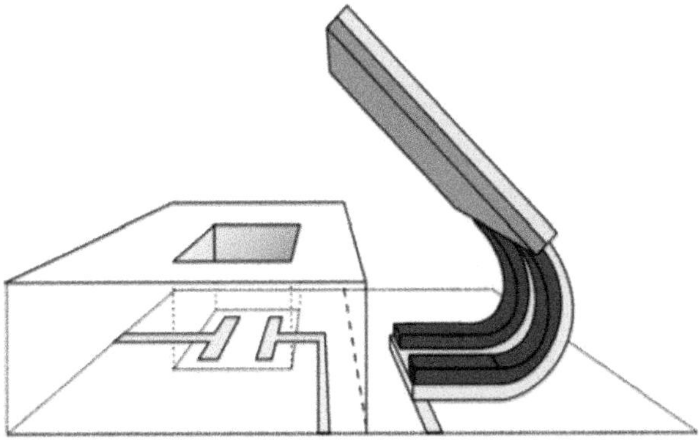

Figure 10.26 Schematic of a closable microvial.
Reproduced with permission from Ref. [86].

The microvial was able to isolate the single cell from the outside environment by closing the lid. The lid was fabricated by a conducting polymer microactuator. The working mechanism of this lid was same as the double-layer artificial muscle, and PPy was used to produce the double-layer lid. By connecting the two layers to electrodes, they could open or close the lid by giving stimulation to the conducting polymer lid.

10.5 Conclusions

Conducting polymers have been widely utilised in biomedical applications [46–49] due to their conductivity, compatibility and low-cost processability. In addition, compared with traditional metal or semiconductor materials, conducting polymers are more biocompatible. These advantages make conducting polymers more attractive to bioengineering researchers. The mechanism of electrical conductivity of conducting polymers is based on the transmission of polarons and bipolarons. The synthesis of conducting polymers can be accomplished by electrochemical polymerisation, which is more straightforward than traditional chemical synthesis. In this chapter, several applications of conducting polymers in biomedical engineering are illustrated with examples. The applications include the use of conducting polymers in biosensors, neural electrodes, drug delivery and bioactuators. However, there are still many studies required to promote relative properties of conducting polymers, and there are a lot of questions remaining to be answered.

References

[1] J.C. Scott, History of conductive polymers, in: Nanostructured Conductive Polymers, 2000, pp. 1–17.

[2] R. Greene, G. Street, L. Suter, Superconductivity in polysulfur nitride (SN) x, Phys. Rev. Lett. 34 (10) (1975) 8–10.

[3] S. Kailas, Chapter 11. Applications and processing of polymers, in: Material Science.

[4] G. Tourillon, F. Garnier, Effect of dopant on the physicochemical and electrical properties of organic conducting polymers, J. Phys. Chem. 87 (13) (1983) 2289–2292.

[5] J. Gardner, P. Bartlett, Application of conducting polymer technology in microsystems, Sensors Actuat. A Phys. A 51 (1995) 57–66.

[6] L. Dai, Chapter 2. Conducting polymers, in: Intelligent Macromolecules for Smart Devices, vol. 1980, 2004, pp. 42–80.

[7] G.B. Street, J.L. Bredas, Polarons, bipolarons, and solitons in conducting polymers, Acc. Chem. Res. 18 (10) (1985) 309–315.

[8] K.M. Molapo, P.M. Ndangili, R.F. Ajayi, G. Mbambisa, S.M. Mailu, N. Njomo, M. Masikini, P. Baker, E.I. Iwuoha, Electronics of conjugated polymers (I): polyaniline, Int. J. Electrochem. Sci. 7 (2012) 11859–11875.

[9] G. Inzelt, Chemical and electrochemical syntheses of conducting polymers, in: Conducting Polymers a New Era in Electrochemistry, Springer Berlin Heidelberg, Berlin, Heidelberg, 2008, pp. 123–136.

[10] G. Sabouraud, S. Sadki, N. Brodie, The mechanisms of pyrrole electropolymerization, Chem. Soc. Rev. 29 (5) (2000) 283–293.

[11] M. Gerard, A. Chaubey, B.D. Malhotra, Application of conducting polymers to biosensors, Biosens. Bioelectron. 17 (5) (May 2002) 345–359.

[12] I.Y. Sapurina, M.A. Shishov, Oxidative polymerization of aniline: molecular synthesis of polyaniline and the formation of supramolecular structures, in: New Polymers for Special Applications, 2012.

[13] E.M. Genies, A. Boyle, M. Lapkowski, C. Tsintavis, Polyaniline: a historical survey, Synthetic. Met. 36 (1990) 139–182.

[14] A. Malinauskas, Chemical deposition of conducting polymers, Polymer (Guildf) 42 (9) (Apr. 2001) 3957–3972.

[15] S. Bhadra, D. Khastgir, N.K. Singha, J.H. Lee, Progress in preparation, processing and applications of polyaniline, Prog. Polym. Sci. 34 (8) (2009) 783–810.

[16] V.G. Kulkarni, L.D. Campbell, W.R. Mathew, Thermal stability of polyaniline, Synth. Met. 30 (1989) 321–325.

[17] B. Wessling, New insight into organic metal polyaniline morphology and structure, Polymers (Basel) 2 (4) (2010) 786–798.

[18] A.J. Epstein, Conducting polymers: electrical conductivity, in: Physical Properties of Polymers Handbook, 2007, pp. 725–755.

[19] A.A. Syed, M.K. Dinesan, Review: polyaniline-a novel polymeric material, Talanta 38 (8) (1991) 815–837.

[20] E.M. Genies, A.A. Syed, C. Tsintavis, Electrochemical study of polyaniline in aqueous and organic medium. Redox and kinetic properties, Mol. Cryst. Liq. Cryst. 121 (1–4) (1985) 181–186.

[21] W.-S. Huang, B.D. Humphrey, A.G. MacDiarmid, Polyaniline, a novel conducting polymer. Morphology and chemistry of its oxidation and reduction in aqueous electrolytes, J. Chem. Soc. Faraday Trans. 1 82 (8) (1986) 2385.

[22] A. Kitani, J. Izumi, J. Yano, Y. Hiromoto, K. Sasaki, Basic behaviors and properties of the electrodeposited polyaniline, Bull. Chem. Soc. Jpn. 57 (8) (1984) 2254–2257.

[23] N. Mermilliod, J. Tanguy, M. Hoclet, A.A. Syed, Electrochemical characterization of chemically synthesized polyanilines, Synth. Met. 18 (1987) 359–364.

[24] A.G. Macdiarmid, J.-C. Chiang, M. Halpern, W.-S. Huang, S.-L. Mu, L.D. Nanaxakkara, S.W. Wu, S.I. Yaniger, 'Polyaniline': interconversion of metallic and insulating forms, Mol. Cryst. Liq. Crys. 121 (1–4) (1985) 173–180.

[25] A.G. MacDiarmid, Polyaniline and polypyrrole: where are we headed? Synth. Met. 84 (1−3) (1997) 27−34.
[26] O.N. Efimov, T. Vernitskaya, Polypyrrole: a conducting polymer; its synthesis, properties and applications, Russ. Chem. Rev. 66 (5) (1997) 443−457.
[27] A.F. Diaz, K.K. Kanazawa, Polypyrrole: an electrochemical approach to conducting polymers, in: Extended Linear Chain Compounds, 1983, pp. 417−441 (LA−English).
[28] E.M. Genies, G. Bidan, A.F. Diaz, Spectroelectrochemical study of polypyrrole films, J. Electroanal. Chem. 149 (1983) 101−113.
[29] K.J. Kim, H.S. Song, J.D. Kim, Mechanism of electropolymerization of pyrrole in acidic aqueous solutions, Bull. Korean Chem. 9 (4) (1988) 248−251.
[30] S. Asavapiriyanont, G.K. Chandler, G.A. Gunawardena, D. Pletcher, The electrodeposition of polypyrrole films from aqueous solutions, J. Electroanal. Chem. 117 (1984) 229−244.
[31] Y. Qlu, J.R. Reynolds, Electrochemically initiated chain polymerization of pyrrole, J. Polym. Sci. Part A Polym. Chem. 30 (7) (1992) 1315−1325.
[32] A.F. Diaz, K.K. Kanazawa, Electrochemical polymerization of pyrrole, J. Chem. Soc. Chem. Commun. 160 (1) (1988) 79−88.
[33] M. Yamaura, K. Sato, T. Hagiwara, K. Iwata, Memory effect of electrical conductivity upon the counteranion exchange of polypyrrole films, Synth. Met. 48 (3) (1992) 337−354.
[34] B.R. Scharifker, E. García-Pastoriza, W. Marino, The growth of polypyrrole films on electrodes, J. Electroanal. Chem. Interfacial Electrochem. 300 (1−2) (1991) 85−98.
[35] G. Kojmehl, G. Chatzitheodorou, Electrical conductivity of poly(2,5-thiophenediyl)-AsF5-complexes, Makromol. Chem. Rapid Commun. 555 (1981) 551−555.
[36] K. Kaneto, K. Yoshino, Y. Inuishi, Electrical and optical properties of polythiophene prepared by electrochemical polymerization, Solid State Commun. 46 (5) (1983) 389−391.
[37] G. Schopf, G. Koßmehl, Chapter 5. Synthesis, in: Polythiophenes-Electrically Conductive Polymers (1997).
[38] R.J. Waltman, J. Bargon, A.F. Diaz, Electrochemical studies of some conducting polythiophene films, J. Phys. Chem. 87 (8) (1983) 1459−1463.
[39] K. Kaneto, K. Yoshino, Y. Inuishi, Electrical properties of conducting polymer, poly-thiophene, prepared by electrochemical polymerization, Jpn. J. Appl. Phys. 21 (Part 2, No. 9) (1982) L567−L568.
[40] M. Sato, S. Tanaka, K. Kaeriyama, Electrochemical preparation of highly conducting polythiophene films, J. Chem. Soc. Chem. Commun. (11) (1985) 713.
[41] Y. Cao, R. Qian, IR and Raman studies of polythiophene prepared by electrochemical polymerization, Solid State Commun. 54 (3) (1985) 211−213.
[42] G. Tourillon, F. Garnier, New electrochemically generated organic conducting polymers, J. Electroanal. Chem. Interfacial Electrochem. 135 (1) (1982) 173−178.
[43] K.-S. Park, S.B. Schougaard, J.B. Goodenough, Conducting-polymer/iron-redox- couple composite cathodes for lithium secondary batteries, Adv. Mater. 19 (6) (Mar. 2007) 848−851.
[44] R. Ko, R.C. Word, M. Godinez, Ultraviolet electroluminescence from ZnO/polymer heterojunction light-emitting diodes, Nano Lett. 5 (2005) 2005−2008.
[45] M.A. Soto-Oviedo, O.A. Araújo, R. Faez, M.C. Rezende, M.-A. De Paoli, Antistatic coating and electromagnetic shielding properties of a hybrid material based on polyaniline/organoclay nanocomposite and EPDM rubber, Synth. Met. 156 (18−20) (Nov. 2006) 1249−1255.

[46] M.R. Abidian, D.C. Martin, Multifunctional nanobiomaterials for neural interfaces, Adv. Funct. Mater. 19 (4) (Feb. 2009) 573–585.
[47] M.R. Abidian, D.C. Martin, Experimental and theoretical characterization of implantable neural microelectrodes modified with conducting polymer nanotubes, Biomaterials 29 (9) (Mar. 2008) 1273–1283.
[48] M.R. Abidian, J.M. Corey, D.R. Kipke, D.C. Martin, Conducting-polymer nanotubes improve electrical properties, mechanical adhesion, neural attachment, and neurite outgrowth of neural electrodes, Small 6 (3) (Feb. 2010) 421–429.
[49] S. Park, G. Yang, N. Madduri, M.R. Abidian, S. Majd, Hydrogel-mediated direct patterning of conducting polymer films with multiple surface chemistries, Adv. Mater. 26 (18) (May 2014) 2782–2787.
[50] K. Gurunathan, A.V. Murugan, R. Marimuthu, U. Mulik, D. Amalnerkar, Electrochemically synthesised conducting polymeric materials for applications towards technology in electronics, optoelectronics and energy storage devices, Mater. Chem. Phys. 61 (3) (Nov. 1999) 173–191.
[51] X.S. Wang, X.Q. Feng, X.W. Guo, Failure behavior of anodized coating-magnesium alloy substrate structures, Key Eng. Mater. 261–263 (2004) 363–368.
[52] X.S. Wang, H.P. Tang, X.D. Li, X. Hua, Investigations on the mechanical properties of conducting polymer coating-substrate structures and their influencing factors, Int. J. Mol. Sci. 10 (12) (2009) 5257–5284.
[53] D.H. Kim, J.A. Wiler, D.J. Anderson, D.R. Kipke, D.C. Martin, Conducting polymers on hydrogel-coated neural electrode provide sensitive neural recordings in auditory cortex, Acta Biomater. 6 (1) (2010) 57–62.
[54] R.A. Green, R.T. Hassarati, J.A. Goding, S. Baek, N.H. Lovell, P.J. Martens, L.A. Poole-Warren, Conductive hydrogels: mechanically robust hybrids for use as biomaterials, Macromol. Biosci. 12 (4) (2012) 494–501.
[55] R.T. Hassarati, W.F. Dueck, C. Tasche, P.M. Carter, L.A. Poole-Warren, R.A. Green, Improving cochlear implant properties through conductive hydrogel coatings, IEEE Trans. Neural Syst. Rehabil. Eng. 22 (2) (2014) 411–418.
[56] D.H. Kim, M. Abidian, D.C. Martin, Conducting polymers grown in hydrogel scaffolds coated on neural prosthetic devices, J. Biomed. Mater. Res. Part A 71 (4) (2004) 577–585.
[57] A.J. Patton, R.A. Green, L.A. Poole-Warren, Mediating conducting polymer growth within hydrogels by controlling nucleation, APL Mater. 3 (1) (2015) 014912.
[58] M. Sasaki, B.C. Karikkineth, K. Nagamine, H. Kaji, K. Torimitsu, M. Nishizawa, Highly conductive stretchable and biocompatible electrode-hydrogel hybrids for advanced tissue engineering, Adv. Healthc. Mater. (2014) 1919–1927.
[59] M. Gao, L. Dai, G.G. Wallace, Biosensors based on aligned carbon nanotubes coated with inherently conducting polymers, Electroanalysis 15 (13) (Aug. 2003) 1089–1094.
[60] G. Yang, K.L. Kampstra, M.R. Abidian, High performance conducting polymer nanofiber biosensors for detection of biomolecules, Adv. Mater. 26 (29) (Aug. 2014) 4954–4960.
[61] L. Groenendaal, G. Zotti, P.-H. Aubert, S.M. Waybright, J.R. Reynolds, Electrochemistry of poly(3,4-alkylenedioxythiophene) derivatives, Adv. Mater. 15 (11) (Jun. 2003) 855–879.
[62] F. Diamond, Electrochemical impedance sensing of DNA hybridization on conducting polymer, J. Phys. Chem. B 109 (28) (2005) 13611–13618.

[63] X. Luo, A.J. Killard, A. Morrin, M.R. Smyth, Enhancement of a conducting polymer-based biosensor using carbon nanotube-doped polyaniline, Anal. Chim. Acta 575 (1) (Aug. 2006) 39–44.

[64] V. Mottaghitalab, G.M. Spinks, G.G. Wallace, The influence of carbon nanotubes on mechanical and electrical properties of polyaniline fibers, Synth. Met. 152 (1–3) (Sep. 2005) 77–80.

[65] R.A. Green, N.H. Lovell, G.G. Wallace, L.A. Poole-Warren, Conducting polymers for neural interfaces: challenges in developing an effective long-term implant, Biomaterials 29 (24–25) (2008) 3393–3399.

[66] X. Cui, V.A. Lee, Y. Raphael, J.A. Wiler, J.F. Hetke, D.J. Anderson, D.C. Martin, Surface modification of neural recording electrodes with conducting polymer/biomolecule blends, J. Biomed. Mater. Res. 56 (2) (Aug. 2001) 261–272.

[67] R.A. Green, P.B. Matteucci, R.T. Hassarati, B. Giraud, C.W.D. Dodds, S. Chen, P.J. Byrnes-Preston, G.J. Suaning, L.A. Poole-Warren, N.H. Lovell, Performance of conducting polymer electrodes for stimulating neuroprosthetics, J. Neural Eng. 10 (1) (Feb. 2013) 016009.

[68] H. Kenneth, D. Gurpreet, Neuroprosthetics: Theory and Practice, 2014.

[69] S.M. Richardson-Burns, J.L. Hendricks, B. Foster, L.K. Povlich, D.-H. Kim, D.C. Martin, Polymerization of the conducting polymer poly(3,4-ethylenedioxythiophene) (PEDOT) around living neural cells, Biomaterials 28 (8) (Mar. 2007) 1539–1552.

[70] M.R. Abidian, K.A. Ludwig, T.C. Marzullo, D.C. Martin, D.R. Kipke, Interfacing conducting polymer nanotubes with the central nervous system: chronic neural recording using poly(3,4-ethylenedioxythiophene) nanotubes, Adv. Mater. 21 (37) (Oct. 2009) 3764–3770.

[71] L. Robert, New methods of drug delivery, Science 249 (4976) (1990) 1527–1533.

[72] A. Grayson, I. Choi, B. Tyler, P. Wang, H. Brem, M. Cima, R. Langer, Multi-pulse drug delivery from a resorbable polymeric microchip device, Nat. Mater. 2 (10) (Oct. 2003) 641–642.

[73] R. Wadhwa, C.F. Lagenaur, X.T. Cui, Electrochemically controlled release of dexamethasone from conducting polymer polypyrrole coated electrode, J. Control. Release 110 (3) (Feb. 2006) 531–541.

[74] M.R. Abidian, D.-H. Kim, D.C. Martin, Conducting-polymer nanotubes for controlled drug release, Adv. Mater. 18 (4) (Feb. 2006) 405–409.

[75] P.M. George, D.A. LaVan, J.A. Burdick, C.-Y. Chen, E. Liang, R. Langer, Electrically controlled drug delivery from biotin-doped conductive polypyrrole, Adv. Mater. 18 (5) (Mar. 2006) 577–581.

[76] Y. Cho, R. Shi, A. Ivanisevic, R. Ben Borgens, A mesoporous silica nanosphere-based drug delivery system using an electrically conducting polymer, Nanotechnology 20 (27) (Jul. 2009) 275102.

[77] A. Ahmed, C. Bonner, T.A. Desai, Bioadhesive microdevices with multiple reservoirs: a new platform for oral drug delivery, J. Control. Release 81 (3) (Jun. 2002) 291–306.

[78] S. Bayliss, L. Buckberry, I. Fletcher, M. Tobin, The culture of neurons on silicon, Sensors Actuators A Phys. 74 (1–3) (Apr. 1999) 139–142.

[79] E. Smela, Conjugated polymer actuators for biomedical applications, Adv. Mater. 15 (6) (Mar. 2003) 481–494.

[80] T.F. Otero, J.M. Sansifiena, Artificial muscles based on conducting polymers, Bioelectrochem. Bioenerg. 38 (1995) 411–414. September 1994.

[81] A. Mazzoldi, D. De Rossi, Conductive polymer based structures for a steerable catheter, Smart Struct. Mater. 3987 (Jun. 2000) 273–280.
[82] S.A. Shabalovskaya, Physicochemical and biological aspects of nitinol as a biomaterial, Int. Mater. Rev. 46 (5) (May 2001) 233–250.
[83] Y. Bar-Cohen, Electroactive Polymer (EAP) Actuators as Artificial Muscles: Reality, Potential, and Challenges, Details Table of Contents, March 2004.
[84] E. Smela, M. Kallenbach, J. Holdenried, Electrochemically driven polypyrrole bilayers for moving and positioning bulk micromachined silicon plates, J. Microelectromech. Syst. 8 (4) (1999) 373–383.
[85] O. Toribio Fernµndez, M.T. Cortøs, Artificial muscles with tactile sensitivity, Adv. Mater. (3) (2003) 279–282.
[86] E.W.H. Jager, C. Immerstrand, H. Peterson, K. Magnusson, O. Ingana, The cell clinic: closable microvials for single cell studies, Biomed. Microdevices (2002) 177–187.
[87] M. Hatamzadeh, A. Mahyar, M. Jaymand, Chemical modification of polyaniline by n-grafting of polystyrenic chains synthesized via nitroxide-mediated polymerization, J. Braz. 23 (6) (2012) 1008–1017.

Biosynthetic conductive polymer composites for tissue-engineering biomedical devices

11

R.A. Green, J.A. Goding
Graduate School of Biomedical Engineering, University of New South Wales, Sydney, NSW, Australia

11.1 Introduction

Conductive polymers (CPs) have been explored over the past 20 years as both an alternative to metallic interfaces within biomedical devices and as a way of imparting electroactivity to normally passive devices (such as tissue scaffolds). While significant advances have been made in understanding CP benefits and limitations, challenges remain that have inhibited the widespread application of CPs to implantable medical devices. There are two key issues that prevent homogenous CPs from performing well in the biological environment: (1) mechanical stability and tuneability [1,2] and (2) persistence of a foreign body response (FBR) [3,4].

Conventional CPs are stiff and friable, with typical moduli of the order of 40–100 MPa [2]. While this is significantly lower than conventional metallic counterparts (platinum having an elastic moduli of >1 GPa), it is still notably higher than that of soft tissue (being in the kPa range). Additionally, concerns have been raised over delamination of CPs when applied as coatings. Studies have shown that material loss can exceed 15% in ASTM tape tests [5,6], and delamination has been reported in materials placed under electrical stimulation [3,7]. Furthermore, although polymer components and fabrication parameters can be varied to obtain some control over mechanical stiffness and adherence of CP coatings [2,8], there is very limited ability to tune the moduli of CPs to match neural tissue [8].

Evidence suggests that CPs are compatible with several cell types [9–12]; however, the vast majority of studies have been in vitro assays. While these studies have provided a number of useful relative findings, which have enabled improvements in CP chemical and topographical compatibility, there is limited understanding of the in vivo response. The few studies that have explored CP performance in vivo have found that the in vitro benefits provided by CPs are not recapitulated in the chronic in vivo environment [3,12,13]. It has been proposed that scar tissue development is the major inhibiting factor. Despite in vitro evidence that neural cells interact well with CPs, in the in vivo environment the inflammation resulting from implantation and ongoing presence of a foreign body results in a chronic inflammatory response. This causes neural cells to regress from the interface and glia to encapsulate the device [12]. Initially, it was proposed that bioactive components could provide a mechanism through which neural cells could be

Biosynthetic Polymers for Medical Applications. http://dx.doi.org/10.1016/B978-1-78242-105-4.00011-0

encouraged to interact with CPs. Several groups incorporated proteins, peptides and growth factors within CP materials [1,5,14]. While this was shown to improve CP cell interactions in vitro and even across acute terms in vivo, it was ultimately unsuccessful in generating chronic-term intimate contact and communication between neural cells and devices [12,15]. Furthermore, the incorporation of these bulky molecules resulted in degradation of CP mechanical and electrical properties [5].

These two key limitations have driven researchers to explore a range of composite CP materials. Composites based on CPs have included blends, hybrids, double networks (DNs) and layered structures that aim to preserve the electrical benefits of CPs but use additional polymer components to impart more control over mechanical and biological properties. It has been proposed that this new range of soft, organic electroactive materials can meet the needs of being more tissue-compatible through proving a softer interface while maintaining the electronic interface between tissues and devices. The addition of alternate polymer components also provides an added mechanism through which biological polymers can be incorporated. This has enabled more flexibility in the way both bound and mobile biomolecules can be incorporated. Furthermore, greater amounts of therapeutic molecules can be provided within these materials without detriment to the mechanical properties. Such composites have included blends of CPs and hydrogels [6,16–18], CPs and elastomers [19], carbon nanotube composites [20–22] and CP nanotubes with gel-like cores [7,23]. Each composite provides some benefits beyond homogenous CPs, but is also associated with trade-offs in other properties. This chapter will seek to explore the associated advantages and disadvantages in each class of composite and elicit the mechanisms through which biological polymers can be included within composites to create multifunctional materials.

11.2 Conductive polymer composites

Several approaches have been used to generate composites of CPs, and most commonly the additional polymer components have been nonconductive. Since the main objective in creating a CP composite is to improve mechanical and biological properties, these nonconductive components have been chosen as they have a material property that can be tailored or used to modify the corresponding CP property. For example, elastomers have been used to impart elasticity to CPs that are prone to brittle fracture [24,25]. While any of the CPs used as homogenous coatings can be used in CP composites, the most commonly employed CP has been the polythiophene variant poly(3,4-ethylene dioxythiophene) (PEDOT) [6,7,17,25]. Other CPs that have been used in composites include polyaniline (PANI) [26] and polypyrrole (PPy) [22].

11.2.1 Conductive hydrogels

Conductive hydrogels (CHs) are a class of composites that combine the electrical functionality of CPs with the mechanical properties and drug-loading capacity of hydrogels [27]. Hydrogels are crosslinked polymer networks that swell in aqueous environments due to their highly hydrophilic nature. Hydrogels have mechanical properties akin to those of neural tissue, generally having elastic moduli in the kPa to MPa range [6,28]. Additionally, unlike CPs, the mechanical properties of hydrogels are easily tailored through the choice of polymer chemistry, macromer concentration, the use of DNs and the method and degree of crosslinking used to form the gel [29,30]. It has been proposed that reducing the stiffness of CP electrode coatings through the use of CH composites will help attenuate the chronic inflammatory response and FBR to implantable electrodes by reducing the strain mismatch at the tissue–electrode interface [6,27]. Green et al. reported a decrease in elastic modulus from 40 MPa for a conventional PEDOT coating down to 2 MPa for a PEDOT-poly(vinyl alcohol) (PVA) CH coating; human neural tissue is commonly reported as having an elastic modulus in the range of 10–250 kPa [6]. The hydrogel component is largely responsible for the mechanical properties of the resulting composite material. Accordingly, researches have investigated methods to use this dependency to control the properties, and in particular the mechanical robustness of CHs. Several researchers have investigated the use of double- and triple-network hydrogels (two or interpenetrating hydrogel networks) to increase the mechanical robustness of the resulting CHs [30–32]. CHs also overcome another key limitation of conventional CP coatings, limited loading capacity [33,34]. Owing to their open, swollen network structures, CHs have large loading capacities, allowing them to accommodate significant volumes of bioactive/drug compounds while maintaining the electrically controlled drug release properties of CPs [35].

Several CH systems have been presented in the literature; a selected summary is provided in Table 11.1. PEDOT, PPy and PANI are heavily favoured choices of CPs for use in CHs due to their well-documented cytocompatibility [36–39]. It should be noted that in Table 11.1 the majority of dopant used in CH systems is in the form of mobile molecules in solution. The use of mobile dopants has been linked to poor integration of the two polymer components [35,40,41]. In a PPy-polyacrylamide system designed for electrochemically controlled drug release, the distribution of PPy within the polyacrylamide network was found to be heterogeneous (semi-IPN) [35]. Integration (or penetration of PPy into the polyacrylamide network) of the two polymer components improved with increasing gel mesh size, tending towards a more homogeneous distribution.

This nature of network distribution is archetypal of many reported CH systems that use mobile dopants, with reports of concentrated CP growth at the working electrode interface and at the exterior surfaces of the gels [35,40,41,45,52]. This pore-filling style of growth is indicative of a lack of interaction between the CP and hydrogel. There has been minimal confirmation of totally interpenetrating networks (IPNs) with many reports of poor network integration, which is critical to fully realising the potential of this class of composite. The degree of polymer network integration is dependent upon the fabrication technique, namely the manner in which the CP component is doped [6].

The conventional fabrication route for producing CHs is the electrochemical deposition of the CP component within a preformed hydrogel matrix to create an IPN of the two polymer components, as shown in Figure 11.1. However, several

Table 11.1 Review of conductive hydrogel systems

Hydrogel	CP	Dopant	References
Polyacrylamide	PPy	pTS, $NaNO_3$	[40]
Polyacrylamide	PPy	Potassium persulfate	[35]
Polyacrylate	PPy	$FeCl_3$	[42]
Poly(2-hydroxyethyl methacrylate)	PPy	NaH_2PO_4, KCl	[43]
Poly(hydroxyethylmethacrylate-co-3-sulfopropylmethacrylate)	PPy	Sulfopropyl-methacrylate[a]	[44]
Poly(acrylic acid)	PEDOT	PSS	[31]
Poly(vinyl alcohol)/poly(acrylic acid)	PEDOT	PSS	[32]
Agarose	PEDOT	KNO_3	[45]
Poly(vinyl alcohol)/heparin	PEDOT	Heparin[a]	[6]
Polyacrylamide	PEDOT:PSS (Baytron-P)	Sodium persulfate	[46]
Poly(2-acrylamido-2-methyl propanesulphonic acid)	PANI	HCl	[47]
Poly(acrylic acid)	PANI	Acrylic acid[a], HCl	[48]
PANI-phytic acid	PANI	Phytic acid[a]	[49]
Chitosan	PANI	Ammonium persulfate	[50]
Chitosan	PANI	HCl	[51]

[a]Signifies the dopant molecule was covalently incorporated within the hydrogel network.

other fabrication approaches have been utilised, including the co-polymerisation of both CP and hydrogel components simultaneously, and using the CP itself to form a hydrogel [49]. For a conventional CH, the gel component is covalently or physically crosslinked from an aqueous solution containing the hydrogel monomer/macromer. The gel is then allowed to equilibrate in a CP precursor solution containing the CP monomer and dopant. A galvanostatic or potentiostatic current is then used to electrochemically deposit the CP component within the hydrogel network. Because the dopant in solution is mobile, electrodeposition will tend to be concentrated at the surface of the working electrode where the oxidation potential is highest, resulting in minimal network integration, as illustrated in Figure 11.2. Minimal integration of the polymer networks may negatively affect the performance of the electrodes by increasing the distance between the electrically active surface and the target cells

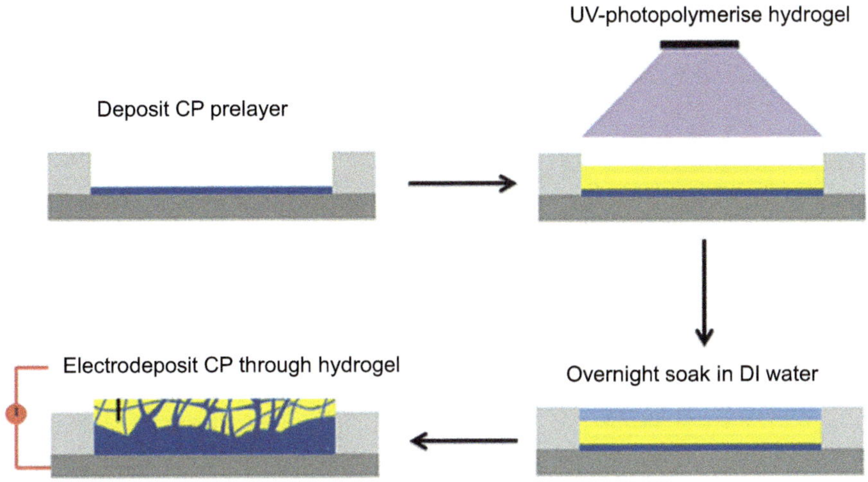

Figure 11.1 Standard fabrication method for conductive hydrogels.
Adapted from Green et al. [27].

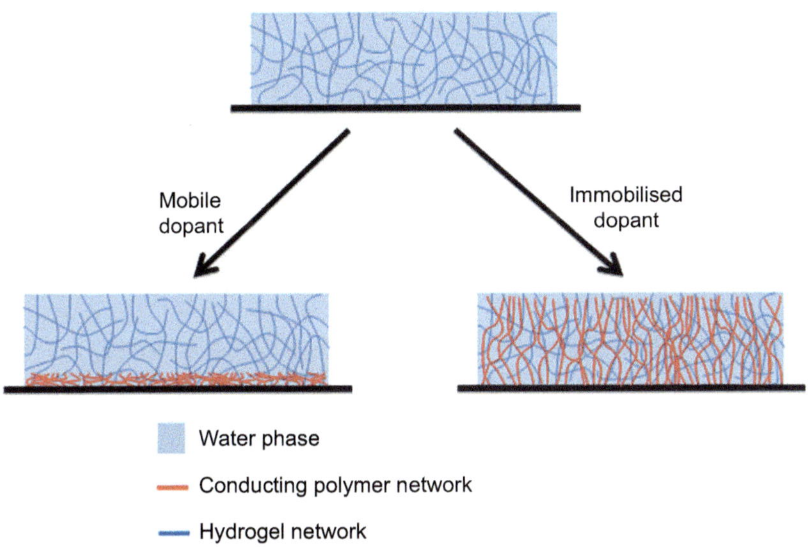

Figure 11.2 The role of dopant mobility in the formation of chapter IPNs.

for stimulation as well as compromising the efficiency of the electrochemical actuation used for controlled drug release.

An approach for encouraging interaction between the two polymer components, and hence the formation of totally IPNs is the use of immobilised dopant, as shown in Figure 11.2. CH systems that utilised immobilised dopant guide the growth of the CP component by covalently incorporating the dopant within the hydrogel network.

Since dopant is required for the growth of the CP, CP growth cannot be concentrated at the working electrode as is the case with the use of mobile dopant. Systems that utilised immobilised dopants have been shown to produce CHs with a high degree of network penetration [16,44,53]. Other approaches used to promote the formation of IPNs include the use of conductive particles or 'pre-polymerised' CP to act as nucleation seeds and ensure homogenous distribution of CP throughout the CH [54].

Early reports of CHs focused on static, nondegradable polymer systems. More recently, the concept of degradable conductive hydrogels (DCHs) has garnered increasing research focus due to their potential for use in nerve-guidance devices and cardiac patches. DCHs are systems in which one or both of the polymer components are degradable under physiological conditions. Conducting polymers are not inherently biodegradable. However, several strategies have been devised to impart erodibility such as the introduction of hydrolysable side-groups to the monomer or the use of CP nanoparticles and short-chain CP oligomers [55,56]. The two most common approaches to creating DCHs are the incorporation of PPy nanoparticles or functionalising the hydrogel component with analine tetramers. PPy nanoparticles, created via microemulsion chemical oxidation techniques, loaded within a poly(D,L-lactide) hydrogel at 5 wt%, resulted in a DCH capable of sustaining a biologically meaningful DC current in physiological conditions for 1000 h [57]. The conductivity of the PPy-poly(D,L-lactide) CH was dependent upon the loading of PPy nanoparticles; increasing the PPy loading from 2 to 9 wt% saw a decrease in sheet resistance from 1.8×10^5 Ω/square down to 60 Ω/square. PPy nanoparticles have also been incorporated within chitosan membranes and scaffolds, showing improved biorecognition, resulting in increased Schwann cell adhesion, spreading and proliferation [58,59]. PPy nanoparticles have also been incorporated within polyurethane elastomers; this is discussed in detail in Section 11.2.2 [60]. Although incorporation of CP nanoparticles successfully imparts conductivity, the nondegradable nature of the nanoparticles and the inability of the kidney to clear them raises concerns over their use in clinical application.

Analine oligomers have also been used to impart electrical conductivity to hydrogels [61–66]. Analine oligomers have been incorporated within several hydrogel systems including polycaprolactone [63], polyglycolide [61], poly(lactide)-poly(ethyleneglycol)-poly(lactide) [64], chitosan [65], gelatin [66] and hemicellulose [62]. As the hydrogel degrades, the oligomers are released; due to their small size they are able to be phagocytosized by macrophages and consequently cleared by the kidneys [67,68]. Increasing oligomer content within the CH has been shown to result in increased conductivity and decreased swelling [62–64]; increasing the analine tetramer content within a chitosan-analine CH from 10 to 30 wt% increased the conductivity from 3×10^{-7} to 3×10^{-5} S/cm and decreased the mass swelling ratio at 24 h from 4 down to 1.3 [69]. The use of CP oligomers to create DCHs, commonly involving a single polymerisation step, overcomes the poor processibility of conventional CHs; however, the resulting DCHs have considerably lower conductivity and charge storage capacities compared to conventional CH systems [56].

There are several routes for incorporation of biological factors within CHs. Biological molecules can be incorporated covalently, through modification of the hydrogel or

CP component [6,53]. Alternatively, factors can be incorporated as mobile dopant or nondopant inclusions [26,53,70,71]. CHs retain the electrochemical actuation abilities of conventional CPs, allowing for the electrochemically controlled release of incorporated mobile factors [35,41]. This will be discussed in more detail in Section 11.3.

CHs provide significant benefits compared to conventional CP coatings. The lower elastic modulus of CH materials more closely resembles that of neural tissue, reducing strain mismatch at the neural interface. Additionally, the open, swollen nature of CH networks confer large loading capacities while retaining electrochemically controlled release properties. CHs present a variety of avenues for the incorporation of biological factors, allowing for modifications that alter the body's response to the implanted CH. DCHs overcome many processing limitations associated with CHs and hold great promise for use in tissue-engineering applications such as nerve-guidance devices and cardiac patches; however, as a class of materials they still face significant challenges such as poor electrochemical performance.

11.2.2 Conductive elastomers

Conductive elastomers (CEs) combine the electrical functionality of CPs with the mechanical robustness and flexibility of elastomeric polymers. CEs most commonly use elastomeric polymers such as polydimethylsiloxane (PDMS) [72–75] and polyurethane (PU) [19,60,76–78]. PDMS and PU make ideal composite constituents due to their high tensile strength, flexural fatigue resistance and long history of use as biomaterials, helping CEs overcome the limitations associated with conventional CP materials relating to processability and brittle fracture [79]. Additionally, the PU/PDMS component is electrically insulating, allowing for the formation of conductive tracks within an insulative bulk material. CEs have potential applications as tissue-engineering scaffolds, flexible electrode arrays, biosensors and in optoelectronics. Several fabrication routes for CEs have been reported including single-step co-polymerisations [60,73,80], chemical [19,77] and/or electrochemical [19,72,74,75] polymerisation of CPs within elastomeric networks and incorporation of CP nanoparticles within elastomeric networks [60,78].

One of the major complications facing the development of CEs is the mismatch in mechanical properties, particularly in elasticity, between the two polymer components [19]. When placed under strain, CEs may experience a decrease in conductivity as percolation falls below critical; at higher strains, the mismatch in properties can result in the mechanical failure of the brittle CP component [19]. Broda et al. investigated the mechanical properties of a PPy-PU CE in which PPy nanoparticles were chemically polymerised within a PU network [60]. The PPy-PU CEs, which had PPy content ranging from 1 to 20 wt%, all experienced approximately a 50% reduction in tensile strength from 30 MPa for PU down to 15 MPa for the CEs. Additionally, increasing PPy content resulted in an increased Young's modulus (8 MPa for PU, 25 MPa for 20 wt% PPy-PU) and decreased breaking elongation (750% for PU, 300% for PPy-PU). Similar trends have been reported in other CE systems [75–77]. Sasaki et al. overcame these limitations through the use of a CE–CH composite [19]. In this study, a PEDOT-PU CE was fabricated by spin coating and

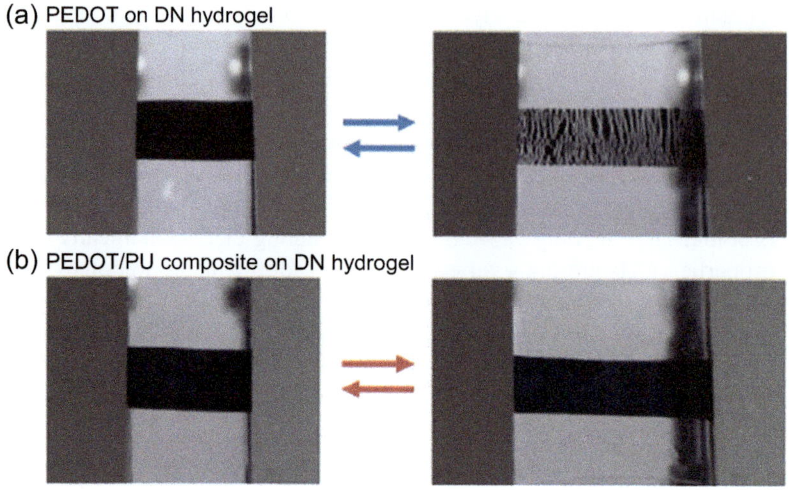

Figure 11.3 Representative images of conducting films at 50% elongation of (a) PEDOT−polyacrylamide composite and (b) PEDOT−PU−polyacrylamide composite. Reproduced with permissions from Sasaki et al., 2014 [19].

thermal treatment of a precursor solution containing EDOT monomer and PU. The PEDOT-PU was then laminated with a polyacrylamide DNs hydrogel followed by electrochemical deposition of PEDOT to bond the PEDOT−PU composite to the hydrogel. The PEDOT−PU−polyacrylamide composite was capable of undergoing strain cycling (refer to Figure 11.3) and autoclaving without significant loss in conductivity or any signs of mechanical failure.

To date, there have been no reports of biosynthetic or bioactive CEs. Owing to the chemical properties of both PU and PDMS, fabrication and processing of CEs typically requires the use of toxic solvents such as tetrahydrofuran and n-heptane [76]. This severely limits the ways in which biological factors could be incorporated within CEs, due to the risk of denaturation. It is the authors' opinion that the most viable routes for incorporation of biological factors include the use of functionalised CPs and post-fabrication modification of CE surfaces. Functionalised CPs, such as carboxylated PEDOT, have been used to incorporate peptides within conventional CP films post-deposition [81]. In a similar fashion, carboxylated PU anionomers could be used to facilitate surface functionalisation with biological molecules [77]. Other potential means to functionalise the surface of CEs include the use of plasma modification such as plasma ion immersion implantation [82,83] as well as more conventional chemical techniques such as surface-initiated atom-transfer radical polymerisation [84−86].

11.2.3 Composite constructs

An alternative approach to the creation of CP-based composites is the fabrication of novel constructs that utilise layered or three-dimensional (3D) forms to fundamentally alter the performance of the base CP component. Examples include bilayered conducting polymers [87–89], nanostructured (nanoporous, nanofibres and nanotubes) CPs [90–92] and polymer brushes [93]. The properties, and hence the potential applications, of these constructs are highly dependent upon their particular 3D structure. Composite constructs have been designed for use as drug-release devices [87,88], neural electrodes [89,93] and nerve guides [90–92].

Bilayered CPs have been used to address limitations with conventional CP coatings for drug release applications. Typically, bilayered CPs will use a conventional CP layer, deposited on top of a bioactive CP layer. The bottom layer acts as a reservoir for an incorporated bioactive compound, while the top layer maintains the electrochemical and mechanical integrity of the coating and regulates the release of bioactive compound from the basal layer. Massoumi et al. utilised a bilayer structure of poly (*N*-methylpyrrole)/polystyrenesulfonate (PSS) on top of a layer of PPy/dexamethasone phosphate to regulate the release of dexamethasone phosphate [88]. The bilayered structure was also found to have significantly increased charge storage capacity compared to a single-layer PPy/dexamethasone phosphate coating.

The structuring of CPs at the nanoscale can have significant impact upon their drug release and electrochemical properties. Kang et al. fabricated a nanoporous PPy/PSS with incorporated nerve growth factor (NGF) by electrodepositing on a substrate coated in polystyrene nanospheres [94]. The beads were removed post-deposition by soaking in tetrahydrofuran, creating a highly regular, open porous network. The nanoporous PPy retained its electrochemical properties, and was capable of releasing significantly higher levels of NGF due to increased permeability of the entrapped NGF.

CP nanofibres and nanotubes have been investigated for use in neural engineering applications such as nerve guides. These constructs are typically fabricated using electrospinning techniques of either the CP component to create a CP nanofibre or of a nonconductive polymer that will act as a template for the deposition of CP nanotubes [90–92,95]. CP nanofibres have been shown to have increased CSC and decreased impedance compared to conventional CP coatings due to the large increase in surface area associated with the creation of nanostructures [7,95]. In vitro testing has also demonstrated the ability of CP nanofibres and nanotubes to support the growth of nerve stem cells and PC12 cells [91,92] and to increase neurite outgrowth in culture with dorsal root ganglia [7,90]. CP nanofibres have also been shown to facilitate neural cell alignment, which allows for the directed growth of neural cells, aiding in the repair of damaged nerves [90].

CP nanotubes have also been designed for use in controlled drug-release devices; Abidian et al. designed a hollow PEDOT nanotube capable of electrochemically controlled release of dexamethasone [95]. To fabricate the PEDOT nanotubes, PEDOT was electrochemically deposited around electrospun fibres of degradable poly(lactide-co-glycolide) loaded with dexamethasone. The inner poly(lactide-co-glycolide) (PLGA) template was then removed by soaking in dichloromethane. The incorporated dexamethasone became trapped within the PEDOT nanotubes and experienced only minimal passive release, while still functioning as an effective electrically controlled release device. In further studies, rather than removing the inner PLGA nanofibres, the nanofibres were encapsulated with an alginate hydrogel prior to electrochemical deposition of PEDOT [96]. The subsequent electrode coating consisted of PEDOT nanotubes within a PEDOT-alginate CH, resulting in a significant improvements in charge storage capacity and impedance while maintaining the drug-release properties of the previous system.

The conventional fabrication methods involved in CHs are incapable of producing thin (submircron), strongly adhered coatings. Baek et al. developed a process that enables the fabrication of submicron thickness, hydrophilic, electroactive coatings using surface-initiated atom-transfer radical polymerisation [93]. To fabricate the composite, hydrophilic polymer brushes of poly(2-hydroxyethyl methacrylate) were covalently bound to a gold electrode substrate. PEDOT was then electrochemically deposited around the brushes. The synergistic incorporation of polymer brushes with PEDOT resulted in high charge storage capacity and was found to increase neurite density in culture with PC12 cells. Baek et al. suggests that this technique could form the basis for a new approach to creating biosynthetic CHs, through the use of biological polymer brushes such as amino acids to impart desired bioactivity to the composite coating.

The studies discussed primarily focused on the development of purely synthetic constructs that use hydrophilic polymers in conjunction with CPs. However, unlike CHs there is no integration at the molecular level, but rather regions of bulk CP combined with regions of hydrophilic polymer. Owing to the ease of functionalisation of hydrogels with biological compounds, such as drugs, peptides and proteins, these systems can easily be used in the creation of biosynthetic composites.

11.3 Biological components in CP composites

CP-based materials have been extensively explored for application to implantable electrodes and nerve guides, with more recent applications including cardiac patches and tissue engineering. In all of these applications it is desirable to preserve and support the growth of tissues surrounding the implant. As a result, there have been several studies that explore the delivery of therapeutics to promote tissue interaction [53,97], cellular regeneration [5,11,98] and downregulate inflammation [26,95,99]. Composites have the advantage of being able to incorporate higher amounts of biologicals within polymer systems that are not restricted by the inelastic CP matrix. Additionally, through careful polymer design and fabrication, multiple therapeutic effects can be imparted to the same material [53]. Fabrication choices are largely dictated by the structure of the biological component and whether fixed or mobile presentation of the biomolecule is desired.

11.3.1 Bound biological components

Biomolecules that do not require uptake by cells to enact a biological response can be incorporated into CP composites such that they are presented at the material surface, but not released into the tissue environment. This approach is usually used when cell attachment and tissue integration with a device is desired. Many CPs and CP composites have incorporated cell-attachment proteins that provide a supporting matrix for neural tissues [1,14,15,53]. In homogenous CPs, peptides containing cell attachment sequences such as RGD, YIGSR and YFQRYLI have been incorporated during fabrication as doping molecules [1,100]. This enables them to be included as a component of the polymer system, ionically interacting with the CP backbone. While small synthetic dopants have been shown to have mobility within a CP matrix and can exchange during electrical cycling for other locally available ions, the relatively large size of peptides renders them immobile [1,89]. As a consequence, this approach enables presentation of a stable, long-term bioactive interface. However, it has been shown that in homogenous CPs, the large size of these peptides (up to 12 amino acids) negatively impacts on the mechanical stability of the material [1,5]. When a hydrogel, CNT or elastomer is used to create a composite, this issue can be ameliorated.

Researchers have shown that hydrogels in particular provide many options for engineering tailored solutions for long-term bioactivity in CP composites. The most common way in which biological polymers have been integrated with CPs has been through simple blends. There are several biopolymers, derived from either plant or animal, which have hydrogel properties including collagen, glucomannan, agarose and alginate [17,45,101]. These physical gels have be used as scaffolds in which CPs have been directly polymerised to produce fibrillar constructs [17,18]. Studies by Kim et al. [17] demonstrated that this approach produced composite CPs with substantial improvements in electrical and mechanical properties over homogenous CPs. Sekine et al. [45] and Ido et al. [101] produced flexible patterned tracks of CP within hydrogels. Both studies demonstrated that electroactive cells attached to these biological polymers, but specific activity was not explored [45].

In all of these studies it was necessary to incorporate a mobile dopant during CP polymerisation. As a result, the CP formed at the underlying electrode and had limited penetration into the hydrogel layer [45]. To improve integration and maintain control over composite properties, studies by Green et al. [6] and Cheong et al. [53] have shown that biomolecules including proteins can be covalently linked into a synthetic hydrogel. These proteins were subsequently used to dope the CP component, which was grown through the hydrogel to produce interpenetrating networks of CP and hydrogel or CHs [6].

A number of bioactive proteins have been incorporated using hydrogel polymer crosslinking mechanisms. Heparin, gelatin and sericin have been incorporated within PVA and used to dope PEDOT [6,16,53]. These molecules were shown to provide growth factor presentation, cell attachment and antioxidant capacity, respectively. Combinations of these materials were used and shown to have the activity of each of the component proteins [53]. It is important to note that these molecules are whole proteins, demonstrating that much larger molecules can be incorporated into CP composites than homogenous CPs without detriment to the mechanical properties [6]. However, to achieve crosslinking, the protein required modification to attach methacrylate functional groups that enabled incorporation by photopolymerisation during PVA hydrogel fabrication. It is a clear constraint in the development of biosynthetic CP hybrids, that the biopolymers used to impart bioactivity to materials are limited to those that are compatible with specific polymer synthesis processes. Future approaches in this area may address the challenge of incorporating a wider range of proteins through synthesis without protein modification.

An alternate approach is to surface-modify the composite, which has been a popular approach in the development of biosensors and nerve guides. This technique uses chemical modifiers to produce ionic or covalent bonds between the CP composite and biomolecule. It has been used to present enzymes, growth factors and other proteins to the biological environment [11,102]. Composites of CPs and carbon nanotubes (CNTs) have been used to improve the sensitivity and accuracy of glucose and hydrogen peroxide sensors [103]. To form effective devices, these coatings must present enzymes to the biological environment. Immobilisation of enzymes onto homogenous CPs requires modification of the CP monomer [98], which can be complex and interfere with the electrical and mechanical properties of the CP [11]. A number of chemical modifications have been made to CNTs in particular through use of carboxylated CNTs, which enable more simplistic immobilisation of complex biomolecules without impacting on material properties. Gomez and Schmidt have also demonstrated that polyelectrolytes can be used to immobilise growth factors to the surface of CP composites. It was shown that polyallylamine (PAA) could be photochemically conjugated with NGF and used to produce a covalently bound composite with PPy, shown in Figure 11.4. This composite was shown to effectively guide the outgrowth of neuronal processes along a patterned material.

It is clear that there are multiple mechanisms through which biological components can be immobilised within CP composites. The presence of not only the CP but additional polymers or other components widens the array of potential routes through

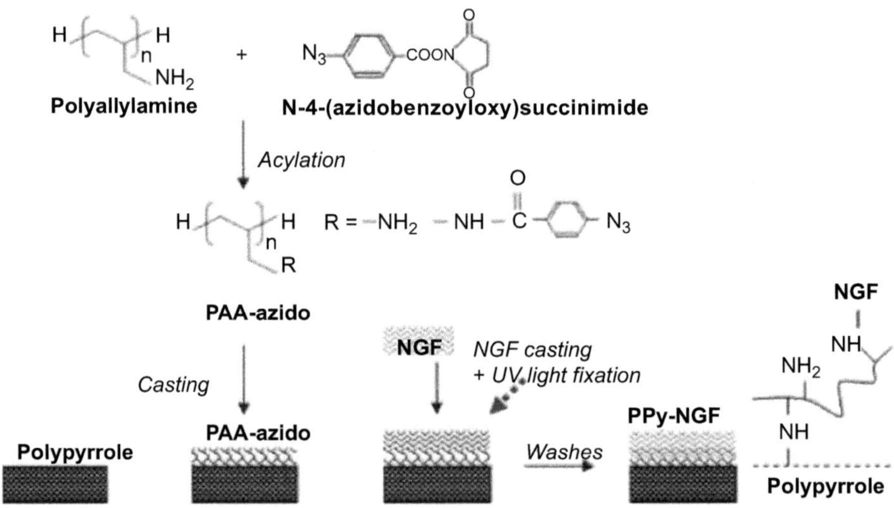

Figure 11.4 Scheme of the NGF immobilisation process. PAA was conjugated to an azido compound (PAA-azido). This conjugate was cast twice on PPy, followed by casting of NGF. UV light exposure promoted the formation of covalent bonds via the azido groups, immobilising NGF to PPy.

Reproduced with permission from Ref. [11].

which conjugation, bonding and formation of polymer networks can be explored. While several systems have been demonstrated, it is clear that there remains a scope for combining a greater array of polymers and biomolecules with CPs. The major challenge in this area is finding systems of nonconductive polymers, CPs and biological polymers that have fabrication and solvent compatibility.

11.3.2 Mobile biologics

Where biologics require uptake by cells, it is necessary that they are first constrained within the polymer matrix or at the surface and then released once in contact with the biological environment. In homogenous CPs, a number of active agents have been explored for cellular regeneration [5,104] and regulation of inflammatory reactions [105]. The most common molecules explored have been growth factors including NGF and brain derived neurotrophic factor (BDNF) [5,104,106], and anti-inflammatories such as dexamethasone and valproic acid [99,105,107]. There are two mechanisms by which mobile factors have been incorporated within CPs: (1) by addition as a dopant, which can be driven out electrically in situ [99,107]; and (2) as an inclusion that is trapped within the matrix during polymerisation and then passively delivered to the tissue by diffusion [5,106,108]. Regardless of the method of incorporation, the mobility of these relatively large reagents has been found to be substantially restricted within the CP matrix [105]. Studies have shown that not only is it difficult to incorporate therapeutic amounts of these biomolecules within a CP, but the mobility required for delivery is also very limited [105,107]. This usually results in very short periods during which the drug is available, and hence has a very limited therapeutic effect [106]. Composites that can incorporate mobile therapeutics, in particular hydrogels, offer a greater range of mechanisms for incorporation of reagents and also present more controlled techniques for delivery. Biological polymers have been incorporated within CP composites through simple entrapment during fabrication, post-fabrication loading of polymers with water-soluble drugs and as a component of a degradable polymer. Two mechanisms have been used to electrically mediate release of mobile biologics from CP composites: (1) electromotive force and (2) electromechanical actuation.

High drug-loading efficiencies and controlled electrical delivery of therapeutics have been demonstrated in CP–hydrogel composites. Tsai et al. [26] entrapped the anti-inflammatory indomethacin in a PVA–PANI composite and found that 65–70% of the drug (provided at 10 mg/mL) was initially loaded within the material [26]. This system offered multiple release mechanisms as the hydrogel component was degradable and electrical cycling of the PANI component actively released the drug through electromotive force. It was shown that drug release could be varied from 12 to 100 h depending on the applied electrical potential, in line with typical therapeutic doses [26]. While complex, this system enabled ratcheting of the therapeutic delivery through control of not only the material properties but also the environment and active release mechanisms. It was shown that contributing factors to the delivery rate of the anti-inflammatory included the degree of PVA crosslinking, the polymeric ratio (PVA: PANI), drug content and the applied electrical potential. However, it should also be noted that high electrical potentials over 1.2 V increased the rate of composite degradation through hydrolysis.

In a CP nanotube composite developed by Abidian et al. [95], it was shown that therapeutic amounts of dexamethasone could be incorporated and delivered in a controlled manner through electro-actuation. In this concept, the dexamethasone was entrapped within a degradable PLGA hydrogel that was electrospun on the surface of a metallic electrode. The spun fibres were then coated with PEDOT through electrodeposition to produce PEDOT nanotubes with drug-loaded hydrogel cores [95]. When diffusion alone was used to deliver the dexamethasone, only 25% of the loaded drug was released after 54 days in a simulated biological environment. Addition of a stimulating voltage resulted in hydrodynamic forces inside the nanotubes, result in expulsion of PLGA degradation products simultaneously with the entrapped dexamethasone. This was shown to significantly increase drug release with each additional stimulation, as shown in Figure 11.5. It was proposed that the dexamethasone was expulsed through the ends of PEDOT nanotubes or through cracks on the surface of the nanotubes created by actuation.

While the use of active CP release mechanisms can enable additional modes of control in these materials, it is also possible for passive release mechanisms to be used. Passive release has advantages in systems that are not actively connected to electrical devices, such as nerve guide scaffolds and cardiac patches. Cheong et al. [53] have shown that NGF can be incorporated with CHs at levels capable of producing neural cell differentiation in vitro. In these studies, it was proposed that the biosynthetic hydrogel PVA-heparin was capable of not only constraining and delivering the NGF, but the covalently bound heparin component may have actively presented the growth factor to the neural cells. While several other polymer systems have been shown to passively degrade and deliver therapeutics at rates controlled through polymer crosslinking, polymer percentages and drug loading [109–111], there is minimal literature combining these with CP approaches. It is expected that future work in drug delivery from CP composites will focus on combining these existing polymer technologies with CPs.

11.4 In vivo application of CP composites

CP composites were first explored in the early 1990s [112,113] and gained greater traction as interest in their potential increased over the successive decades. As a result, several studies investigating functionality and biocompatibility of these materials have been conducted in vitro. This has enabled a greater understanding of CP interactions with specific cells types and design of materials with optimised physicochemical properties. However, it is intended that CP composites augment the performance of medical devices, with a significant focus being on implantable devices. While several studies have investigated the impact of implanting composites of CPs and hydrogels, the approach taken has varied greatly. There is inconsistency in both placement and implant duration of materials between different studies, which prevents commensurate

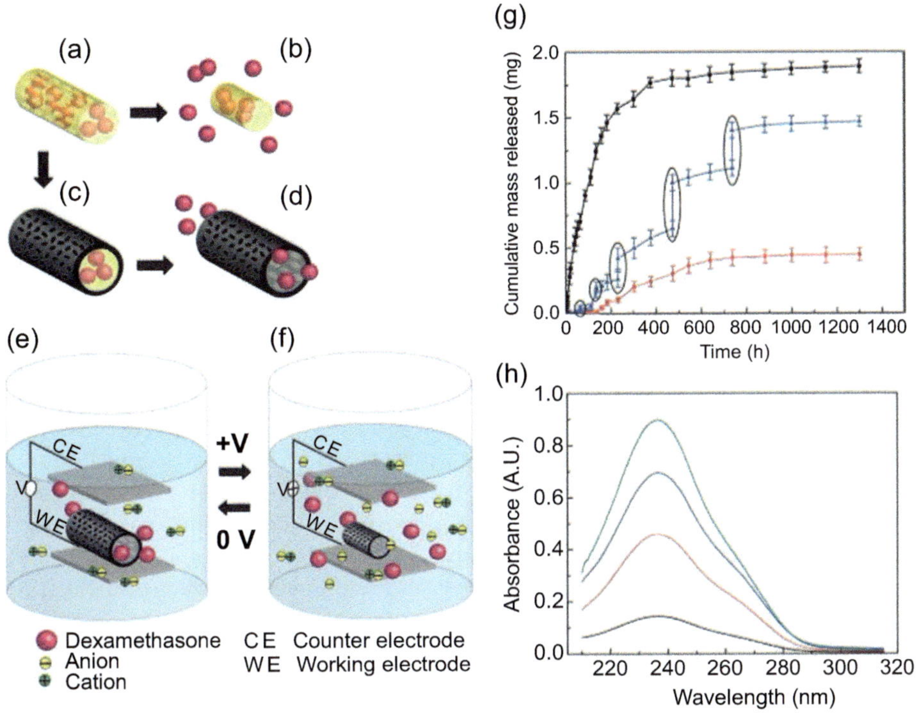

Figure 11.5 Schematic illustration of the controlled release of dexamethasone. (a) Dexamethasone-loaded electrospun PLGA. (b) Hydrolytic degradation of PLGA fibres, leading to release of the drug. (c) Electrochemical deposition of PEDOT around the dexamethasone-loaded electrospun PLGA fibre. (d) This deposition slows down the release of dexamethasone. (e) PEDOT nanotubes in a neutral electrical condition. (f) External electrical stimulation controls the release of dexamethasone from the PEDOT nanotubes due to contraction or expansion of the PEDOT. By applying a positive voltage, electrons are injected into the chains and positive charges in the polymer chains are compensated. To maintain overall charge neutrality, counter-ions are expelled towards the solution and the nanotubes contract. This shrinkage causes the drugs to come out of the ends of tubes. (g) Cumulative mass release of dexamethasone from: PLGA nanoscale fibres (black squares), PEDOT-coated PLGA nanoscale fibres (red circles) without electrical stimulation and PEDOT-coated PLGA nanoscale fibres with electrical stimulation of 1 V applied at the five specific times indicated by the circled data points (blue triangles). (h) UV absorption of dexamethasone-loaded PEDOT nanotubes after 16 h (black), 87 h (red), 160 h (blue) and 730 h (green). The UV spectra of dexamethasone have peaks at a wavelength of 237 nm. (Data are shown with a ± standard deviation; $n = 15$ for each case.) Reproduced with permission from Ref. [95].

literature analysis. The few in vivo studies that have been conducted on CP composites have sought to establish functional efficacy in stimulating devices, efficacy in recording devices and compatibility in tissue-engineered devices.

An assessment of functionality in neural-stimulating devices was conducted by Chikar et al. [100]. In this study, a cochlear implant coating was designed to improve electrical properties and encourage neural regeneration at the device interface. A simplified single electrode array was produced with a layered coating of PEDOT on platinum, which was then dip coated with RGD-functionalised alginate. In some samples the hydrogel coating was also functionalised through loading with BDNF. These electrodes were implanted in the cochlea of four guinea pigs for up to 200 days. All coated devices demonstrated reduced impedance over the implant period compared to uncoated controls. However, despite finding that at 2 weeks the BDNF levels were increased in the perilymph fluid of guinea pigs where BDNF had been incorporated in the coating, there was no significant difference in auditory nerve survival over the implant period. Histology of the implant site and measures of fibrotic encapsulation were not reported in this study.

In a study that sought to establish functionality of CP—hydrogel composites as recording electrodes, Kim et al. [18] implanted PEDOT-alginate coated arrays within the auditory cortex of guinea pigs. There was a clear relationship found between hydrogel thickness and function. Importantly, it was noted that when the hydrogel coating exceeded 30 μm there was a significant drop in both signal-to-noise ratio and detectable units recorded from neural cells. It was proposed that the swelling of the hydrogel component impacted on the proximity of neural tissue, with thicker gels having a more significant impact on function of the device. These studies were conducted across acute time frames and a result did not look at inflammation or other time-dependent cell responses. Ultimately, this study suggested that the utility of CP—hydrogel composites would be largely dependent on the impact of stress and deformation of neural tissues resulting from reswelling of polymer constituents [18].

The potential for inflammatory reactions from CP-composite membranes was investigated by Wang et al. [114]. In this study, PPy/poly(D,L-lactide) (PDLLA) composite and PPy-coated poly(D,L-lactide-co-glycolide) membranes were implanted subcutaneously in rats for up to 4 months. Histology and enzyme analysis at the site was conducted to ascertain the biological response to samples at acute and chronic time points, with chronic reactions shown in Figure 11.6. Each material component was tested individually and in combination, with all samples having mild inflammatory reactions at the 4-month chronic-term time point [114]. This study demonstrates that CP composites have potential as implantable materials. However, it should be noted that the composite used in this study contained degradable elements that are known to be metabolised and cleared from the body. The PPy component was not degraded and remained at the termination of the study. It is likely that alternate polymer combinations will have differing results, and each combination will require in vivo study to investigate tissue reactions.

The few studies that have explored CP composite performance in vivo indicate that while these materials are not toxic, there is scope to further improve performance through control of material properties and form. It is also necessary that future studies look to analyze not only implant functionality but also histology and impacts on tissues. Ideally, these studies should be conducted in the same tissue in which the final device is intended to operate, to more accurately depict specific cell responses. As the variety and scope of CP composites continue to grow, it will be important to perform comparative studies that enable systematic and accurate assessment of material performance.

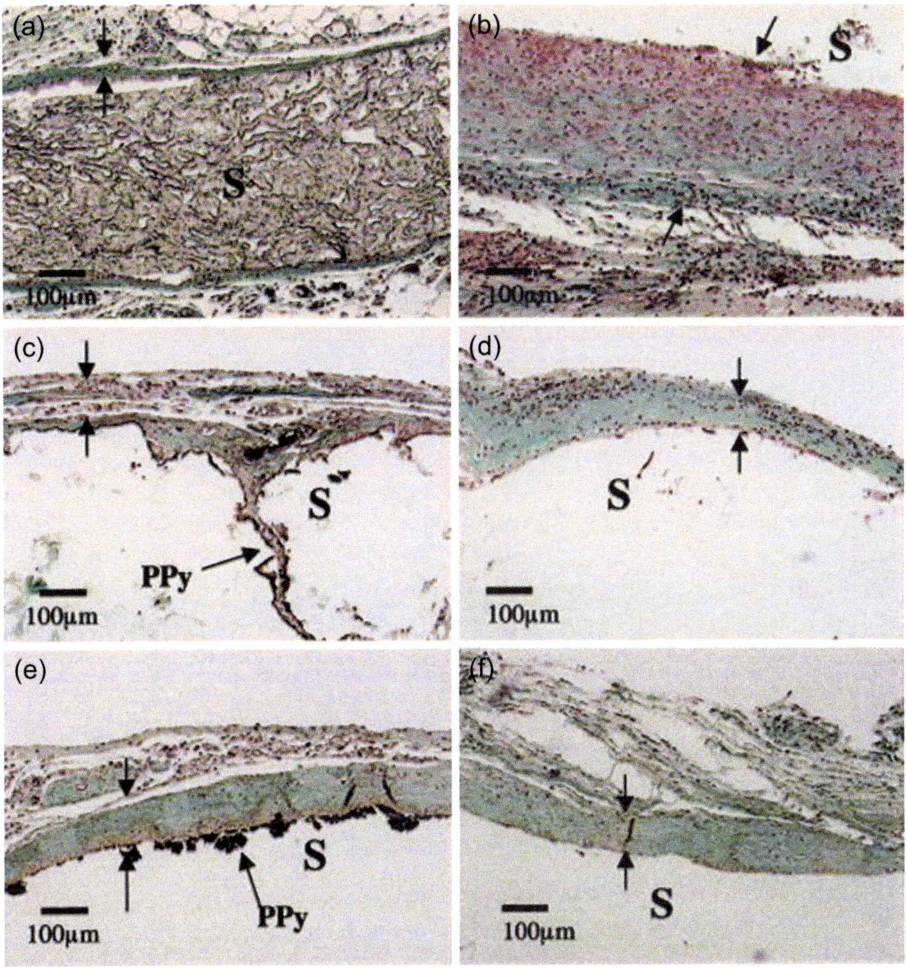

Figure 11.6 Masson's trichrome-stained samples explanted at 60 days, showing by arrows the thin dense capsules associated with the ePTFE and the biodegradable membranes, and the thick dense capsule surrounding the rubber membrane. (a) ePTFE. (b) Rubber. (c) PPy-coated DLPLG. (d) DLPLG. (e) PPy/PDLLA. (f) PDLLA composite. (S, sample side.) Reproduced with permission from Ref. [114].

11.5 Summary and future directions

Conductive composites based on CPs have enabled the development of a range of materials for biomedical applications that can be tailored to improve material properties critical to long-term performance of implantable devices. Nonconductive polymers can be used to impart tailored presentation of biomolecules and improve the brittle mechanical properties of CPs. Additionally, CPs have been used to successfully impart conductivity to hydrogel and elastomeric polymers. While there have been significant challenges in producing interpenetrating networks of CPs, several approaches have yielded materials with bulk characteristics that indicate the presence of each of the component polymers. True interpenetrating networks, such as DNs, where one network is a CP have not yet been realised; however, it is expected that IPNs would provide optimal materials with the highest electroactivity.

While in vitro testing has been used extensively to probe cytocompatiblity, there is a clear need for translational studies that demonstrate both safety and efficacy in the in vivo environment. This is particularly important to demonstrate that the polymers being blended with CPs are successfully mediating the mechanical properties, translating into a reduction in scar tissue formation at the device interface. Additionally, the incorporation of biomolecules used to drive cell interactions with tissues needs to be assessed across chronic time frames within the biological environment where multiple cell types are present.

While composite CPs have been shown to improve the properties of homogenous CPs and used to coat metal electrodes, their development as stand-alone materials could provide new and flexible ways of fabricating fully polymeric devices. It is expected that future directions in CP technologies will yield new techniques of creating devices that are printed, with both insulating and conductive components produced in a single run. These fully polymeric devices will also provide a platform technology for producing devices in which cells can be incorporated during printing, to provide functional biological interfaces.

References

[1] R.A. Green, N.H. Lovell, L.A. Poole-Warren, Biomaterials 30 (2009) 3637.

[2] R.T. Hassarati, J.A. Goding, S. Baek, A.J. Patton, L.A. Poole-Warren, R.A. Green, J. Polym. Sci. B Polym. Phys. 52 (2014) 666.

[3] S. Venkatraman, J. Hendricks, Z.A. King, A.J. Sereno, S. Richardson-Burns, D. Martin, J.M. Carmena, IEEE Trans. Neural Syst. Rehabil. Eng. 19 (2011) 307.

[4] A.L. Kip, B.L. Nicholas, D.J. Mike, M.R.-B. Sarah, L.H. Jeffrey, R.K. Daryl, J. Neural Eng. 8 (2011) 14001.

[5] R.A. Green, N.H. Lovell, L.A Poole-Warren, Acta Biomater. 6 (2010) 63.

[6] R.A. Green, R.T. Hassarati, J.A Goding, S. Baek, N.H. Lovell, P.J. Martens, L.A. Poole-Warren, Macromol. Biosci. 12 (2012) 494.

[7] M.R. Abidian, J.M. Corey, D.R. Kipke, D.C. Martin, Small 6 (2010) 421.

[8] R.A. Green, R.T. Hassarati, L. Bouchinet, C.S. Lee, G.L.M.M. Cheong, J.F. Yu, C.W. Dodds, G.J. Suaning, L.A. Poole-Warren, N.H. Lovell, Biomaterials 33 (2012) 5875.

[9] A.S. Widge, M. Jeffries-El, X. Cui, C.F. Lagenaur, Y. Matsuoka, Biosens. Bioelectron. 22 (2007) 1723.

[10] D.H. Kim, S.M. Richardson-Burns, J.L. Hendricks, C. Sequera, D.C. Martin, Adv. Funct. Mater. 17 (2006) 1.

[11] N. Gomez, C.E. Schmidt, J. Biom. Mater. Res. A 81A (2007) 135.

[12] X. Cui, V.A. Lee, Y. Raphael, J.A. Wiler, J.F. Hetke, D.J. Anderson, D.C. Martin, J. Biomed. Mater. Res. 56 (2001) 261.

[13] K.A. Ludwig, J.D. Uram, J. Yang, D.C. Martin, D.R. Kipke, J. Neural Eng. 3 (2006) 59.
[14] W.R. Stauffer, X.T. Cui, Biomaterials 27 (2006) 2405.
[15] X. Cui, J. Wiler, M. Dzaman, R.A. Altschuler, D.C. Martin, Biomaterials 24 (2003) 777.
[16] R.T. Hassarati, W.F. Dueck, C. Tasche, P.M. Carter, L.A. Poole-Warren, R.A. Green, IEEE Trans. Neural Syst. Rehabil. Eng. 22 (2014) 411.
[17] D.H. Kim, M. Abidan, D.C. Martin, J. Biomed. Mater. Res. 71 (2004) 577.
[18] D.-H. Kim, J.A. Wiler, D.J. Anderson, D.R. Kipke, D.C. Martin, Acta Biomater. 6 (2010) 57.
[19] M. Sasaki, B.C. Karikkineth, K. Nagamine, H. Kaji, K. Torimitsu, M. Nishizawa, Adv. Healthc. Mater. 3 (2014) 1919.
[20] R.A. Green, C.M. Williams, N.H. Lovell, L.A Poole-Warren, J. Mater. Sci. Mater. Med. 19 (2008) 1625.
[21] N.G. Sahoo, Y.C. Jung, H.H. So, J.W. Cho, Synth. Met. 157 (2007) 374.
[22] X.L. Cui, M.H. Engelhard, Y.H. Lin, J. Nanosci. Nanotechnol. 6 (2006) 547.
[23] M.R. Abidian, D.C. Martin, Biomaterials 29 (2008) 1273.
[24] M. Seki, M. Shibata, T. Kobayashi, R. Yosomiya, Polym. Polym. Compos. 5 (1997) 337.
[25] T.S. Hansen, K. West, O. Hassager, N.B. Larsen, Adv. Funct. Mater. 17 (2007) 3069.
[26] T.-S. Tsai, V. Pillay, Y.E. Choonara, L.C. du Toit, G. Modi, D. Naidoo, P. Kumar, Polymers (Basel) 3 (2011) 150.
[27] R.a Green, S. Baek, L.a Poole-Warren, P.J. Martens, Sci. Technol. Adv. Mater. 11 (2010) 014107.
[28] K.S. Anseth, C.N. Bowman, L. Brannon-Peppas, Biomaterials 17 (1996) 1647.
[29] P. Martens, J. Blundo, A. Nilasaroya, R.A. Odell, J. Cooper-white, L.A. Poole-warren, 37 (2007) 2641.
[30] T. Dai, X. Qing, H. Zhou, C. Shen, J. Wang, Y. Lu, Synth. Met 160 (2010) 791.
[31] T. Dai, X. Qing, Y. Lu, Y. Xia, Polymer (Guildf) 50 (2009) 5236.
[32] Y. Lu, Y. Li, J. Pan, P. Wei, N. Liu, B. Wu, J. Cheng, C. Lu, L. Wang, Biomaterials 33 (2012) 378.
[33] J. Goding, L. Poole-Warren, R. Green, P. Martens, Ther. Deliv. 3 (2012) 1.
[34] J. Goding, L. Poole-Warren, P. Martens, R. Green, in: D.W. Hutmacher, W. Chrzanowski (Eds.), Biointerfaces Where Material Meets Biology, Royal Society of Chemistry, 2014, pp. 192–220.
[35] R.C. Barthus, L.M. Lira, S.I.C. De Torresi, 19 (2008) 630.
[36] J.M. Fonner, L. Forciniti, H. Nguyen, J.D. Byrne, Y.-F. Kou, J. Syeda-Nawaz, C.E. Schmidt, Biomed. Mater. 3 (2008) 034124.
[37] P.M. George, A.W. Lyckman, D.A. LaVan, A. Hegde, Y. Leung, R. Avasare, C. Testa, P.M. Alexander, R. Langer, M. Sur, Biomaterials 26 (2005) 3511.
[38] R. Balint, N.J. Cassidy, S.H. Cartmell, Acta Biomater. 10 (2014) 2341.
[39] N.K. Guimard, N. Gomez, C.E. Schmidt, Prog. Polym. Sci. 32 (2007) 876.
[40] B.C. Kim, G.M. Spinks, G.G. Wallace, R. John, Polymer, 41 (2000) 1783–1790.
[41] L.M. Lira, S.I. Córdoba de Torresi, Electrochem. Commun. 7 (2005) 717.
[42] J. Lin, Q. Tang, J. Wu, Q. Li, Journal of Applied Polymer Science, 116 (3) (2010) 1376–1383.
[43] S. Brahim, A. Guiseppi-Elie, Electroanalysis 17 (2005) 556.
[44] G. Justin, A. Guiseppi-Elie, Biomacromolecules 10 (2009) 2539.
[45] S. Sekine, Y. Ido, T. Miyake, K. Nagamine, M. Nishizawa, J. Am. Chem. Soc. 132 (2010) 13174.
[46] F.A. Aouada, M.R. Guilherme, G.M. Campese, E.M. Girotto, A.F. Rubira, E.C. Muniz, Polym. Test 25 (2006) 158.

[47] S.K. Siddhanta, R. Gangopadhyay, Polymer (Guildf) 46 (2005) 2993.
[48] Y. Xia, H. Zhu, Soft Matter 7 (2011) 9388.
[49] L. Pan, G. Yu, D. Zhai, H.R. Lee, W. Zhao, N. Liu, H. Wang, B.C.-K. Tee, Y. Shi, Y. Cui, Z. Bao, Proc. Natl Acad. Sci. U.S.A. 109 (2012) 9287.
[50] Y.A. Ismail, J. Chang, S.R. Shin, R.S. Mane, S.-H. Han, S.J. Kim, J. Electrochem. Soc. 156 (2009) A313.
[51] A. Tiwari, S. Gong, Electroanalysis 20 (2008) 1775.
[52] Y. Lu, D. Wang, T. Li, X. Zhao, Y. Cao, H. Yang, Y.Y. Duan, Biomaterials 30 (2009) 4143.
[53] G.L. Mario Cheong, K.S. Lim, A. Jakubowicz, P.J. Martens, L.A. Poole-Warren, R.A. Green, Acta Biomater. 10 (2014) 1216.
[54] A.J. Patton, R.A. Green, L.A. Poole-Warren, APL Mater, 31 (2015) 014912.
[55] M.R. Abidian, E.D. Daneshvar, B.M. Egeland, D.R. Kipke, P.S. Cederna, M.G. Urbanchek, Adv. Healthc. Mater. 1 (2012) 762.
[56] B. Guo, L. Glavas, A.-C. Albertsson, Prog. Polym. Sci. 38 (2013) 1263.
[57] G. Shi, M. Rouabhia, Z. Wang, L.H. Dao, Z. Zhang, Biomaterials 25 (2004) 2477.
[58] J. Huang, X. Hu, L. Lu, Z. Ye, Q. Zhang, Z. Luo, J. Biomed. Mater. Res. A 93 (2010) 164.
[59] Y. Wan, H. Wu, D. Wen, Macromol. Biosci. 4 (2004) 882.
[60] C.R. Broda, J.Y. Lee, S. Sirivisoot, C.E. Schmidt, B.S. Harrison, J. Biomed. Mater. Res. A 98 (2011) 509.
[61] C. Ding, Y. Wang, S. Zhang, Eur. Polym. J. 43 (2007) 4244.
[62] W. Zhao, L. Glavas, K. Odelius, U. Edlund, A.-C. Albertsson, Polymer (Guildf) 55 (2014) 2967.
[63] B. Guo, A. Finne-Wistrand, A.-C. Albertsson, J. Polym. Sci. A Polym. Chem. 49 (2011) 2097.
[64] B. Guo, A. Finne-Wistrand, A.-C. Albertsson, Chem. Mater. 23 (2011) 1254.
[65] B. Guo, A. Finne-Wistrand, A.-C. Albertsson, Biomacromolecules 12 (2011) 2601.
[66] Y. Liu, J. Hu, X. Zhuang, P. Zhang, Y. Wei, X. Wang, X. Chen, Macromol. Biosci. 12 (2012) 241.
[67] N. Nasongkla, B. Chen, N. Macaraeg, M.E. Fox, J.M.J. Fréchet, F.C. Szoka, J. Am. Chem. Soc. 131 (2009) 3842.
[68] T.J. Rivers, T.W. Hudson, C.E. Schmidt, Adv. Funct. Mater. 12 (2002) 33.
[69] J. Han, L. Wang, R. Guo, Macromol. Rapid Commun. 32 (2011) 729.
[70] P. Chansai, A. Sirivat, S. Niamlang, D. Chotpattananont, K. Viravaidya-Pasuwat, Int. J. Pharm. 381 (2009) 25.
[71] Y. Li, K.G. Neoh, E.T. Kang, J. Biomed, Mater. Res. A 73 (2005) 171.
[72] R. Ofek Almog, H. Ben-Yoav, Y. Sverdlov, T. Shmilovich, S. Krylov, Y. Shacham-Diamand, J. Mol. Opt. Phys. 2012 (2012) 1.
[73] B. Ustamehmetoğlu, N. Kızılcan, Ö. Demir, Pigment Resin Technol. 41 (2012) 179.
[74] M. Yasuzawa, S. Inoue, S. Imai, Int. J. Mod. Phys. B 17 (2003) 1217.
[75] G. Cakmak, Z. Kucukyavuz, S. Kucukyavuz, J. Appl. Polym. Sci. 93 (2004) 736.
[76] H. Deligöz, B. Tieke, Macromol. Mater. Eng. 291 (2006) 793.
[77] G. Robila, I. Diaconu, T. Buruiana, E. Buruiana, P. Coman, J. Appl. Polym. Sci. 75 (2000) 1385.
[78] F. Keohan, X.F. Wei, A. Wongsarnpigoon, E. Lazaro, J.E. Darga, W.M. Grill, J. Biomater. Sci. Polym. Ed. 18 (2007) 1057.
[79] Q. Chen, S. Liang, G.A. Thouas, Prog. Polym. Sci. 38 (2013) 584.

[80] N. Kızılcan, N.K. Öz, B. Ustamehmetoğlu, A. Akar, Eur. Polym. J. 42 (2006) 2361.
[81] L.K. Povlich, J.C. Cho, M.K. Leach, J.M. Corey, J. Kim, D.C. Martin, Biochim. Biophys. Acta 1830 (2013) 4288.
[82] M.M. Bilek, D.R. McKenzie, Biophys. Rev. 2 (2010) 55.
[83] J. Wang, P. Yang, H. Sun, J.Y. Chen, Y.X. Leng, G.J. Wan, N. Huang, in: 30th International Conference. Plasma Science 2003. ICOPS 2003, IEEE Conference Record - Abstracts, IEEE, 2003, p. 282.
[84] Z. Zhang, J. Wang, Q. Tu, N. Nie, J. Sha, W. Liu, R. Liu, Y. Zhang, J. Wang, Colloids Surf. B. Biointerfaces 88 (2011) 85.
[85] F.J. Xu, Z.H. Wang, W.T. Yang, Biomaterials 31 (2010) 3139.
[86] C. Lu, N. Zhou, D. Xu, Y. Tang, S. Jin, Y. Wu, J. Shen, Appl. Surf. Sci. 258 (2011) 618.
[87] B. Massoumi, A. Entezami, Eur. Polym. J. 37 (2001) 1015.
[88] B. Massoumi, A. Entezami, J. Bioact. Compat. Polym. 17 (2002) 51.
[89] J.H. Collier, J.P. Camp, T.W. Hudson, C.E. Schmidt, J. Biomed. Mater. Res. 50 (2000) 574.
[90] J. Xie, M.R. Macewan, S.M. Willerth, X. Li, D.W. Moran, S.E. Sakiyama-Elbert, Y. Xia, Adv. Funct. Mater. 19 (2009) 2312.
[91] Y. Liu, X. Liu, J. Chen, K.J. Gilmore, G.G. Wallace, Chem. Commun. (Camb) (2008) 3729.
[92] L. Ghasemi-Mobarakeh, M.P. Prabhakaran, M. Morshed, M.H. Nasr-Esfahani, S. Ramakrishna, Biomaterials 29 (34) (2008) 4532–4539.
[93] S. Baek, R. Green, A. Granville, P. Martens, L. Poole-Warren, J. Mater. Chem. B 1 (2013) 3803.
[94] G. Kang, R. Ben Borgens, Y. Cho, Langmuir 27 (2011) 6179.
[95] M.R. Abidian, D.-H.H. Kim, D.C. Martin, Adv. Mater. 18 (2006) 405.
[96] M.R. Abidian, D.C. Martin, Adv. Funct. Mater. 19 (2009) 573.
[97] M. Nishizawa, T. Kamiya, H. Nozaki, H. Kaji, Langmuir 23 (2007) 8304.
[98] J.Y. Lee, J.-W. Lee, C.E. Schmidt, J. R Soc. Interface (2008) 1, http://dx.doi.org/10.1098/rsif.2008.0403.
[99] R. Wadhwa, C.F. Lagenaur, X.T. Cui, J. Control. Release 110 (2006) 531.
[100] J.A. Chikar, J.L. Hendricks, S.M. Richardson-Burns, Y. Raphael, B.E. Pfingst, D.C. Martin, Biomaterials 33 (2012) 1982.
[101] Y. Ido, D. Takahashi, T. Miyake, K. Nagamine, M. Nishizawa, 62nd Annu. Meet. Int. Soc. Electrochem. (2011).
[102] Z. Wang, S. Liu, P. Wu, C. Cai, Anal. Chem. 81 (2009) 1638.
[103] D.W. Hatchett, M. Josowicz, Chem. Rev. 108 (2008) 746.
[104] B.C. Thompson, S.E. Moulton, J. Ding, R. Richardson, A. Cameron, S. O'Leary, G.G. Wallace, G.M. Clark, J. Control. Release 116 (2006) 285.
[105] J.A. Goding, A.D. Gilmour, P.J. Martens, L.A. Poole-Warren, R.A. Green, J. Mater. Chem. B 3 (2015) 5058–5069.
[106] R.T. Richardson, A.K. Wise, B.C. Thompson, B.O. Flynn, P.J. Atkinson, N.J. Fretwell, J.B. Fallon, G.G. Wallace, R.K. Shepherd, G.M. Clark, S.J. O'Leary, Biomaterials 30 (2009) 2614.
[107] G. Stevenson, S.E. Moulton, P.C. Innis, G.G. Wallace, Synth. Met. 160 (2010) 1107.
[108] A.J. Evans, B.C. Thompson, G.G. Wallace, R. Millard, S.J. O'Leary, G.M. Clark, R.K. Shepherd, R.T. Richardson, J. Biomed. Mater. Res. A 91A (2009) 241.
[109] X. Xu, W.-C. Yee, P.Y.K. Hwang, H. Yu, A.C.A. Wan, S. Gao, K.-L. Boon, H.-Q. Mao, K.W. Leong, S. Wang, Biomaterials 24 (2003) 2405.

[110] S.E. Sakiyama-Elbert, J.A. Hubbell, J. Control. Release 69 (2000) 149.
[111] J. Kundu, L.A. Poole-Warren, P. Martens, S.C. Kundu, Acta Biomater. 8 (2012) 1720.
[112] K. Gilmore, A.J. Hodgson, B. Luan, C.J. Small, G.G. Wallace, Polym. Gels Networks 2 (1994) 135.
[113] A. Andreatta, P. Smith, in: Goteborg, Sweden, 1992, pp. 1017–1022.
[114] Z. Wang, C. Roberge, L.H. Dao, Y. Wan, G. Shi, M. Rouabhia, R. Guidoin, Z. Zhang, J. Biomed. Mater. Res. A 70A (2004) 28.

Degradable conjugated conducting polymers and nerve guidance

12

M. Asplund[1,2]
[1]Freiburg Institute for Advanced Studies, Albert-Ludwigs Universität, Freiburg, Germany;
[2]IMTEK, Albert-Ludwigs Universität, Freiburg, Germany

12.1 Introduction

This chapter outlines the most important routes to synthesise and process conjugated polymers (CPs) into materials specially designed for neural tissue engineering. The focus of this chapter will be on the most commonly described materials – polyaniline (PANI), polypyrrole (PPy) and poly(3,4-ethylenedioxythiophene) (PEDOT) – but also various derivatives and copolymers based on this class of materials will be discussed. Within other fields of applications for conducting polymers, for example, solar cells, microelectrodes and printed electronics, these materials are well known as thin films or coatings but rarely come in the form of stand-alone structural materials that are needed for tissue engineering. Therefore, various techniques to deposit, blend or form conducting polymers on/into three-dimensional (3D) structures are outlined in detail in Section 12.3. Closely related to this topic is of course the biodegradability of the resulting material. CPs themselves are not biodegradable, something that can be addressed either by allowing only a fraction in the resulting scaffold, or by synthesising new families of conducting polymers. The latter will be discussed in detail in Section 12.4. Even if electrical conductivity is the main challenge for these materials, it is equally important to investigate the possibilities to provide biomolecular and topographical cues for guidance, especially without compromising the conducting properties. Some possible routes to do so are outlined in Section 12.5.

The main work within this field is invested into materials design. Many of the studies include data from cell-culture studies to preliminary confirm material functionality and compatibility with cells. However, only few studies go into detail on the effect stimulation has on the cells in question and what this means for future design of materials and devices. In Section 12.6, a handful of studies that show biological results beyond the point of cytotoxicity testing will briefly be discussed. Finally, some future trends and remaining challenges will be brought to light in Section 12.7.

It is difficult to list scaffold requirements in terms of numbers, since it is to large extent unclear what will in the end be a successful strategy to assist regeneration. While some authors investigate cylindrical scaffolds, others use membranes as stimulation surfaces. It is naturally a different situation to pass current via the surface of a

Biosynthetic Polymers for Medical Applications. http://dx.doi.org/10.1016/B978-1-78242-105-4.00012-2

membrane rather than through a complete 3D object. Therefore, it is also a vital part of this research to simultaneously test materials in the real settings to ensure that polymer design focuses on the right questions. Some comments on how to do so are included in Section 12.7.

12.2 Material challenges in neural engineering

A highly desired target in tissue engineering is to present a solution for the repair of severed nerves. Tubes, or porous cylindrical scaffolds, could potentially offer guidance and support for regenerating axons and ensure that fibrous tissue does not infiltrate and interfere with the healing process. In many cases, however, passive support is not sufficient for successful regeneration, but there is a need for actively encouraging and steering this process. The presentation of bioactive species patterned throughout the 3D scaffold, together with electrical stimulation, accordingly offers a promising strategy for extending the possibilities of neural repair. For supporting continuous stimulation of the tissue, the scaffold would therefore have to be either a 3D porous conductor or at least comprise conductive domains. The ideal scaffold would in addition have to be bioresorbable, offering guidance and support during healing but progressively degrading without further interference with the regenerated tissue.

From the requirements listed above it is obvious that conventional metallic conducting materials cannot offer a full solution. For this reason, CPs have since the early 1990s gained significant attention as candidates for electrically conducting nerve-guidance structures.[27,46,80,81,96,97] The versatility of these polymers and their composites make it possible to address all points on the wish list. After nearly two decades of research within this field, a broad set of techniques developed and refined for processing conducting polymers into scaffolds and channels with topographical and biochemical guidance cues for nerve regeneration can be found in the literature. Biodegradability has been addressed with various strategies, aiming for decomposition of either the separate components of a composite material or the polymer backbone itself.

12.3 Processing of conducting polymers for the generation of 3D scaffolds

For tissue engineering purposes it is essential to establish routes for processing conducting polymer-based materials into porous scaffolds. In general, efforts within conducting polymer research have been aiming towards high and stable conductivity in the thin-film format rather than the formation of 3D conducting objects. This means that there is a need for a new set of methods for generation of conducting polymers in the 3D format. In general, this can be done by forming two-phase materials where the conducing polymer phase is mixed with a nonconducting structural material that adds mechanical stability and bulk. Biodegradability is accomplished by dissolution of the structural phase and ideally the leftover CP phase will not need further dissolution to be cleared out from the tissue. The structural phase can be a fibrous structure, for instance formed by electrospinning (Section 12.3.4); a gel; or other spongy or porous constructs. Often, the formation of the nonconducting phase is separated from the conducting polymer deposition, which is done in a subsequent step through wet chemical polymerisation, vapour-phase polymerisation (VPP) (Section 12.3.3) or electrodeposition (Section 12.3.2). In addition, it is possible to start by forming the conducting phase in a separate step and mixing in the conducting polymer fragments while synthesising the scaffold, such as is done with emulsion polymerisation (Section 12.3.1). Some authors do indeed present processes where the formation of both phases takes place simultaneously, although the majority of papers separate the two. A few authors in addition develop one-component versions of conducting polymer materials that are more easily processable into structural objects and whose polymer backbone can be chopped up in smaller pieces by the biological environment.[7,63] It is not our intention to take a standpoint in placing one of these techniques in front of another but rather acknowledging the fact that there is a variety of ideas to choose from. Further work is needed for tuning each process to its optimal performance so that the resulting material fulfils all possible requirements of the resorbable conducting nerve graft.

12.3.1 Emulsion polymerisation for nanoparticle composites

Various methods in the literature address the formation of conducting particles for inclusion in composite materials. An early paper by Kim et al. describes the preparation of processable hydrogel composites from PPy colloids and poly(ethylene)/poly(ε-caprolactone) (PCL) multiblock copolymers.[46] Subsequently, emulsion polymerisation of PPy for the generation of 3D biodegradable scaffolds has been employed by several authors.[8,40,82–84,94] The general principle is to allow the polymerisation to take place in a water-in-oil emulsion leading to the formation of PPy particles that can be mixed with a nonconducting structural element. This can either be done by allowing this element to be part of the polymerisation solution itself, as for poly-D,L-lactic acid (PDLA)[84] or polyurethane,[8] or by extracting the conducting nanoparticles for subsequent mixing with the structural phase as shown for poly(L-lactic acid) (PLLA),[82,83] chitosan,[40,94] and chitosan-g-polycaprolactone (CPC).[94] For the latter, chemical polymerisation of the pyrrole (Py) monomer is performed in a water-in-oil emulsion system by adding iron chloride ($FeCl_3$) oxidant and stirring vigorously. The PPy nanoparticles are extracted by solution casting and solvent evaporation.

The conductivity of emulsion-polymerised composites is highly dependent on the proportion of colloids included in the matrix. Kim et al. report conductivities up to $8.5 * 10^{-5}$ S/cm for the highest proportion studied, 30 wt% PPy. However, such a high particle content is rather unrealistic keeping in mind that the PPy particles themselves are not biodegradable. In the continued work by Shi et al. proportions were kept in the range of 5 wt% and conductivity was still found sufficient for supporting stimulation in cell-culture models.[83,84] It is worth noting that the arrangement of the nanoparticles within the supporting matrix has substantial influence on the resulting

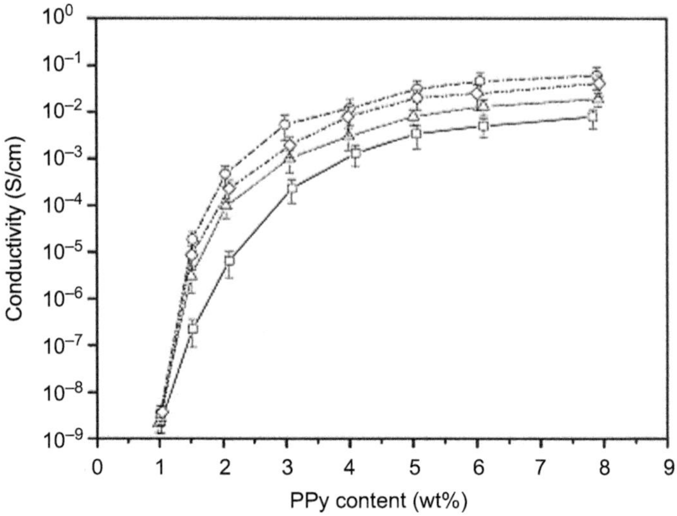

Figure 12.1 Measured conductivity nanoparticle-based composites depending on the wt% of PPy included in the structural chitosan-based matrix. PPy together with regular chitosan is shown in boxes, and the composites CPC-A:PPy/CPC-B:PPy and CPC-C PPy are represented as diamonds, circles and triangles, respectively. Arrangement of PCL side chains on the chitosan backbone influenced crystallinity of the matrix and thereby also particle distribution.
Reprinted from Ref. 94, Copyright 2010, with permission from Elsevier.

conducting properties. Shi et al. report that the nanoparticles aggregated to form a network of microdomains. They proposed a model where overall conductivity of the composite would depend on conductivity of individual particles, contact between particles, size of particle domains and the connectivity between different domains in the network. Furthermore, the number of domains exposed on the surface, accessible to the interconnection device, would matter for the conductivity measurement.[84] Comparing different particle-based materials in terms of conductivity versus PPy load is therefore important to gain insight into the efficiency of the particle distribution in a specific composite.[84,94] An example of such a measurement can be seen in Figure 12.1 comparing performance of a chitosan–PPy composite to the CPC-PPy counterparts. The latter, having a more beneficial dispersion of particles in the material, displays a rise in conductivity by one order of magnitude for the same PPy load (5 wt% PPy at both samples). The structural change was attributed to the fact that PCL side chains introduced to the chitosan backbone for the CPC copolymer prevented the formation of a crystalline structure of the non-conducting phase.[94] These results clearly point to the significance of controlling the particle arrangement within the composite.

12.3.2 Electrodeposition

There are several reasons why electrodeposition is an attractive route for conducting polymer generation. It allows for well-defined growth of highly conducting polymer coatings on metallised surfaces. Furthermore, it introduces the ability to entrap biologically relevant ions in the material (Section 12.5.2), and through the tight interconnection formed to the working electrode (WE), the redox state of the formed polymer can easily be controlled. A standard three-electrode system, comprises WE, counter electrode (CE) and reference electrode (RE), is used to electrochemically oxidise the monomer in an electrolyte in order to induce polymerisation on the surface of the WE. The growth rate can conveniently be controlled by current density and, by keeping track of the charge consumed in the reaction, it is also possible to estimate the mass of the formed material. Electropolymerisation is, however, mainly associated with the formation of thin coatings on metallic electrodes rather than the production of bulk material. The possibility of using a hydrogel scaffold to guide electroformation of the polymer was pointed out already in the early 1990s,[27] and work has been continued by several groups over the years.[1,47,48] In principle, the WE is embedded in a hydrogel matrix that is soaked in the monomer solution within the deposition cell. If contact between WE and gel is sufficiently tight, the polymer infiltrates the gel as it grows, creating an interpenetrating network of conducting fibres inside the hydrogel (Figure 12.2). The conducting polymer network was found not to interfere with the hydration properties of the hydrogel and was estimated to occupy less than 5 wt% of the resulting material.[27] In comparison to the particle-dispersion composites, the efficiency in terms of conducting polymer content versus conductivity can be expected to be high, since the continued growth requires a nondisrupted connection to the previously formed chains. Thus, the growing structure will infiltrate the support matrix in a bottom-up manner.[1]

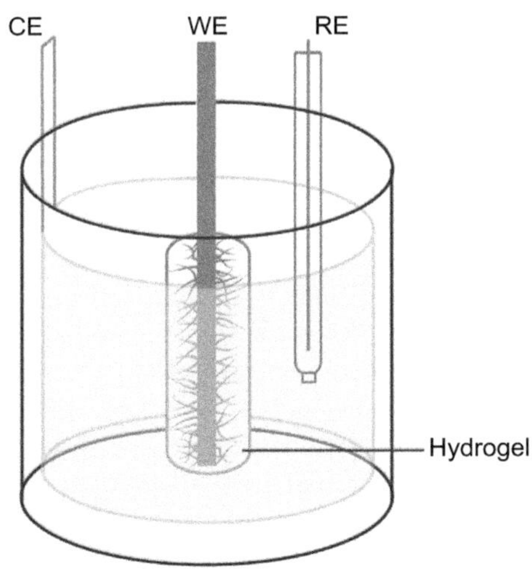

Figure 12.2 Example of a three-electrode setup for electrodeposition of conducting polymer in a hydrogel support matrix using a wire WE. A cylindrical CE provides a homogenous field distribution and the reference electrode RE enables stable maintenance of a well-defined deposition potential.

A clear drawback of this method is the difficulty in scaling-up production. Electrodeposition is a time-consuming process; to give some point of reference, 4.5 h was needed to form 36 cm^3 of conducting gel composite.[27] More recent work reports deposition times of 30 min per fabricated scaffold.[1] It might therefore not be the method of choice for the preparation of substantial quantities of material intended for further processing. The conducting polymer in the gel will in addition not be homogenously distributed over the bulk. The growth pattern depends on the electrical field distribution – that is, it is determined by the geometry of the setup – and is also clearly directional with higher density of formed conducting polymer closer to the WE. Recent work from Green et al. suggests that if anionic counter-ions are immobilised within the hydrogel, this can serve the dual purpose of acting as counter-ion in the deposition process and as a scaffold for the electropolymerisation.[31,62] It is suggested that the balancing of charge, provided by the anionic hydrogel, facilitates the polymer chain formation within the complete hydrogel. The resulting polymer network is thereby truly interpenetrating and not in the same way confined to the space closest to the WE. They report on the deposition within a photo-cross-linked network of polyvinyl alcohol and heparin, but suggest that the principle could likely be extended to other hydrogel-ionic systems.

The benefit of having the tight interconnection to the WE, which naturally results from the deposition process, should not be overlooked. Preferably, the polymerisation should be performed directly from the electrode of the final device intended for implantation. If not, the polymer gel has to be reconnected to a second device, an approach that is likely more challenging when it comes to accomplishing a stable contact. Furthermore, electropolymerisation offers the additional possibility to use separate WEs and deposition steps, thus controlling the formation of polymer at specific locations in a nonconducting gel matrix. This process can, for instance, be used to deposit polymer only at specific spots in the gel, forming separate conducting regions that are not short circuited and can be individually controlled from the separate WEs.

To shape the electrostatically grown material during deposition it is also possible to use solid templates that are subsequently solubilised or otherwise removed. George et al. describe a process where electrodeposition on metallic wires is used to form tubular structures suitable for nerve guidance. PPy, deposited as a coating on the wire, is delaminated from the wire template by applying a reversed potential that induces swelling of the polymer.[24] Kang et al. used self-assembled polystyrene colloids on indium tin oxide (ITO) WEs as sacrificial templates to produce nanoporous surfaces.[45] Furthermore, an electrospinning process has been used to deposit aligned and well-separated nanofibres of poly(D,L-lactide) (PDLLA)[a]-poly(lactide-co-glycolide) (PLGA) on top of large WEs made from metallised Mylar. The conducting polymer was subsequently grown around these fibres so that they were embedded but not fully covered. In this case, the fibres remained in the material, providing topographical features for guidance and as a biodegradable component of the resulting device.[72]

[a] Abbreviation PLA used instead of PDLLA in original paper.

12.3.3 In situ and VPP on nonconducting constructs

The principle of using a complete scaffold of a nonconducting material, and integrating the conducting polymer through a separate chemical polymerisation step, can be applied to a variety of scaffolds using wet chemical in situ or VPP processes. Such methods can readily be applied to a multitude of materials that are already well known as valid tissue engineering biomaterials. The main objective is that the scaffold can maintain its favourable physical properties and that the conducting polymer simply adds electrical conductivity on top of that. A lot of important work in this direction is performed using electrospun nanofibrous networks as base material, but the general method applies to various types of scaffolds.[44,54,55,60,86,100,101] Some further examples that can be found in literature are acellularised tissue constructs,[69] hydrogels,[78] or membranes from PDLLA-co-epsiloncaprolactone (PDLLA/CL), polycaprolactone fumarate (PCLF),[77,105] or PDLLA.[95] Since the family of electrospun materials is discussed in detail in a separate Section (12.3.2), this section will briefly describe the general methods exemplified with some other scaffold materials that have been presented in literature.

For performing in situ and/or VPP, a chemical oxidiser is brought in contact with the monomer to be polymerised. The essential difference between the two processes is that for the latter, the monomer is introduced as a vapour and interacts with an oxidiser adsorbed at the surface of the scaffold, rather than allowing the reaction to take place in a solvent bath. Commonly used oxidisers within both reaction types are $FeCl_3$ and iron tosylate ($Fe(TOs)_3$).

General points to consider when polymerising in preformed scaffold structures is that the matrix used must be sufficiently permeable for monomer and oxidant to ensure that the polymerisation takes place within the bulk material, not just as a surface process.[69] Since porosity is decisive for function of the scaffold, it is indeed also essential to tune the polymerisation not to add too much bulk within the pores of the scaffold. Furthermore, it is important that any remaining reactants can be cleaned out from the constructs so as not to impair the biocompatibility of the resulting scaffold.

12.3.3.1 Vapour-based processes

Zhang et al.[105] used a VPP process to coat PDLLA/CL membranes. Therefore membranes were spray-coated with a solution of ethanol, $FeCl_3$, polystyrene sulphonate (PSS) or butane sulphonic acid. Following this, the membranes were exposed to Py fumes using a nitrogen flow for distributing the fumes to the sample. Similarly, Wan et al. immersed polylactide (PLA) membranes in the $FeCl_3$ solution and introduced them into a chamber containing Py vapour. With optimised deposition parameters, conductivities of membranes ranged up to 0.001 S/cm and contained ~2–3 wt% of PPy.[95]

12.3.3.2 Wet chemical in situ polymerisation

Peramo et al. used an acellularised tissue construct (mouse abdominal muscle) as base scaffold and formed PEDOT within this matrix using chemical oxidation of ethylene dioxythiophene (EDOT) by $FeCl_3$ in ethanol. PEDOT infiltrated the filaments in the construct, filling out voids throughout the bulk material. Unfortunately, the deposition of PEDOT made the construct stiff and brittle, which might limit the usefulness of this particular composite material. Runge et al. performed polymerisation on biodegradable PCLF membranes and scaffolds. The constructs were first soaked in benzoyl peroxide, dried, and submerged in a bath of Py and naphthalene-2-sulphonic acid sodium salt. The PPy content could be controlled by varying the polymerisation time and the concentration of benzoyl peroxide in solution. Conductivities ranged up to 0.006 S/cm depending on the PPy content, which ranged from 5 to 14 wt%. In a subsequent study, the composites were found to perform well with respect to mechanical properties, cell compatibility and ability to deliver relevant electrical stimulation to PCS.[65] The same group performed additional work in this direction using instead a hydrogel, oligo(polyethylene glycol fumarate), as base material. The materials were found suitable to support PC12 cells in culture, meaning that the cleaning steps for eluting toxic monomer and oxidant were successful.[78]

12.3.4 Electrospinning

Over the last decade, electrospinning has emerged as one of the most important techniques for generating multiporous scaffolds for tissue engineering purposes. In short, the electrospinner uses an electrostatic field to draw a thin flow of solution from a polymer liquid. The solution to be spinned is exposed at the tip of a capillary, and when the electrostatic pulling forces overcome the surface tension of the liquid, a jet is drawn from the liquid surface (Figure 12.3). As the liquid jet dries in flight, a continuous fibre is formed, which can be in the size range from tens of nanometres up to tens of microns

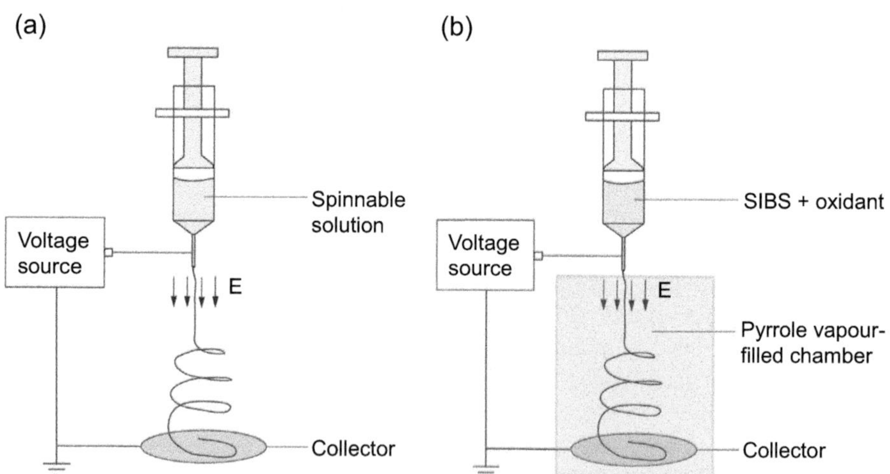

Figure 12.3 (a) Principle of electrospinning. (b) Specialty version of electrospinning, where polymerisation of PPy takes place in parallel with the spinning process as suggested by Liu and co-workers.[60]

in diameter. Nanofibres can be collected in an aligned or randomly organised manner forming a nonwoven mesh of a 3D and highly porous character. Such meshes, or aligned fibre collections, are attractive for several purposes. Aligned fibres provide topographical cues for regenerating axons. Furthermore, they have a high surface-area-to-volume ratio, and meshed fibre collections build up networks of interconnected pores in which neurons can be cultured in a 3D manner. The electrospinning process readily lends itself to a variety of polymer materials, including several biodegradable polymers. Unfortunately, most conducting polymer materials cannot easily be processed into spinnable polymer solutions but must be integrated into the electrospun networks by tricks or additional process steps. Fortunately, several possibilities to do so are already presented in literature, and some examples will be outlined in the following section. Three possible pathways in which electrospun nanofibrous conducting polymer scaffolds can be generated are:

1. Spinning a blend of a conducting polymer and a nonconducting spinnable polymer solution.
2. Spinning a blend of spinnable polymer solution and precursor for the conducting polymer.
3. Spinning a nonconducting material and subsequently covering it with the conducting polymer through an additional process step.

Each of these points will be elaborated upon next.

1. For CPs based on thiophenes, Breukers et al. report an ester-functionalised thiophene material, poly(octanoic acid 2-thiophen-3-yl-ethyl ester) poly(OTE), that was spinnable from a blend of organic solvents.[7] The majority of work in this direction, however, reports electrospinning of conducting scaffolds from blends of PANI, using various structural polymers such as gelatin,[58] poly(L-lactide-co-ε-caprolactone) (PLCL),[43] PDLA,[64] PLLA,[70] or a mix of PCL and gelatin (PG)[26] in the polymer blend. The formed fibre networks were found to be homogenous, biodegradable and able to support the growth of various cell types. On one hand the reported conductivities of these nanofibrous films can still be considered to be modest (0.008–0.04 S/cm) even though they in general could be increased with increasing proportion of PANI in the blend. On the other hand, the electrospinning process itself was challenging at the higher concentrations of PANI.[26] There was also an inverse relationship between the diameter of the formed fibres and the proportion of PANI included in the blend: increasing PANI concentration correlated with decreasing diameters,[26,58,70] and reduced elasticity of the resulting fibres.[26,43] The optimal proportions of the blend accordingly need to be tuned with regard to the desired fibre diameter, mechanical properties and the polymers involved. It should be mentioned that the electrospinning technique has provided fibrous materials of much higher conductivity (in range 0.1 S/cm) in the cases where the final biological application did not limit the chemistry involved in the process.[66]
2. As an alternative to direct electrospinning of the conducting polymer itself, spinning a blend of the precursor and a nonconducting spinnable polymer solution is an additional possibility. Thus, the conducting polymer is still formed in parallel with the electrospinning process, creating a composite fibre in a one-step process. Two excellent examples are the electrospinning VPP polymerisation process described by Liu and co-workers and similarly the incorporation of the PPy precursor in a poly(vinyl pyrrolidone) (PVP) blend as described by Srivastava et al.[60,86] The former report electrospinning of the base material poly(styrene-ß-isobutylene-ß-styrene) (SIBS), a nonbiodegradable block copolymer. By mixing in the oxidant $Fe(TOs)_3$ directly into the SIBS and performing the electrospinning in a closed box containing the Py vapour, they performed a VPP process in parallel with electrospinning

(see Figure 12.3(b)). By this process, a thin shell (in the range of 20 nm) of PPy was efficiently deposited along the surface of individual fibres. Similarly, Srivastava et al. use a one-step procedure to electrospin a blend of Py, $FeCl_3$ and PVP, allowing PPy to form within the spun fibres. This technique led to a uniform, continuous conducting phase formed within the fibre, providing conductivities in the range of 0.0001 S/cm. The same group also attempted a two-step procedure, including only the oxidiser in the spinnable blend and providing the monomer through a VPP step. The process was similar to the VPP process described above, although the polymerisation was not simultaneous with the spinning process itself. It was found that the polymerisation on the surface of the fibre inhibited further diffusion of the monomer into the bulk of the material, which led to an unsatisfactory yield of the polymer and low conductivities in comparison to the other technique.

3. In addition to the specialised electrospinning protocols described above, it naturally suggests itself to spin a nonconducting fibre scaffold from a more conventional electrospinning blend and use an additional process step, for example, VPP, for subsequently covering the fibrous network with conducting polymer. Ideally, the process would lead to a thin and continuous coating of conducting polymer, a 'core-sheath,' completely enclosing the fibres yet retaining the attractive nanofibrous and porous structure.[54,100] The choice of core fibres and the process for coating these varies. Several authors use modifications on a standard aqueous in situ polymerisation process to coat electrospun fibres of PCL,[100] PLLA[b] nanofibres,[44,100] and poly(lactic-co-glycolic acid) (PLGA).[54,55] $FeCl_3$ or ammonium peroxydisulphate (APS) are used as oxidants and sodium *para*-toluene sulphonate Na(pTS) or H_2SO_4 as counterions.[101] As expected it was found that reactant concentration and time for reactions was decisive for the quality of the fibre coating.[54] Ideally, for optimised conductivity and retained fibrous morphology, the fibres should be enclosed by a thin and uniform PPy shell. If the reaction parameters are not properly tuned, aggregates in solution lead to nonuniform coatings or incomplete coverage of the fibre structure, which in turn leads to poor conductivity and disrupted topography (see Figure 12.4). With optimised processes, uniform coatings with thicknesses in the range of 50–100 nm were obtained on various fibres of diameters in the range 0.2–0.4 μm.

12.4 Biodegradable conducting polymers

It is necessary that a material intended as nervous tissue scaffold can maintain a certain mechanical strength over the first time of regeneration. The purpose of the scaffold is partially to ensure an open lumen that can be infiltrated by the regenerating tissue and preventing the wrong cells from entering, meaning mechanical integrity of the implanted scaffold must be maintained over a significant time frame of implantation, possibly several months.[84] It should also be taken into account that the implantation procedure itself can be expected to further stress the material.[26] On the other hand, once regeneration is complete, the scaffold should ideally be completely resorbed, since remaining material might risk interfering with normal functions of the regenerated nerve and effect chronic inflammation in the tissue. The two properties – mechanical integrity versus biodegradability – are, however,

[b] Abbreviation PLA used by original author Ref. 100.

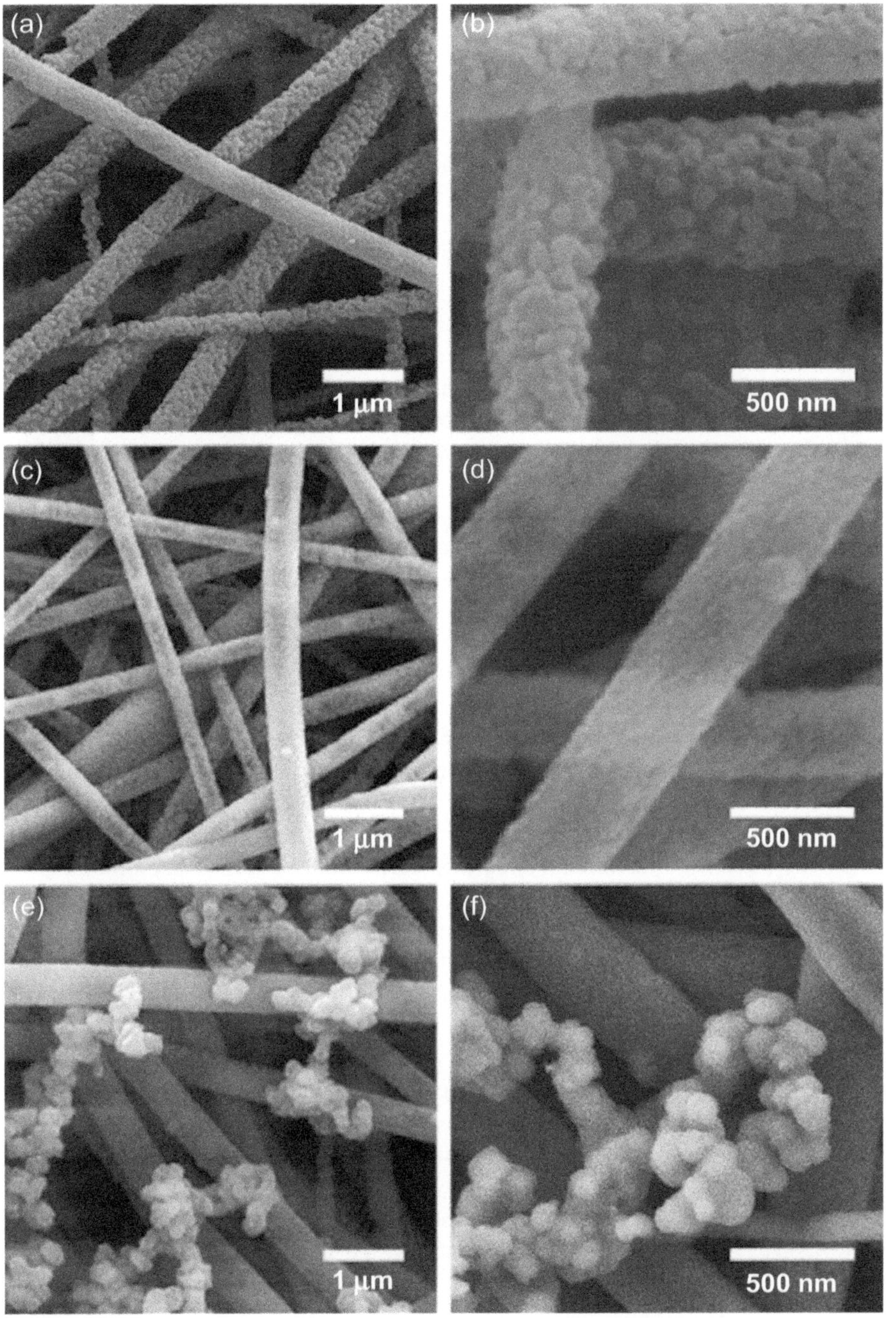

Figure 12.4 Scanning electron microscopy (SEM) micrographs showing polymer coverage for different process parameters of the wet chemical polymerisation process (a, c, e) in low magnification, and (b, d, f) in high magnification. PLGA fibres were coated with PPy from a solution containing Py, pTS and $FeCl_3$. (a, b) show the incomplete coverage resulting from an insufficient reaction time; (c, d) show the cohesive coating accomplished under optimised reaction conditions and (e, f) show PPy aggregates that appeared when the reactant concentration was too high.

not easily combined. Furthermore, conducting polymers such as PPy, PANI and PEDOT are not considered to be biodegradable themselves. This can to some extent be circumvented through fabrication of composites, where the conducting polymer phase is present in small fractions in an otherwise biodegradable scaffold. If the polymer fragments are sufficiently small, it is expected that their influence will be insignificant and/or they could hopefully be excreted through circulatory systems even though they cannot be degraded.[84,95] Again, this leads to a trade-off: on one hand, the CP content of the material should be kept low with respect to biodegradability, and on the other hand, there is a need for a certain amount of CP to be present to maintain good conducting properties. Balancing conductivity versus mechanical properties and biodegradability is therefore challenging but essential.

This chapter already provides detailed information on a variety of methods for making composites of nonconducting materials together with micro- and nanosized particles or fragments of PPy, PEDOT and PANI. Therefore, this section will focus explicitly on papers that take a molecular design approach to the bioresorbable conducting polymer material, attempting to make the polymer backbone itself biodegradable in contrast to only degrading the structural framework of a composite.

Early on, Rivers et al. addressed this issue by employing a strategy in which pyrrole-thiophene oligomers were synthesised and connected by ester linkages.[75] Ester linkages are known to be degradable by enzymes normally present during the wound healing reaction. The polymer chains would thus decompose into oligomer fragments over the time course of implantation. Resulting films displayed conductivities in the range of 10^{-4} S/cm. Degradation in the presence of the enzyme esterase confirmed that the main concept, the cleavage of the ester linkage, worked according to plan. In vivo experiments over 30 days (in rodents) further confirmed this finding, and the inflammatory reaction surrounding the implanted material was mild and comparable to that of PLGA controls. Unfortunately, to accomplish conductivity, the material had to be doped and the doping process itself turned out to cause toxicity of the resulting material.[34] Continued work on ester-linked oligomers from the same group led to the development of 5,5‴-bis(hydroxymethyl)-3,3‴-dimethyl-2,2′:5′,2″:5″,2‴-quaterthiophene-co-adipic acid polyester (QAPE) doped with $Fe(ClO_4)_3$. A schematic of the material is given in Figure 12.5. Electroactivity of the formed material was confirmed by cyclic voltammetry, although it could only be reported as 'moderately electroactive' even in its doped state.[34]

Further work on PPy co-polymers addresses the synthesis of block co-polymers with segments of poly(ethyl 2-cyanoacrylate) or PCL.[19] The resulting materials were processable from liquid dispersion and could be laminated onto a biodegradable poly(3-hydroxybutyrate-co-3-hydroxyvalerate) substrate. Films were highly conducting and their compatibility with nerve tissue was confirmed.

In an effort to produce a one-component thiophene-based conducting, and yet biodegradable, scaffold material, Mawad et al. synthesised poly(3-thiopheneacetic acid) (PTAA) crosslinked into hydrogels using 1,1′-carbonyldiimidazole.[63] Depending on swelling, conductivities ranged up to 80 μS/cm in neutral solutions. The gel is expected to be degraded by hydrolysis.

A line of work addresses the issue of biodegradability using block-copolymers based on aniline oligomers, commonly aniline pentamer (AP). A biocompatible triblock copolymer based on AP and PLA was synthesised according to PLA-b-AP-b-PLA.[41]

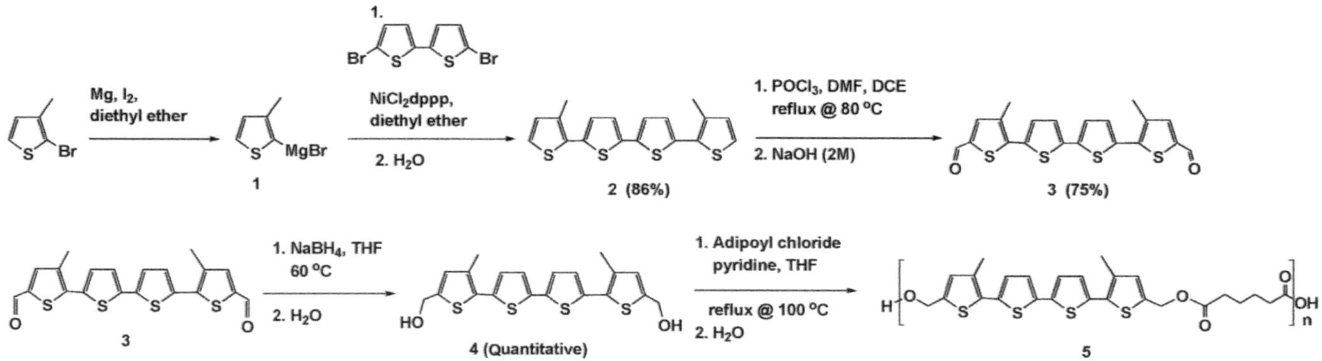

Figure 12.5 Schematic of the synthesis of the ester-linked thiophene oligomer material QAPE presented by Guimard et al. Reprinted with permission from Ref. 34, Copyright 2009, American Chemical Society.

The PLA is expected to provide flexible and biodegradable segments to the polymer backbone.[41,42] The measured conductivity was on the order of 10^{-6} S/cm, on one hand substantially lower than that of AP itself, but on the other hand a significant increase in comparison to the pure PLA. To improve mechanical properties of the AP-based materials, a similar system, but using alternant multiblocks of PLA and AP, was synthesised.[42] A schematic of the process and the expected macroscopic morphology of the resulting material can be seen in Figure 12.6. The conductivity of the new system was in the range of 10^{-5}–10^{-6} S/cm, which is only a slight improvement upon what could be accomplished for the previous material. Mechanical properties were, however, significantly improved by the structural change. More recently, AP has also been combined with poly(glycine ethyl ester) phosphazene yielding a biodegradable material with conductivities on the order of 20 μS/cm.[102,103]

Further work on AP includes carboxyl-capped AP (CCAP). This has, for instance, been used for crosslinked chitosan gels, synthesised by condensation polymerisation between carboxylic acid terminal groups on the AP chain and amino groups of the chitosan.[39] Similarly, and to completely exclude the need for organic solvents, further work with this methodology proceeded to hydrogels of AP and gelatin.[61]

Continued work on AP has focused on synthesis of CCAP into branched copolymers with PCL, the rationale being to increase conductivity by increasing the order of the AP segments within the material.[35] It was shown that the highly ordered hyperbranched versions yielded materials with higher conductivity than their linear copolymer counterparts (Figure 12.7). Conductivities of scaffolds of this material were on the order of 10^{-5} S/cm.[36] This work states an important point for future development within this field.

Taking control of the 3D arrangement of the conducting sequences in the individual copolymer chains offers solutions to the dilemma of combining biodegradability with higher conductivity. In general, the higher the content of CP, the higher conductivity can be expected. On the other hand problems arise as a result of the increased proportion of nondegradable polymer fragments. By transferring from systems of randomly organised material to a highly controlled 3D structure, it can be ensured that the included CP is used as efficiently as possible, yielding higher conductivity for the same mass percent of conducting material included. Recent work points in the direction that AP is indeed toxic to certain cells and might influence the cellular

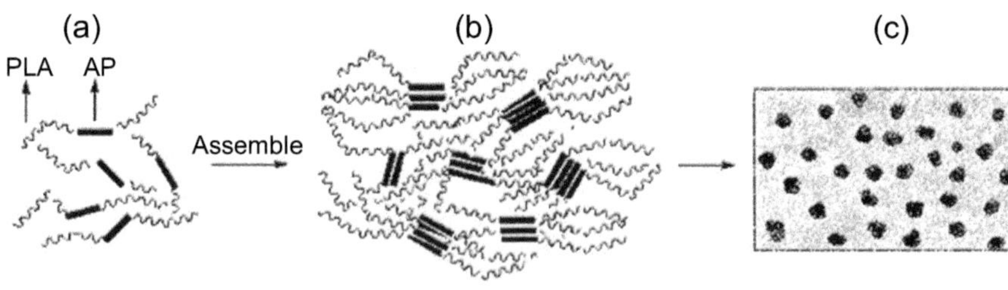

Figure 12.6 (a) Schematic showing the structure of the PLA AP copolymer system suggested by Huang et al. (b–c) Proposed organisation of the segments within the formed material. Reprinted from Ref. 41, Copyright (2007), with permission from Elsevier.

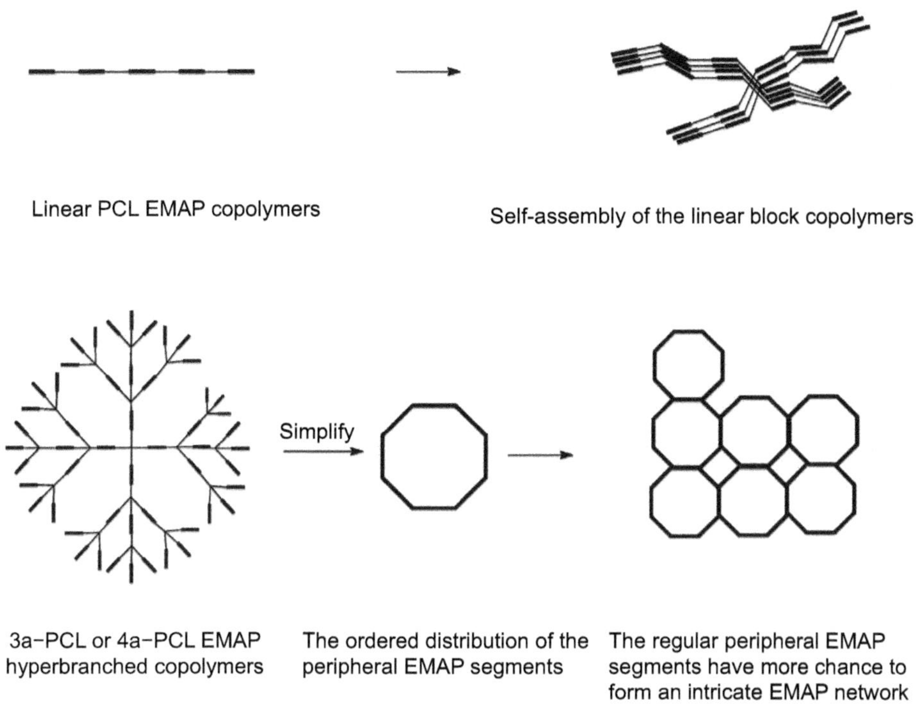

Figure 12.7 Arrangement of AP segments in materials based on linear versus hyperbranched PCL emeraldine state AP (EMAP) copolymers as shown in Guo et al. The ordered distribution of AP in the hyperbranched versions would be the rationale behind the higher conductivity measured for this material in comparison to the linear versions of corresponding EMAP content. Reprinted with permission from Ref. 35, Copyright 2010, American Chemical Society.

behaviour,[89,102,104] further stressing the importance of keeping the AP content low.[104] This point can in fact be generalised to comprise also the composite materials where the conducting phase is introduced as nano- or micro-sized particles.[94] PPy nanoparticles were found cytotoxic to several cell types at higher concentrations.[92] Elevating conductivity of the biodegradable material can therefore not solely be addressed by increasing the conducting polymer content.

12.5 Biomolecular and topographical guidance

For increasing the probability to successfully heal damaged nerves, the regenerating fibres have to be encouraged to grow in a favourable manner. The fibres need to be guided and also biochemically supported. While electrical stimulation poses one possibility to do so, the combination with topographical and biochemical guidance cues in addition to this is essential for accomplishing the most beneficial result.[28] Inclusion or attachment of biomolecules is of interest for two quite different reasons. Either the biomolecule can be immobilised on the surface to modulate cellular adhesion, or it can be included in the polymer bulk for subsequent delivery to the surrounding fluid and cells at appropriate time points. Both functions can provide biomolecules for guidance and support of neural regeneration. A problematic issue with nerve guidance channels is that fibrous tissue, surrounding the regenerating fibres, occupies space within the channel that would be needed for more constructive neural regeneration. Surfaces that promote neural attachment to the channel walls, and prevent ingrowth of thick fibrous tissue into the lumen, would therefore be a significant improvement.[77]

In vitro, effects are commonly evaluated in terms of orientation and length of neurites, and number of neurite-bearing cells. It is indicated in literature that topography and biomolecules address these measures differently. While topography has been found to influence the axon initiation, and also orientation of axons, the biomolecules have been shown to be more efficient in promoting longer axons.[28,29] Therefore, both types of guidance might be needed and should preferably be combined with stimulation. There is a wide range of literature reviewing the influence of neurotrophic factors, guidance cues and topography alone.[57,76] A detailed insight into the underlying mechanisms is beyond the scope of this chapter, but this text is focused on methods for combining these features with the conducting polymer. A few biological results will also be presented here as well as in Section 12.6.

12.5.1 Micro- and nano-topography for guiding regeneration

Whereas a groove with a depth of several microns can constrain the cell mechanically to stay in a certain orientation, shallow structures influence the cell by a mechanism denoted contact guidance.[73] During development, axons use other axons for guidance, and similarly a regenerating axon can climb along the natural scaffold given by the damaged nerve to find its way.[16] It therefore makes sense to mimic this topographical structure for the control of neural outgrowth.

As already discussed (Section 12.3.4), electrospinning is an efficient technique for the formation of 3D constructs of aligned fibres. Diameters can be in the range of 60 nm–30 μm,[58,72] and a rotating drum collector can be used to control alignment. The difference in biological response to aligned versus randomly organised fibres clearly points in the direction that the impact of topographical guidance should not be neglected. From the scanning electron microscopy micrograph in Figure 12.8, an example of cells that are clearly influenced by the aligned topography can be seen. A promoting effect on neurite outgrowth in terms of neurite length and percentage of neurite-bearing cells has been found when electrical stimulation was applied and especially when presented in combination with aligned fibres.[54] Protruding neurites have also been found to preferably follow the alignment of the individual electrospun fibres.[60] From atomic force microscopy (AFM) images, it could be confirmed that filopodia projected from the growth cone and made contact with the surface of the fibre, which is in accordance with the contact guidance mechanism.

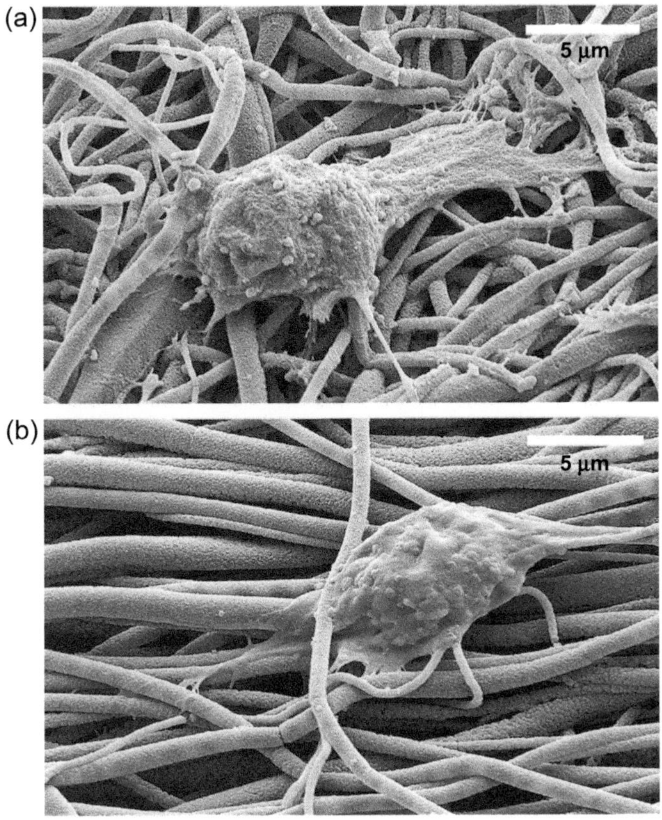

Figure 12.8 Morphology of PC12 cells on top of randomly organised (a) versus aligned (b) nanofibres.
Reprinted from Ref. 54, Copyright 2009, with permission from Elsevier.

The combination of electrodeposited PPy and aligned PLA-PLGA fibres on gold/Mylar electrodes, already described in Section 12.3.2, show an alternative method to accomplish aligned topography.[72] Also here axonal growth and Schwann cell migration followed the presented fibre lines. Templated electropolymerisation can in general be a useful route to control topography of the electropolymerised material.[45] Furthermore, Gomez et al. used an electropolymerisation-based technique to form PPy with microchannels (1–2 μm width, 400–800 nm depth).[28] E-beam-lithography was used to pattern the WE with an insulating layer leaving conducting lines open for electropolymerisation. The presence of microchannels was found to increase the number of hippocampal neurons presenting axons after 20 h in culture, and in addition influenced the orientation of axonal outgrowth. Axons preferably grew either along the channels or with a perpendicular orientation.[28] This technique offers a straightforward route to fabricate various patterns and test their effect in vitro, which is important to cast light on how the combined effect of topography and stimulation influences the cells. Realistically, the process might be difficult to use as basis for the patterning of 3D scaffolds.

12.5.2 Entrapment of biomolecular cues for guidance

By exchanging the counter-ion in the polymerisation process for a biologically relevant molecule, composite materials can be formed. If the biomolecule is of appropriate chemistry and charge, the electropolymerisation can be driven without introducing additional ionic species in the supporting electrolyte, meaning a substantial amount of the biological ion can be directly entrapped in the polymer matrix. In theory, the mass of counter-ions incorporated, m_{CI}, could thus be calculated from the following equation:

$$m_{CI} = \frac{nQM_w}{q_e N_A} \qquad [12.1]$$

where Q is charge consumed for electrodeposition, M_W is molar weight, q_e is elementary charge, n is molecular charge of the counter-ion and N_A is the Avogadro's number. For many substances there is, however, a need to include additional ions, commonly PSS or pTS, to ensure an efficient polymerisation. Naturally this also means a lower fraction of biomolecule per charge is included in the composite. The ionic entrapment approach was discovered early within the field of conducting polymer-based biosensors[9,91] and has since then been extensively studied for the formation of composites for tissue engineering and within the area of neural electrodes.[3] The approach can be used to accomplish both biofunctionalisation of the surface and drug delivery. In general, a large biomolecule can be entrapped in the polymer matrix in such a manner that it is accessible on the surface of the material, yet mechanically restricted so it cannot readily leave the matrix. In contrast to this, small- and medium-sized ionic species trapped in the polymer during synthesis can be released upon redox as a combined effect of electrostatic repulsion and mechanical actuation.

The combination of PPy or PEDOT with the glycosaminoglycans such as heparin and hyaluronic acid (HA) has been studied by several authors.[4,13,21,22,38,106] In the right combination, it has been shown that such composites can be of high quality from the electrochemical perspective, functioning comparable to the conventional PPy/PSS and PEDOT/PSS counterparts. For instance, PPy/HA films prepared in this manner have been shown to promote vascularisation in rodents, which is attributed to the immobilised HA.[13] PPy/heparin composites have been shown appropriate to support growth of endothelial cells and for culture and stimulation of PC12 cells.[22] As an additional feature, the amount of heparin exposed on the surface can be influenced by the oxidation state of the polymer, making the biochemistry of the surface electrochemically switchable.[21,38,68] Based on this, it is of significant interest to in turn use the composite surface for binding of growth factors that have a heparin-binding domain, as shown for neural stem cells by Herland et al.[38] In this case, the oxidation state dependence can be used to hide/expose growth factors by the redox functionality, yielding a certain temporal control useful for steering stem-cell differentiation.

Several authors studied the inclusion of peptides or proteins in the polymer films, showing that cells can indeed interact also with the entrapped fragments. The inclusion of proteins in general had a stronger influence on the electrochemical properties than for the glycosaminoglycans.[4] It can also be assumed that entrapment does not simply occur due to electrostatic binding, but passive adsorption to the surface is partly responsible. Included peptides/proteins have, for instance, been silk-like polymer fibronectin fragments, various laminin peptides,[14,15,32,87] fibrinogen,[4] and collagen.[49] Furthermore, small proteins, such as growth factors, can be controllably released from the polymer matrix, as shown for neurotrophin-3 (NT3),[74,90] neural growth factor (NGF),[45,49] and brain-derived neurotrophic factor (BDNF).[20]

There has been an extensive interest in the release of the anti-inflammatory drug dexamethasone for the local treatment of inflammation surrounding neural implants. Several authors show the inclusion of the ionic pre-drug dexamethasone sodium phosphate, providing promising data concerning the electrically triggered release of this drug from PPy.[2,93] Furthermore, release of adenosine triphosphate (ATP) from PEDOT/ATP systems has been studied as an agent for delivery of ATP to PC12 cells.[99]

It is worth mentioning a few studies offering specialty versions of the same basic concept, which allow for species to be incorporated and/or released that could not readily be included by the simple electropolymerisation step. One such example is ion exchange. In this, the polymer is electropolymerised with a more conventional counter-ion, for instance pTS, which by subsequent polarisation steps is eluted into solution and replaced by another ion electrostatically driven into the polymer. For instance, this process is shown for ATP[98] and glutamate.[12] Another innovative approach is presented by Song and Toste, who show that, using first poly-L-glutamic acid as counter-ion, a surface presenting a high concentration of carboxylic acid groups can be formed.[85] This surface can in turn be used to covalently bind polylysine and laminin through amide-coupling reactions. Similarly, George et al. showed that PPy, with biotin incorporated as dopant, could be used for binding of biotinylated NGF through biotin–streptavidin coupling chemistry.[23] The material was tested for controlled delivery of the thereby-bound NGF to PC12 cells. Abidian et al. suggest a combination between nanofibres and electropolymerisation.[2] The electrodeposited polymer forms a shell around the nanofibres spun from a mixture of PLLA and the drug dexamethasone. The PLLA fibres were subsequently dissolved and eluted through the polymer, leaving only the PEDOT shell containing the drug. Release from the resulting surface could then be triggered by redox activation of the polymer shell. An alternative, and generally useful, approach to controlled release from PPy films is presented by Li et al.[59] A polyvinyl alcohol heparin-containing gel was chemically bound to the surface, and electrical activation of the PPy film was used to drive release from the gel. The recent work by Green et al. regarding the electropolymerisation in polyvinyl alcohol gels with immobilised anions further widens the possibilities for using electrochemical methods for entrapments and delivery.[31] This technique can support both incorporation of mobile substances in the gel (demonstrated for NGF in the study) and covalently bound proteins.[62] These papers all address the important issue of finding a more general approach than what can readily be accomplished relying solely on inclusion by the electropolymerisation reaction.

It should be noted that much of the work on electropolymerised biomolecular conducting polymer composites is related to neural electrodes rather than tissue engineering. There is a significant overlap between the two, meaning protocols and ideas would be largely transferrable. To summarise: The approach of electrostatically binding relevant biological molecules through the electropolymerisation reaction has some clear pros and cons. On the positive side, the process is simple, most of the time one-step, and performs well in aqueous solutions for a wide variety of charged biomolecules. The thereby-formed electroactive composite can to some extent present a surface whose properties can be biochemically switched upon redox. Drug release from the surface can be electrochemically triggered, offering a convenient route for temporal control of release. On the downside, and as already discussed in Section 12.3.2, electrochemical methods are rather inefficient for bulk fabrication of 3D scaffolds. Furthermore, for the inclusion of biomolecules, the WE has to be immersed in an electrolyte partly based on this substance, meaning a substantial amount of biomolecule is needed for the process even if only a tiny fraction can be efficiently entrapped. For expensive biomolecules, this method might therefore not be justifiable from an economical point of view. If entrapment has to take place simultaneously with the polymer formation, this also limits the technique used for polymer synthesis itself, leaving out many attractive possibilities to control morphology, mechanical properties and biodegradability.

12.5.3 Attachment of biomolecular cues to CP surfaces

Several methods presented in the literature address the chemical binding of biomolecules to the polymer after its formation. The biomolecules will then be confined to the surface rather than distributed throughout the bulk. A clear benefit is that the biofunctionalisation of the polymer is separated from the polymerisation, meaning that the synthesis route can be chosen freely and with respect to the optimisation of other properties. However, it is also essential to ensure that the surface modification process itself does not degrade the conducting polymer or otherwise interfere with its function as a conductor. It should furthermore be noted that functionalisation of the monomer itself can be expected to have a major influence on the electrochemistry of the resulting material.[53] A possible route to circumvent this is to apply layers of materials where the bulk-conducting polymer is optimised with regard to conductivity and only the outer layer is made from the special version, which allows for facile biofunctionalisation.[53,56]

De Giglio et al. studied the grafting of L-cysteine and then later developed RGD-grafted PPy through the same route, suggesting cysteine can be bound to the surface through sulphur atoms interacting with the PPy backbone.[17,18] A multistep process for the covalent attachment of HA to PPy films was described by Cen et al.[10] where ultraviolet illumination was used to graft-copolymerise 2-hydroxyethyl acrylate (HEA) with PPy films. The resulting films were silanized, introducing amine functional groups to which HA could be covalently anchored in a subsequent immersion step. Bioactivity of the films was confirmed in a concomitant paper using PC12 cells as model system.[11]

An unconventional approach was presented by Sanghvi et al., using phage display to identify a peptide that would naturally bind to a PPy system.[79] From this method, a peptide sequence (T59 peptide), which would naturally bind to the PPy/Cl complex, could be selected. This peptide then formed the basis for a strategy where a cell-adhesive sequence could in turn be joined to the T59 peptide, yielding a cell-adhesion–promoting peptide extended with a PPy binding sequence. It could be confirmed that PC12 cells responded to the thereby immobilised adhesion peptide (GRGDS), thus showing that the T59 peptide indeed was efficient as a bifunctional linker.

With the ambition to develop a robust and general scheme for surface immobilisation of biological molecules, modification of the monomer itself has also been addressed. Py has, for example, been functionalised with a carboxylic acid.[53] PPy-COOH could then readily be prepared using either electrochemical or chemical routes, yielding surfaces available for covalent attachment of various peptides. Once again, the GRGDS sequence[c] was used as model to confirm that covalent conjugation to the carboxylic acid was possible and that cultured cells could interact with the thereby immobilised peptide. Conductivity of the resulting polymer was unfortunately significantly lowered by the functionalisation of the monomer. In further work from the same group, copolymers were synthesised from pristine pyrrole and pyrrole-N-hydroxyl succinimidyl ester. The copolymer version, exposing a high number of ester functional groups, could then be functionalised with amine-bearing compounds, as for instance NGF. At the same time, the negative influence on conductivity was not as pronounced as what is commonly encountered for versions where only functionalised monomers are included in the conducting material.

Yet another generally useful possibility for covalent grafting of biological molecules was investigated by Gomez and Schmidt.[30] The PPy surface was covered with polyallylamine functionalised with an arylazido side group. NGF could subsequently be tethered to this surface using a photolinking process. The thereby-immobilised NGF was active and accessible for cultured cells. It was reported that the influence of this surface treatment on conductivity was less pronounced than what was encountered using monomer functionalisation strategies. Over shorter time periods (2 days), the response of the PC12 cells to the immobilised NGF was similar to what was encountered with solubilised NGF. Interestingly, the combination with electrical stimulation from the surface further increased the length of formed neurites in comparison to unstimulated controls.

Even if the majority of papers until now focused on biofunctionalisation of PPy, the functionalisation of oligoaniline has also been addressed.[37] Based on amino-capped aniline trimers, an electroactive silsesquioxane precursor was developed that allowed

[c] GRGDSP.

the self-assembly of monolayers. The monolayers exposed a surface that could readily be used for covalent attachment of amino acids or phospholipids.

12.6 Biological performance of CPs for neural regeneration

It is not the intention of this chapter to penetrate deeply into the complex subject of the possible mechanisms of the biological response to electrical stimulation, but rather focus on the materials that can offer a platform for such investigations. It is, however, worth including some short words on the reported effects that have been accomplished using these materials together with the intended biological targets. Especially since the development of these materials is a prerequisite for the biological investigations and the two lines of research therefore go hand in hand.

The vast majority of studies evaluate effects in cell culture models, for instance PC12 or dorsal root ganglions (DRGs). Effects are commonly evaluated in terms of orientation and length of neurites and number of neurite-bearing cells, all being measures that are relevant in terms of evaluating guidance strategies. Few researchers get the opportunity to evaluate their materials on actual regenerating nerves, and since much work on the materials remains, optimisation in vitro is in most cases still a necessity before proceeding to more realistic conditions.

In early work, Schmidt et al. concluded that stimulation (steady potential of 100 mV) from PPy films could induce a significant increase in neurite length for PC12 cells cultured on top of the films.[80] This result has later been confirmed by many others,[65,68] and also been shown with PLLA/PANI or PANI/PG nanofibre scaffolds for neural stem cells.[26,70] In further work, it could be concluded that increased absorption of fibronectin to the surface would be partly responsible for the effect.[50] An upregulation of mitochondrial activity and increased cytokine secretion has also been observed upon stimulation of human cutaneous fibroblasts from PPy/PLLA membranes.[82,83] Furthermore, stimulation of Schwann cells on PPy/chitosan membranes resulted in increased secretion of NGF and BDNF.[40] The rate of axonal growth from DRG neurons and Schwann cell migration was increased by stimulation from PPy surfaces with aligned fibres.[72]

A handful of studies address the combined effects of electrical stimulation and biomolecular and/or topographical features. Gomez et al. state that they see an additive effect of electrical stimulation and the chemical stimulation given by their NGF functionalised surfaces (Section 12.5).[30] This has also been shown by others studying NGF-PPy/PLGA scaffolds where NGF presentation is combined with stimulation and submicron fibres.[55] Furthermore, using similar PPy–PLGA without NGF, it was seen that stimulation using aligned fibres rather than randomly oriented counterparts led to both longer neurites and a larger proportion of neurite-bearing cells.[54]

Some important steps towards in vivo work have been taken in recent years. In rodents, nerve guidance channels based on PPy biodegradable composites[105] or electropolymerised PPy[24] were implanted as replacement and for guidance of transected sciatic nerves. No stimulation was applied, but an encouraging finding was that the regenerated tissue displayed the 'characteristic structure' of a native axon.[105]

In summary, these biological results further emphasise the benefits of offering combinations of biomolecular treatment strategies and materials capable of supporting stimulation simultaneously with topographical guidance, stressing the need to find a material solution that offers a solution to all. Much of the research concerning studying actual effects of these scaffolds, especially in vivo, remains for future work.

12.7 Future trends and remaining challenges

12.7.1 New directions

In this chapter, a wide variety of ideas has been presented, each addressing one or several of the topics of biofunctionalisation, patterning and biodegradation. Many of these ideas have great potential for the future, and thus far, reports only scratched the surface of what can potentially be accomplished. It is worth mentioning a few of these where a closer look would be worthwhile for predicting the next generation of materials.

On the biofunctionalisation side, a topic where interesting future results would be expected to follow is to use the redox control functionality of the polymer for temporal control of the biochemical treatment of the regenerating nerve. A few papers that go in this direction have already been mentioned,[38,68] and it would be an exciting development if future work could make more out of this additional possibility offered by the conducting polymers. The right biochemical treatment for initiation of regeneration might in fact not at all be optimal for support at later stages, wherefore a polymer that reveals different cues at different time points is expected to be an improvement. Furthermore, it can be expected that more work goes into the direction of including cells themselves in the matrix of the implants. It has been shown that cells can indeed be cultured within conducting polymer matrices. Using seed cells in combination with conducting polymer scaffolds could be a possible route to modulate the cellular microenvironment by stimulation using the receptacle seed cells as intermediate agents. For instance, it has been shown that olfactory ensheathing cells significantly increased their expression and secretion of many important neurotrophic factors in response to stimulation from PPy-based materials.[71]

Regarding the development of biodegradability, it is expected that the conclusions regarding the beneficial outcome on conductivity from controlling the organisation of polymer chains within the composite will guide the way for future work.[35,36,94] Some authors point out that nanosized particles and fragments from the conducting polymers are toxic to cells.[92,104] Therefore, in order to accomplish biodegradable materials of acceptable conductivities, every effort in the direction of optimising performance without increasing conducting polymer content will be needed.

On the processing technology and patterning side, more work is needed on synthesis of materials that can more easily be processed into 3D objects and that carry anchors for easy and general functionalisation. Good examples are the ester-functionalised thiophene versions[7] or the single-component hydrogels based on covalently crosslinked PTAA.[63] Ideally, with such development, the processing technique could be chosen more freely and be tuned with the optimal chemistry for accomplishing other qualities.

12.7.2 Remaining challenges

From the literature reviewed in this chapter, it is clear that, as a result of the last two decades of work within this field, there is already an exciting library of methods that can be applied to provide conducting polymer-based scaffolds with topographical and biochemical guidance on top of their inherent conducting properties. A challenge that to a large extent remains is the combination of all these beneficial properties into one material. The combined effects of stimulation, biochemical treatment and topographical guidance should be investigated more thoroughly to find the right balance. It might not always be possible to optimise materials with respect to all three qualities, but trade-offs could be necessary in the materials design. It is therefore an important piece of information to learn what is sufficiently good and how these three routes to influence regeneration affect and complement each other.

12.7.3 Devices for electrical stimulation

A topic slightly on the side of the conducting polymer development track is solving the problem of interconnecting these materials to the driving electronics. There is still a concerning lack of studies addressing stimulation from the herein described scaffolds or membranes in situ. It is only in such studies that performance can truly be evaluated and proper feedback be given to point the way for further materials development. To continue in the wording of the previous section, 'sufficiently good' needs to be replaced by actual figures and numbers.

A substantial reason for this gap in research is that it is technically challenging to make these interconnects in a way that they do not interfere with the experiment themselves. All the effort that goes into the development of soft, biodegradable, porous polymers will be made in vain if the interconnection device itself is bulky and stiff. In fact, a rigid interconnection device will induce detrimental strain on materials, and on surrounding tissue, due to the micromotion that follows from the natural movements of the patient or animal. This effect is well known from literature on cortical silicon microfabricated implants[52,89] and might even mask the positive effects on neural regeneration, making the experiment difficult to evaluate.

To address this issue, much technology can be directly transferred from the world of flexible, microfabricated electronic devices intended for neuroprosthetic systems. Substantial effort has gone into the development of microelectrode arrays fabricated from highly flexible materials such as polydimethyl siloxane (PDMS), polyimide and Parylene-C.[51,67] Furthermore, stretchable cables have been developed for connecting such flexible foil electrodes. A remaining challenge is the implementation of implantable counterparts to the stimulation devices often used for activation of the polymers in vitro. While the petri dish can readily be connected to electrochemical instruments such as potentiostats/galvanostats, offering the superior control of a three-electrode system, there is currently no standard instrument that allows the researcher to perform the same kind of measurements in the implanted situation. A non-implantable system will always risk interfering with normal tissue development due to tethering forces arising from cables attached to percutaneous ports.[6]

In summary, there is a wide range of highly interesting materials that would deserve further evaluation in real tissue and with active stimulation applied. Progress within this field is in fact highly dependent on such studies being performed. Unfortunately, up to this point, the devices to do so have simply not been there yet. On the positive side, the technology needed to fabricate these devices is to large extent already developed for other purposes. Future work should therefore go into the direction of technology transfer.

12.8 Sources for further information

There is a selection of reviews that could be consulted to find more information within the topic of conducting polymers for neural tissue engineering. Guimard et al. present an extensive overview of the role of conducting polymers within the broader biomedical field, that is, biosensors, tissue engineering and neural probes.[33] A few more recent reviews concentrate explicitly on the tissue-engineering applications for the conducting polymers.[5,25] Furthermore, there are plenty of common denominators with the field of conducting polymers for neural electrodes and, especially for exploring the drug delivery capabilities, a closer look at this topic of research is recommended.[3] It has been a conscious decision within this chapter to focus on results directly related to the conducting polymer approach to tissue engineering rather than the general field of neural scaffolds. A few exceptions to this have been made in appropriate places. However, for a deeper understanding of the design requirements of scaffolds, and for finding inspiration for new ideas that should be integrated with the conducting scaffolds, a broader literature review is highly recommended. A few suggestions on the way would be the excellent reviews by Li et al.[57] regarding the possible strategies for accomplishing guidance (electrical, molecular, physical, topographical), by Straley et al. regarding biomaterial design possibilities to accommodate these strategies, and by Roach et al. focusing explicitly on surface techniques to modulate tissue regeneration.[76,88]

Abbreviations

PANI	polyaniline	p. 299
PPy	polypyrrole	p. 299
PEDOT	poly(3,4 ethylenedioxythiophene)	p. 299
CP	conducting polymer/conjugated polymer	p. 299
PCL	poly(ethylene)/poly(ε-caprolactone)	p. 301
PLLA	poly(L-lactic acid)	p. 301
CPC	chitosan-g-polycaprolactone	p. 301
Py	pyrrole	p. 301
($FeCl_3$)	iron chloride	p. 301
PDLA	poly-D,L-lactic acid	p. 301
wt%	weight percentage	p. 301
WE	working electrode	p. 303
CE	counter electrode	p. 303
RE	reference electrode	p. 303
PDLLA	poly(D,L-lactide)	p. 304
ITO	indium tin oxide	p. 304
VPP	vapour-phase polymerisation	p. 305
PDLLA/CL	poly(D,L-lactide)-co-epsiloncaprolactone	p. 305
PCLF	polycaprolactone fumarate	p. 305
$Fe(TOs)_3$	iron tosylate	p. 305
PSS	polystyrene sulphonate	p. 305
EDOT	ethylene dioxythiophene	p. 306
PLA	polylactide	p. 305
poly(OTE)	poly(octanoic acid 2-thiophen-3-yl-ethyl ester)	p. 306
PLCL	poly(L-lactide-co-ε-caprolactone)	p. 308
PVP	poly(vinyl pyrrolidone)	p. 308
SIBS	poly(styrene-ß-isobutylene-ß-styrene)	p. 308
APS	ammonium peroxydisulphate	p. 308
pTS	para-toluene sulphonate	p. 309
H_2SO_4	sulphuric acid	p. 308
PLGA	poly(lactide-co-glycolide)	p. 304
SEM	scanning electron microscope	Figure 12.4

QAPE	5,5‴-bis(hydroxymethyl)-3,3‴-dimethyl-2,2′:5′,2″:5″,2‴-quaterthiophene-co-adipic acid polyester	p. 310
$Fe(ClO_4)_3$	iron(III) perchlorate	p. 310
PTAA	poly(3-thiopheneacetic acid)	p. 310
AP	aniline pentamer	p. 310
CCAP	carboxyl-capped aniline pentamer	p. 310
AFM	atomic force microscope	p. 314
N_A	Avogadro's number	p. 314
HA	hyaluronic acid	p. 315
NT3	neurotrophin-3	p. 315
NGF	nerve growth factor	p. 315
BDNF	brain-derived neurotrophic factor	p. 315
ATP	adenosine triphosphate	p. 315
RGD	arginylglycylaspartic acid	p. 316
HEA	2-hydroxyethyl acrylate	p. 316
GRGDS	Gly-Arg-Gly-Asp-Ser peptide	p. 317
PPyCOOH	carboxylated polypyrrole	p. 319
DRGs	dorsal root ganglions	p. 318
OECs	olfactory ensheathing cells	p. 320
PDMS	polydimethyl siloxane	p. 321

References

1. Abidian MR, Daneshvar ED, et al. Hybrid conducting polymer-hydrogel conduits for axonal growth and neural tissue engineering. *Adv Healthc Mater* 2012;**1**(6):762–7.
2. Abidian MR, Kim DH, et al. Conducting-polymer nanotubes for controlled drug release. *Adv Mater* 2006;**18**(4):405–9.
3. Asplund M, Nyberg T, et al. Electroactive polymers for neural interfaces. *Polym Chem* 2010;**1**(9):1374–91.
4. Asplund M, von Holst H, et al. Composite biomolecule/PEDOT materials for neural electrodes. *Biointerphases* 2008;**3**(3):83–93.
5. Bendrea A-D, Cianga L, et al. Review paper: progress in the field of conducting polymers for tissue engineering applications. *J Biomater Appl* 2011;**26**(1):3–84.
6. Biran R, Martin DC, et al. The brain tissue response to implanted silicon microelectrode arrays is increased when the device is tethered to the skull. *J Biomed Mater Res Part A* 2007;**82A**(1):169–78.

7. Breukers RD, Gilmore KJ, et al. Creating conductive structures for cell growth: growth and alignment of myogenic cell types on polythiophenes. *J Biomed Mater Res Part A* 2010;**95A**(1):256–68.
8. Broda CR, Lee JY, et al. A chemically polymerized electrically conducting composite of polypyrrole nanoparticles and polyurethane for tissue engineering. *J Biomed Mater Res Part A* 2011;**98A**(4):509–16.
9. Bull RA, Fan FR, et al. Polymer-films on electrodes: 13. Incorporation of catalysts into electronically conductive polymers - iron phthalocyanine in polypyrrole. *J Electrochem Soc* 1983;**130**(7):1636–8.
10. Cen L, Neoh KG, et al. Surface functionalization of electrically conductive polypyrrole film with hyaluronic acid. *Langmuir* 2002;**18**(22):8633–40.
11. Cen L, Neoh KG, et al. Assessment of in vitro bioactivity of hyaluronic acid and sulfated hyaluronic acid functionalized electroactive polymer. *Biomacromolecules* 2004;**5**(6): 2238–46.
12. Che J, Xiao Y, et al. Electro-synthesized PEDOT/glutamate chemically modified electrode: a combination of electrical and biocompatible features. *Polym Int* 2008;**57**(5): 750–5.
13. Collier JH, Camp JP, et al. Synthesis and characterization of polypyrrole-hyaluronic acid composite biomaterials for tissue engineering applications. *J Biomed Mater Res* 2000; **50**(4):574–84.
14. Cui X, Lee VA, et al. Surface modification of neural recording electrodes with conducting polymer/biomolecule blends. *J Biomed Mater Res* 2001;**56**(2):261–72.
15. Cui XY, Martin DC. Electrochemical deposition and characterization of poly(3,4-ethylenedioxythiophene) on neural microelectrode arrays. *Sens Actuators B Chem* 2003;**89**(1–2):92–102.
16. Curtis A, Wilkinson C. Topographical control of cells. *Biomaterials* 1997;**18**(24): 1573–83.
17. De Giglio E, Sabbatini L, et al. Synthesis, analytical characterization, and osteoblast adhesion properties on RGD-grafted polypyrrole coatings on titanium substrates. *J Biomater Sci Polym Ed* 2000;**11**(10):1073–83.
18. De Giglio E, Sabbatini L, et al. Development and analytical characterization of cysteine-grafted polypyrrole films electrosynthesized on Pt- and Ti-substrates as precursors of bioactive interfaces. *J Biomater Sci Polym Ed* 1999;**10**(8):845–58.
19. Durgam H, Sapp S, et al. Novel degradable co-polymers of polypyrrole support cell proliferation and enhance neurite out-growth with electrical stimulation. *J Biomater Sci Polym Ed* 2010;**21**(10):1265–82.
20. Evans AJ, Thompson BC, et al. Promoting neurite outgrowth from spiral ganglion neuron explants using polypyrrole/BDNF-coated electrodes. *J Biomed Mater Res Part A* 2009;**91A**(1):241–50.
21. Garner B, Georgevich A, et al. Polypyrrole-heparin composites as stimulus-responsive substrates for endothelial cell growth. *J Biomed Mater Res* 1999;**44**(2):121–9.
22. Garner B, Hodgson AJ, et al. Human endothelial cell attachment to and growth on polypyrrole-heparin is vitronectin dependent. *J Mater Sci Mater Med* 1999;**10**(1): 19–27.
23. George PM, LaVan DA, et al. Electrically controlled drug delivery from biotin-doped conductive polypyrrole. *Adv Mater* 2006;**18**(5):577–81.
24. George PM, Saigal R, et al. Three-dimensional conductive constructs for nerve regeneration. *J Biomed Mater Res Part A* 2009;**91A**(2):519–27.

25. Ghasemi-Mobarakeh L, Prabhakaran MP, et al. Application of conductive polymers, scaffolds and electrical stimulation for nerve tissue engineering. *J Tissue Eng Regen Med* 2011;**5**(4):E17–35.
26. Ghasemi-Mobarakeh L, Prabhakaran MP, et al. Electrical stimulation of nerve cells using conductive nanofibrous scaffolds for nerve tissue engineering. *Tissue Eng Part A* 2009; **15**(11):3605–19.
27. Gilmore K, Hodgson AJ, et al. Preparation of hydrogel conducting polymer composites. *Polym Gels Networks* 1994;**2**(2):135–43.
28. Gomez N, Lee JY, et al. Micropatterned polypyrrole: a combination of electrical and topographical characteristics for the stimulation of cells. *Adv Funct Mater* 2007;**17**(10): 1645–53.
29. Gomez N, Lu Y, et al. Immobilized nerve growth factor and microtopography have distinct effects on polarization versus axon elongation in hippocampal cells in culture. *Biomaterials* 2007;**28**(2):271–84.
30. Gomez N, Schmidt CE. Nerve growth factor-immobilized polypyrrole: bioactive electrically conducting polymer for enhanced neurite extension. *J Biomed Mater Res Part A* 2007;**81A**(1):135–49.
31. Green RA, Hassarati RT, et al. Conductive hydrogels: mechanically robust hybrids for use as biomaterials. *Macromol Biosci* 2012;**12**(4):494–501.
32. Green RA, Lovell NH, et al. Cell attachment functionality of bioactive conducting polymers for neural interfaces. *Biomaterials* 2009;**30**(22):3637–44.
33. Guimard NK, Gomez N, et al. Conducting polymers in biomedical engineering. *Prog Polym Sci* 2007;**32**(8–9):876–921.
34. Guimard NKE, Sessler JL, et al. Toward a biocompatible and biodegradable copolymer incorporating electroactive oligothiophene units. *Macromolecules* 2009;**42**(2):502–11.
35. Guo B, Finne-Wistrand A, et al. Enhanced electrical conductivity by macromolecular architecture: hyperbranched electroactive and degradable block copolymers based on poly(epsilon-caprolactone) and aniline pentamer. *Macromolecules* 2010;**43**(10): 4472–80.
36. Guo BL, Sun Y, et al. Electroactive porous tubular scaffolds with degradability and non-cytotoxicity for neural tissue regeneration. *Acta Biomater* 2012;**8**(1):144–53.
37. Guo Y, Li M, et al. Electroactive oligoaniline-containing self-assembled monolayers for tissue engineering applications. *Biomacromolecules* 2007;**8**(10):3025–34.
38. Herland A, Persson KM, et al. Electrochemical control of growth factor presentation to steer neural stem cell differentiation. *Angew Chem* 2011;**123**(52):12737–41.
39. Hu J, Huang LH, et al. Electroactive aniline pentamer cross-linking chitosan for stimulation growth of electrically sensitive cells. *Biomacromolecules* 2008;**9**(10):2637–44.
40. Huang J, Hu X, et al. Electrical regulation of Schwann cells using conductive polypyrrole/chitosan polymers. *J Biomed Mater Res Part A* 2010;**93A**(1):164–74.
41. Huang L, Hu J, et al. Synthesis and characterization of electroactive and biodegradable ABA block copolymer of polylactide and aniline pentamer. *Biomaterials* 2007;**28**(10): 1741–51.
42. Huang L, Zhuang X, et al. Synthesis of biodegradable and electroactive multiblock polylactide and aniline pentamer copolymer for tissue engineering applications. *Biomacromolecules* 2008;**9**(3):850–8.
43. Jeong SI, Jun ID, et al. Development of electroactive and elastic nanofibers that contain polyaniline and poly(L-lactide-co-epsilon-caprolactone) for the control of cell adhesion. *Macromol Biosci* 2008;**8**(7):627–37.

44. Jin L, Feng Z-Q, et al. A novel fluffy conductive polypyrrole nano-layer coated PLLA fibrous scaffold for nerve tissue engineering. *J Biomed Nanotechnol* 2012;**8**(5):779–85.
45. Kang G, Ben Borgens R, et al. Well-ordered porous conductive polypyrrole as a new platform for neural interfaces. *Langmuir* 2011;**27**(10):6179–84.
46. Kim BC, Spinks G, et al. Preparation and characterisation of processable conducting polymer-hydrogel composites. *React Funct Polym* 2000;**44**(1):31–40.
47. Kim BC, Spinks GM, et al. Electroformation of conducting polymers in a hydrogel support matrix. *Polymer* 2000;**41**(5):1783–90.
48. Kim DH, Abidian M, et al. Conducting polymers grown in hydrogel scaffolds coated on neural prosthetic devices. *J Biomed Mater Res Part A* 2004;**71A**(4):577–85.
49. Kim DH, Richardson-Burns SM, et al. Effect of immobilized nerve growth factor on conductive polymers: electrical properties and cellular response. *Adv Funct Mater* 2007; **17**(1):79–86.
50. Kotwal A, Schmidt CE. Electrical stimulation alters protein adsorption and nerve cell interactions with electrically conducting biomaterials. *Biomaterials* 2001;**22**(10):1055–64.
51. Lacour SP, Benmerah S, et al. Flexible and stretchable micro-electrodes for in vitro and in vivo neural interfaces. *Med Biol Eng Comput* 2010;**48**(10):945–54.
52. Lee H, Bellamkonda RV, et al. Biomechanical analysis of silicon microelectrode-induced strain in the brain. *J Neural Eng* 2005;**2**(4):81–9.
53. Lee JW, Serna F, et al. Carboxylic acid-functionalized conductive polypyrrole as a bioactive platform for cell adhesion. *Biomacromolecules* 2006;**7**(6):1692–5.
54. Lee JY, Bashur CA, et al. Polypyrrole-coated electrospun PLGA nanofibers for neural tissue applications. *Biomaterials* 2009;**30**(26):4325–35.
55. Lee JY, Bashur CA, et al. Nerve growth factor-immobilized electrically conducting fibrous scaffolds for potential use in neural engineering applications. *IEEE Trans Nanobioscience* 2012;**11**(1):15–21.
56. Lee JY, Lee J-W, et al. Neuroactive conducting scaffolds: nerve growth factor conjugation on active ester-functionalized polypyrrole. *J R Soc Interface* 2009;**6**(38):801–10.
57. Li GN, Hoffman-Kim D. Tissue-engineered platforms of axon guidance. *Tissue Eng Part B Rev* 2008;**14**(1):33–51.
58. Li MY, Guo Y, et al. Electrospinning polyaniline-contained gelatin nanofibers for tissue engineering applications. *Biomaterials* 2006;**27**(13):2705–15.
59. Li Y, Neoh KG, et al. Controlled release of heparin from polypyrrole-poly(vinyl alcohol) assembly by electrical stimulation. *J Biomed Mater Res A* 2005;**73**(2):171–81.
60. Liu Y, Liu X, et al. 3D bio-nanofibrous PPy/SIBS mats as platforms for cell culturing. *Chem Commun* 2008;**28**(32):3729–31.
61. Liu YD, Hu J, et al. Synthesis and characterization of novel biodegradable and electroactive hydrogel based on aniline oligomer and gelatin. *Macromol Biosci* 2012;**12**(2): 241–50.
62. Mario Cheong GL, Lim KS, et al. Conductive hydrogels with tailored bioactivity for implantable electrode coatings. *Acta Biomater* 2014;**10**(3):1216–26.
63. Mawad D, Stewart E, et al. A single component conducting polymer hydrogel as a scaffold for tissue engineering. *Adv Funct Mater* 2012;**22**(13):2692–9.
64. McKeon KD, Lewis A, et al. Electrospun poly(d,l-lactide) and polyaniline scaffold characterization. *J Appl Polym Sci* 2010;**115**(3):1566–72.
65. Moroder P, Runge MB, et al. Material properties and electrical stimulation regimens of polycaprolactone fumarate-polypyrrole scaffolds as potential conductive nerve conduits. *Acta Biomater* 2011;**7**(3):944–53.

66. Norris ID, Shaker MM, et al. Electrostatic fabrication of ultrafine conducting fibers: polyaniline/polyethylene oxide blends. *Synth Met* 2000;**114**(2):109–14.
67. Ordonez J, Schuettler M, et al. Thin films and microelectrode arrays for neuroprosthetics. *Mrs Bull* 2012;**37**(6):590–8.
68. Park K-H, Jo EA, et al. Heparin/Polypyrrole (PPy) composite on gold-coated matrix for the neurite outgrowth of PC 12 cells by electrical stimulation. *Biotechnol Bioprocess Eng* 2007;**12**(5):463–9.
69. Peramo A, Urbanchek MG, et al. In situ polymerization of a conductive polymer in acellular muscle tissue constructs. *Tissue Eng Part A* 2008;**14**(3):423–32.
70. Prabhakaran MP, Ghasemi-Mobarakeh L, et al. Electrospun conducting polymer nanofibers and electrical stimulation of nerve stem cells. *J Biosci Bioeng* 2011;**112**(5):501–7.
71. Qi F, Wang Y, et al. Electrical regulation of olfactory ensheathing cells using conductive polypyrrole/chitosan polymers. *Biomaterials* 2013;**34**(7):1799–809.
72. Quigley AF, Razal JM, et al. A conducting-polymer platform with biodegradable fibers for stimulation and guidance of axonal growth. *Adv Mater* 2009;**21**(43):4393–7.
73. Rajnicek A, Britland S, et al. Contact guidance of CNS neurites on grooved quartz: influence of groove dimensions, neuronal age and cell type. *J Cell Sci* 1997;**110**(23): 2905–13.
74. Richardson RT, Thompson B, et al. The effect of polypyrrole with incorporated neurotrophin-3 on the promotion of neurite outgrowth from auditory neurons. *Biomaterials* 2007;**28**(3):513–23.
75. Rivers TJ, Hudson TW, et al. Synthesis of a novel, biodegradable electrically conducting polymer for biomedical applications. *Adv Funct Mater* 2002;**12**(1):33–7.
76. Roach P, Parker T, et al. Surface strategies for control of neuronal cell adhesion: a review. *Surf Sci Rep* 2010;**65**(6):145–73.
77. Runge MB, Dadsetan M, et al. The development of electrically conductive polycaprolactone fumarate-polypyrrole composite materials for nerve regeneration. *Biomaterials* 2010;**31**(23):5916–26.
78. Runge MB, Dadsetan M, et al. Development of electrically conductive oligo(polyethylene glycol) fumarate-polypyrrole hydrogels for nerve regeneration. *Biomacromolecules* 2010;**11**(11):2845–53.
79. Sanghvi AB, Miller KPH, et al. Biomaterials functionalization using a novel peptide that selectively binds to a conducting polymer. *Nat Mater* 2005;**4**(6):496–502.
80. Schmidt CE, Shastri VR, et al. Stimulation of neurite outgrowth using an electrically conducting polymer. *Proc Natl Acad Sci USA* 1997;**94**(17):8948–53.
81. Shastri VR, Schmidt CE, et al. Polypyrrole - a potential candidate for stimulated nerve regeneration. In: Cotell CM, Meyer AE, Gorbatkin SM, Grobe GL, editors. *Thin films and surfaces for bioactivity and biomedical applications*, vol. 414. Pittsburgh: Materials Research Society; 1996. p. 113–8.
82. Shi G, Rouabhia M, et al. Electrical stimulation enhances viability of human cutaneous fibroblasts on conductive biodegradable substrates. *J Biomed Mater Res Part A* 2008; **84A**(4):1026–37.
83. Shi G, Zhang Z, et al. The regulation of cell functions electrically using biodegradable polypyrrole-polylactide conductors. *Biomaterials* 2008;**29**(28):3792–8.
84. Shi GX, Rouabhia M, et al. A novel electrically conductive and biodegradable composite made of polypyrrole nanoparticles and polylactide. *Biomaterials* 2004;**25**(13):2477–88.
85. Song HK, Toste B, et al. Micropatterns of positive guidance cues anchored to polypyrrole doped with polyglutamic acid: a new platform for characterizing neurite extension in complex environments. *Biomaterials* 2006;**27**(3):473–84.

86. Srivastava Y, Marquez M, et al. Multijet electrospinning of conducting nanofibers from microfluidic manifolds. *J Appl Polym Sci* 2007;**106**(5):3171–8.
87. Stauffer WR, Cui XT. Polypyrrole doped with 2 peptide sequences from laminin. *Biomaterials* 2006;**27**(11):2405–13.
88. Straley KS, Foo CWP, et al. Biomaterial design strategies for the treatment of spinal cord injuries. *J Neurotrauma* 2010;**27**(1):1–19.
89. Subbaroyan J, Martin DC, et al. A finite-element model of the mechanical effects of implantable microelectrodes in the cerebral cortex. *J Neural Eng* 2005;**2**(4):103–13.
90. Thompson BC, Moulton SE, et al. Optimising the incorporation and release of a neurotrophic factor using conducting polypyrrole. *J Control Release* 2006;**116**(3):285–94.
91. Umana M, Waller J. Protein-modified electrodes - the glucose-oxidase polypyrrole system. *Anal Chem* 1986;**58**(14):2979–83.
92. Vaitkuviene A, Kaseta V, et al. Evaluation of cytotoxicity of polypyrrole nanoparticles synthesized by oxidative polymerization. *J Hazard Mater* 2013;**250**:167–74.
93. Wadhwa R, Lagenaur CF, et al. Electrochemically controlled release of dexamethasone from conducting polymer polypyrrole coated electrode. *J Control Release* 2006;**110**(3): 531–41.
94. Wan Y, Gao J, et al. Biodegradability of conducting chitosan-g-polycaprolactone/ polypyrrole conduits. *Polym Degrad Stab* 2010;**95**(10):1994–2002.
95. Wan Y, Wen DJ. Preparation and characterization of porous conducting poly(DL-lactide) composite membranes. *J Membr Sci* 2005;**246**(2):193–201.
96. Wang XD, Gu XS, et al. Evaluation of biocompatibility of polypyrrole in vitro and in vivo. *J Biomed Mater Res Part A* 2004;**68A**(3):411–22.
97. Williams RL, Doherty PJ. A preliminary assessment of poly(pyrrole) in nerve guide studies. *J Mater Sci Mater Med* 1994;**5**(6–7):429–33.
98. Xiao Y, Che J, et al. Preparation of nano-tentacle polypyrrole with pseudo-molecular template for ATP incorporation. *J Biomed Mater Res Part A* 2007;**80A**(4):925–31.
99. Xiao YH, Li CM, et al. Adenosine 5'-triphosphate incorporated poly(3,4-ethylenedioxythiophene) modified electrode: a bioactive platform with electroactivity, stability and biocompatibility. *J Appl Electrochem* 2008;**38**(12):1735–41.
100. Xie J, MacEwan MR, et al. Conductive core-sheath nanofibers and their potential application in neural tissue engineering. *Adv Funct Mater* 2009;**19**(14):2312–8.
101. Yu Q-Z, Dai Z-w, et al. Fabrication of high conductivity dual multi-porous poly(L-lactic acid)/polypyrrole composite micro/nanofiber film. *Mater Sci Eng B Adv Funct Solid State Mater* 2011;**176**(12):913–20.
102. Zhang Q, Yan Y, et al. The synthesis and characterization of a novel biodegradable and electroactive polyphosphazene for nerve regeneration. *Mater Sci Eng C Mater Biol Appl* 2010;**30**(1):160–6.
103. Zhang QS, Yan YH, et al. Synthesis of a novel biodegradable and electroactive polyphosphazene for biomedical application. *Biomed Mater* 2009;**4**(3):035008.
104. Zhang XY, Qi HX, et al. Cellular responses of aniline oligomers: a preliminary study. *Toxicol Res* 2012;**1**(3):201–5.
105. Zhang Z, Rouabhia M, et al. Electrically conductive biodegradable polymer composite for nerve regeneration: electricity-stimulated neurite outgrowth and axon regeneration. *Artif Organs* 2007;**31**(1):13–22.
106. Zhou D, Too CO, et al. Synthesis and characterisation of polypyrrole/heparin composites. *React Funct Polym* 1999;**39**(1):19–26.

Index

Note: Page numbers followed by "f", "t" and "b" indicate figures, tables and boxes, respectively.

CPI Antony Rowe
Chippenham, UK
2015-12-23 16:49